Study Guide

to
Treatments
of Psychiatric
Disorders,
Second Edition

Study Guide

to Treatments of Psychiatric Disorders, Second Edition

Sarah D. Atkinson, M.D.
Medical Director, Adolescent Inpatient Unit and
Crisis Intervention Unit
Genesee Hospital
Rochester, New York

Glen O. Gabbard, M.D.
Callaway Distinguished Professor of
Psychoanalysis and Education
Karl Menninger School of Psychiatry
The Menninger Clinic
Topeka, Kansas;
Clinical Professor of Psychiatry,
University of Kansas School of Medicine
Wichita, Kansas

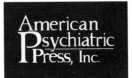
American Psychiatric Press, Inc.

Washington, DC
London, England

Note: The authors have worked to ensure that all information in this book concerning drug dosages, schedules, and routes of administration is accurate as of the time of publication and consistent with standards set by the U.S. Food and Drug Administration and the general medical community. As medical research and practice advance, however, therapeutic standards may change. For this reason and because human and mechanical errors sometimes occur, we recommend that readers follow the advice of a physician who is directly involved in their care or the care of a member of their family.

Books published by the American Psychiatric Press, Inc., represent the views and opinions of the individual authors and do not necessarily represent the policies and opinions of the Press or the American Psychiatric Association.

American Psychiatric Press, Inc.
1400 K Street, N.W., Washington, DC   20005

Contents

Section 12: Sleep Disorders

Section 13: Disorders of Impulse Control

Introduction

This study guide is designed as a companion text to the two-volume *Treatments of Psychiatric Disorders*, Second Edition, and to some extent may also be used in conjunction with the *Synopsis of Treatments of Psychiatric Disorders, Second Edition*. We recognize that an extraordinary amount of information is contained in both the two-volume text and the synopsis. A study guide is a succinct way to organize the voluminous material into quantities that can be assimilated easily.

Moreover, this text identifies the key points in each chapter through the selection of specific questions. In most cases, we have expanded on these points by elaborating on material from the text in the answer key provided at the end of each chapter. When no elaboration is necessary, we have simply provided answers without comment.

An obvious use of this study guide is as a tool to help one prepare for examinations that test one's knowledge of psychiatric treatment. The formats of the questions in the study guide follow those in the Psychiatry Resident In-Training Examination (PRITE), the American Board of Psychiatry and Neurology examinations for certification in general, child, and adolescent psychiatry, and the United States Medical Licensing Medical Examination (USMLE). This study guide also may be used to help one prepare for examinations in undergraduate and graduate courses in psychology, medical school courses in psychiatry, and postgraduate seminars, whether or not *Treatments of Psychiatric Disorders*, Second Edition, or the synopsis is assigned as a text. Neither of us are involved in creating or contributing questions for any of the aforementioned national examinations, but we are familiar with the exams and have constructed the questions accordingly.

Psychiatric treatment of complex disorders and syndromes is pluralistic. Many of these disorders may be effectively treated by several different modalities. We recognize that each treatment that is recommended or discussed may be supported by varying degrees of empirical research. Some types of treatment may be more controversial than others. The questions and answers in this study guide are culled from the opinions of experts who have written chapters in the two-volume textbook. We are aware, of course, that other experts may disagree, and we anticipate that some readers may disagree with some of the answers provided in this text.

We had to be selective in designing the questions in the study guide; thus, the reader must realize that it is not in and of itself a textbook and should not be used as such. The study guide should be regarded as an adjunct volume to the textbook and the synopsis. The material in the study guide may be used to supplement readings in clinical and didactic curricula. To receive maximum benefit from the study guide, the reader should keep these guidelines in mind.

We would like to acknowledge the support of Dr. Carol Nadelson, Ms. Claire Reinburg, and Mr. Greg Kuny of American Psychiatric Press throughout the duration of this project. We would particularly like to express our gratitude to Mrs. Faye Schoenfeld for her editorial assistance in the preparation of this manuscript.

Sarah D. Atkinson, M.D.
Glen O. Gabbard, M.D.

SECTION 1

General Considerations in Psychiatric Treatment

CHAPTER 1

The Multiaxial System in Psychiatric Treatment

■ **DIRECTIONS: For statements 1–1 through 1–5, indicate whether the statement is true or false.**

1–1. _____ A multiaxial evaluation involves assessing patients on each of the five axes of DSM-IV.

1–2. _____ The first modern proposal for a multidimensional approach to diagnosis came in 1967 from the World Health Organization.

1–3. _____ The first appearance of a multiaxial system in the *Diagnostic and Statistical Manual of Mental Disorders* occurred in 1980 with the publication of the third edition.

1–4. _____ Mental retardation was first added to Axis II in 1980 with the publication of DSM-III.

1–5. _____ In DSM-IV, Axis I includes pervasive developmental disorders, specific developmental disorders, and mental retardation.

■ **DIRECTIONS: For questions 1–6 through 1–10, select the single best answer.**

1–6. Axis III in DSM-IV was changed from "Physical Disorders and Conditions" to "General Medical Conditions" because

1. Some of the Axis III conditions were not physical.

2. The word *physical* seemed to imply that conditions on Axis I and Axis II do not have "physical" components.

3. The term *general* connotes the nonspecific nature of many of the physical conditions.

4. The new terminology is more consistent with international nomenclature.

1–7. The main difference in Axis IV between DSM-III-R and DSM-IV is that

1. Psychosocial and environmental problems are listed in the form of a checklist rather than numerical coding of multiple stressors as in DSM-III-R.

2. More psychosocial stressors were added in DSM-IV.

3. Both environmental and intrapsychic stressors are included in DSM-IV.

4. A different numerical rating system—one starting at zero and going up to 100—was implemented in DSM-IV.

1–8. Axis V of DSM-IV includes which of the following changes?

1. Vocational assessment is required, and the numerical system is no longer used.

2. Marital assessment was added, and the range of the score was expanded up to 200.

3. Only the current level of functioning is used routinely, and scores on the Global Assessment of Functioning (GAF) Scale range to 100 instead of 90.

4. The scale begins at 10, and a third level of functioning score was added.

1–9. Axis II disorders may present special problems in treatment planning. Which of the following is **not** an influence on the treatment plan frequently formulated for patients with Axis II conditions?

1. Poor adherence to treatment regimens

2. Poorer response to treatment

3. Improved medication compliance

4. Altered course of comorbid Axis I condition

1–10. Which of the following statements is **true** regarding Axis V?

1. The GAF Scale on Axis V measures only psychological, not social or occupational, functioning at the time of the initial assessment.

2. There has been extensive research using the Axis V measure.

3. Axis V is not useful because, as studies have shown, measures of functional impairment have virtually no correlation with symptom severity or Axis I diagnosis.

4. The GAF Scale on Axis V shows promise as an instrument to monitor the patient's progress throughout the course of treatment.

■ **ANSWERS:**

1–1. **True** In DSM-IV, each patient must be assessed on Axis I (clinical disorders and other conditions that may be a focus of clinical attention), Axis II (personality disorders and mental retardation), Axis III (general medical conditions), Axis IV (psychosocial and environmental problems), and Axis V (global assessment of functioning).

1–2. **False** The first modern proposal for a multidimensional approach to diagnosis came from Essen-Möller and Wohlfahrt in 1947. They suggested having two dimensions: one for describing etiology and one for prescribing symptomatology. This proposal evolved into the "biaxial system" approved in 1952 by the Danish Psychiatric Association.

1–3. **True** DSM-III was the first official manual to incorporate all five axes of the current multiaxial system.

1–4. **False** Mental retardation was not added to Axis II until 1987, with the publication of DSM-III-R.

1–5. **False** Pervasive developmental disorders and specific developmental disorders are included on Axis I of DSM-IV. (In DSM-III-R, these disorders were included on Axis II.) However, mental retardation continues to be coded on Axis II, along with personality disorders.

1–6. **Answer: 2.** In DSM-III-R, the use of the word *physical* could have been construed as implying that certain psychiatric disorders were not "physical." Because of the increasing knowledge of the biological components of the major mental disorders, in DSM-IV, Axis III was changed to "General Medical Conditions."

1–7. **Answer: 1.** Whereas DSM-III-R provided for numerical coding of multiple stressors, DSM-IV provides a listing of psychosocial and environmental problems in the form of a checklist. The main advantage of this style is the simplicity in allowing the notation of a variety of problems.

1–8. **Answer: 3.** Whereas in DSM-III-R the GAF Scale ended at 90 ("Absent or minimal symptoms"), in DSM-IV the scale ranges up to 100 ("Superior functioning . . . No symptoms"). Also in DSM-IV, only the current level of functioning is used routinely, although a rating of the highest level of functioning in the past year can also be made if appropriate to do so in the given setting. In contrast, in DSM-III-R, both the current level of functioning and the highest level of functioning in the past year were recorded.

1–9. **Answer: 3.** Personality disorders may influence adherence to treatment regimens, response to treatment, and the course of treatment. However, there are no data suggesting improved medication compliance. It has been shown, for example, that patients with coexisting major depressive disorder and a personality disorder have a poorer response to treatment than patients with major depressive disorder alone. The course of treatment may be more severe for a depressed patient if there is a comorbid Axis II disorder. Patients with personality disorders may also miss more appointments and not take medications as directed.

1–10. **Answer: 4.** The GAF Scale on Axis V can be used to rate the patient's psychological, social, and occupational functioning at the time of the initial assessment. Some studies have found that measures of functional impairment may be correlated with symptom severity or Axis I diagnosis and thus may provide additional information to clinicians. There has been little research done on the Axis V measure, but its use in monitoring the patient's clinical progress throughout the course of treatment seems to have the most promise at this time.

CHAPTER 2

Mind and Brain in Psychiatric Treatment

■ **DIRECTIONS: For questions 2–1 through 2–5, match the author who has examined the mind-body problem with his theory.**

2–1.	René Descartes	a.	Neural Darwinism
2–2.	William James	b.	Substance dualism
2–3.	Gerald Edelman	c.	Biological naturalism
2–4.	Marshall Edelson	d.	Mind-body problem redefined as a relationship between two disciplines
2–5.	John Searle	e.	Consciousness as a process rather than a substance

■ **DIRECTIONS: For questions 2–6 through 2–9, indicate**

A if answers 1, 2, and 3 are correct.
B if answers 1 and 3 are correct.
C if answers 2 and 4 are correct.
D if only answer 4 is correct.
E if all are correct.

2–6. Which of the following biochemical changes have been associated with the early separation of infant rhesus monkeys from their mothers?

1. Higher levels of plasma cortisol and ACTH (adrenocorticotropic hormone)
2. Higher cerebrospinal fluid (CSF) levels of norepinephrine
3. Higher levels of 3-methoxy-4-hydroxyphenylglycol (MHPG)
4. Lower levels of MHPG

2–7. According to the studies of Jerome Kagan and his colleagues, children who were born with a temperament characterized by behavioral inhibition to the unfamiliar

1. Clearly belong to a qualitative distinct category of infants born with a lower threshold for limbic hypothalamic arousal in response to unexpected environmental changes.

    2. Did not necessarily grow up to be shy.

    3. Required some form of chronic environmental stress to activate the original temperamental disposition and lead to shy, quiet, and timid behavior.

    4. Develop social phobia.

2–8. In a study of 1,018 pairs of female twins, Kendler and co-workers examined the relationship between parental loss before age 17 years and adult psychopathology. These investigators found that

    1. There was no association between panic disorder as an adult and loss as a child.

    2. Maternal separation early in life was much more strongly associated with later development of panic disorder than was paternal separation.

    3. Parental death could not be linked with adult manifestations of panic disorder.

    4. The impact of parental loss was three times greater for panic disorder than for major depression.

2–9. The fact that only 23.6% of persons exposed to traumatic events experience symptoms of posttraumatic stress disorder (PTSD) may indicate which of the following?

    1. There is increased genetic vulnerability to psychiatric illness in some individuals.

    2. The same stressor has different meanings to different individuals.

    3. Old traumas may be reawakened by present-day circumstances.

    4. There is no basis for connecting trauma with symptomatology.

■ **DIRECTIONS: For questions 2–10 through 2–13, select the single best answer.**

2–10. In determining whether psychotherapy or pharmacotherapy is the treatment of choice for a particular disorder, which of the following considerations is most useful?

    1. Psychotherapy is the treatment of choice for "psychological" disturbances.

    2. Pharmacotherapy is the treatment of choice for "biological" disturbances.

    3. Effective treatments do not directly depend on etiology, so generalizations are ill-advised.

    4. Psychotherapy should only be used for treatment of patients with personality disorders.

2–11. Group therapy has been shown to prolong life in the treatment of which of the following medical conditions?

    1. Metastatic breast cancer

    2. Hodgkin's disease

    3. Lung cancer

    4. Metastatic bowel cancer

2–12. Analysis of the data from the National Institute of Mental Health (NIMH) Treatment of Depression Collaborative Research Program provided which of the following predictors of differential treatment outcome?

1. Relatively mild impairment and cognitive dysfunction predicted superior response to interpersonal psychotherapy (IPT).

2. Relatively mild impairment and cognitive dysfunction predicted superior response to cognitive-behavior therapy (CBT).

3. Relatively limited social dysfunction predicted superior response to imipramine.

4. Relatively limited social dysfunction predicted superior response to CBT.

2–13. According to the American Psychiatric Association (APA) Practice Guideline on Depression (1993), psychotherapeutic management is

1. Unnecessary in most cases.

2. An essential component of every psychopharmacological treatment plan.

3. Necessary only when psychotherapy is a treatment of choice.

4. Rarely useful.

■ **ANSWERS:**

2–1. René Descartes: **b**

2–2. William James: **e**

2–3. Gerald Edelman: **a**

2–4. Marshall Edelson: **d**

2–5. John Searle: **c**

2–6. **Answer: B (1 and 3).** When infant rhesus monkeys were separated from their mothers at 6 months of age, they manifested higher levels of plasma cortisol and ACTH than peers who continued to be reared by their own mothers. In addition, they also manifested lower CSF levels of norepinephrine and higher levels of MHPG.

2–7. **Answer: A (1, 2 and 3).** Kagan and his colleagues demonstrated the interaction between constitutional temperament and environment by studying cohorts of children using a longitudinal design. The authors compared consistently inhibited children with those who were consistently uninhibited. Children who were behaviorally inhibited clearly belonged to a qualitatively distinct category of infants apparently born with a lower threshold for limbic hypothalamic arousal in response to unexpected changes in the environment or novel events that could not be assimilated easily. Kagan and colleagues termed this temperamental disposition "behavioral inhibition to the unfamiliar." In addition, they noted that some form of chronic environmental stress was necessary to activate the original temperamental disposition and thereby lead to an end result of shy, quite, and timid behavior at 2 years of age. Otherwise, the shyness did not become a prominent personality trait.

2–8. **Answer: C (2 and 4).** In the study by Kendler and co-workers involving 1,018 pairs of female twins, the findings suggest that early parental loss may trigger inherited neurophysiological vulnerability. The authors observed that panic disorder was significantly and strongly associated with both parental death and separation. Moreover, maternal separation early in life was much more strongly associated with development of panic disorder later in life than was paternal separation. Contrary to conventional wisdom, the impact of parental loss was three times greater for panic disorder than for major depression.

2–9. **Answer: A (1, 2, and 3).** The diathesis-stress model of illness implies that environmental trauma interacts with genetic vulnerability and that specific stressors have highly personal meanings to victims of trauma. Certain individuals may have increased genetic vulnerability to psychiatric illness and to trauma. Also, the same stressor may have different meanings to different individuals; the meaning a traumatic experience has for a person may be shaped, in part, by past traumas that are reawakened by the current trauma. In one study, the risk for developing PTSD could be linked to early separation from parents, neuroticism, family history of anxiety, and preexisting anxiety or depression.

2–10. **Answer: 3.** Although there was a time in psychiatry when psychotherapy would be the treatment of choice for so-called psychological disturbances and pharmacotherapy would be the treatment of choice for so-called biological disturbances, such distinctions are no longer clear-cut. Effective treatments do not necessarily elucidate or depend on a specific etiology. Recent investigations demonstrate that psychosocial and psychopharmacological interventions may have similar effects on brain functioning. Each patient must be carefully assessed as an individual, and the treatment plan must be individualized accordingly.

2–11. **Answer: 1.** In a study by Spiegel and co-workers, metastatic breast cancer patients who received standard medical treatment and also underwent supportive-expressive group psychotherapy lived an average of 18 months longer than a randomly assigned control sample who received standard treatment but no therapy. Forty-eight months after the onset of the study, all the control patients had died, but a third of the psychotherapy treatment sample were still living. A support-group protocol for malignant melanoma patients was also shown to produce favorable mortality rates and more lengthy remissions than occurred in a control group without the support group.

2–12. **Answer: 2.** Sotsky and co-workers found that relatively mild impairment and cognitive dysfunction predicted superior response both to CBT and to imipramine. Relatively limited social dysfunction predicted superior response to IPT. Also, significant vocational impairment predicted superior response to imipramine. High severity of and impairment from depression predicted superior response both to imipramine and to IPT.

2–13. **Answer: 2.** The APA Practice Guideline on Depression suggests that psychotherapeutic management is an essential component of every treatment plan involving the prescription of medication.

CHAPTER 3

Gender Issues in
Psychiatric Treatment

■ **DIRECTIONS: For statements 3–1 through 3–4,
indicate whether the statement is true or false.**

3–1. _____ A substantial body of literature suggests that therapists are not entirely free of bias involving sex role expectations.

3–2. _____ Less serious psychopathology has been attributed to men who express nontraditional attitudes, such as dependency, compared with women who do so.

3–3. _____ Men's physical complaints are more likely than those of women to be labeled psychogenic.

3–4. _____ A woman's choosing to be treated by a woman may represent the patient's wish to restore her relationship with her mother.

■ **DIRECTIONS: For questions 3–5 through 3–8, indicate**

    A if answers 1, 2, and 3 are correct.

    B if answers 1 and 3 are correct.

    C if answers 2 and 4 are correct.

    D if only answer 4 is correct.

    E if all are correct.

3–5. A man may seek treatment from a woman

    1. To avoid a competitive or authoritarian relationship with a man.

    2. To avoid the risk of homosexual feelings being evoked.

    3. Because he has had poor relationships with women in the past and wants to work these out with a woman.

    4. Because his expectations are that a woman will provide the cure for his problems with intimacy.

3–6. In current thinking, the role played by the real attributes of the therapist, such as age, race, and gender, can be summarized in which of the following statements?

    1. Transference is not based on real aspects of the therapist.

    2. Whereas gender may be important in psychotherapy, age and race are not.

3. Age, race, and gender are thought to play a minor role in the therapist-patient relationship.

4. Real attributes of the therapist, such as age, race, and gender, are thought to have a significant influence on the development of the transference.

3–7. A transfer or reassignment from a therapist of one gender to a therapist of the opposite gender

1. May be a way of avoiding responsibility for failure or dealing with the embarrassment of a negative outcome.

2. Is useful because gender itself is a highly significant variable in the majority of cases in which treatment is not successful.

3. May be useful if a sexual interaction has occurred with a previous therapist.

4. Should only be done if an erotic transference develops.

3–8. Which of the following statements are **true** regarding gender and group psychotherapies?

1. The more women talk in group situations, the more they tend to be ignored.

2. In female-led groups, men tend to experience a sense of loss of control.

3. In group situations, men are more likely to respond negatively to female leaders while positively reinforcing and reassuring male leaders who say the same things.

4. No distinctions have been noted between male-led and female-led groups.

■ **DIRECTIONS: For questions 3–9 through 3–12, select the single best answer for each question.**

3–9. The most important determinant of gender identity is

1. Anatomical genital differences.

2. Chromosomal constellations.

3. Prenatal factors.

4. How the parents relate to the infant regarding male and female roles.

3–10. The concept of gender identity is defined as

1. The cultural construct referring to the expectations, attitudes, and behaviors that are considered appropriate for each gender in a particular culture.

2. The internalized sense of maleness or femaleness.

3. The attractiveness assigned to persons of the same sex and to those of the opposite sex.

4. The sex of the child according to chromosomal constellations.

3–11. Which of the following disorders is **not** more commonly diagnosed in women than in men?

1. Depression

2. Agoraphobia

3. Antisocial personality disorder

4. Borderline personality disorder

3–12. Which of the following statements is **true** regarding menopause?

1. Menopause may cause depression.

2. Estrogen replacement therapy may alleviate depression.

3. Women who become depressed at the time of menopause are generally those who have had depressions at other times in their lives.

4. Responses to menopause are not influenced by cultural expectations.

■ **ANSWERS:**

3–1. **True** Numerous studies have demonstrated that therapists are subject to the same sex role stereotypes and biases as other segments of society.

3–2. **False** Men who express dependency or other nontraditional attitudes are often viewed as having more serious psychopathology than women who exhibit the same traits.

3–3. **False** Although women tend to come to see physicians earlier in the course of an illness than do men, their complaints are less likely to be taken seriously. Women's complaints are often pejoratively labeled as psychogenic. Women receive a diagnosis later and have different treatments prescribed as well compared with men.

3–4. **True** Although patients give many reasons for their choice of those who provide care for them, some of these reasons include stereotyped views about gender differences. Male therapists may be regarded by female patients as more likely to perpetuate patriarchal values. A female patient who chooses a female therapist, on the other hand, may unconsciously be wishing to restore the relationship with her mother or to develop a relationship with the therapist that is better than the original mother-daughter relationship.

3–5. **Answer: E (All).** The reasons that a man chooses a woman as a therapist are complicated and may involve particular forms of resistance to the therapy. Stereotypes and expectations about women often underlie the choice of a female therapist by a male. Some male patients may believe they can avoid competitiveness with a woman. Others fear that homosexual feelings would arise with a male therapist. Still others secretly believe that their problems with intimacy will be solved by having a female therapist. Finally, some may be motivated because of a past history of poor relationships with women and a wish to work these difficulties out with a female therapist.

3–6. **Answer: D (Only 4).** For many years, transference was thought to be only minimally affected by real attributes of the therapist. In recent years, a consensus has developed that real attributes of the therapist (reality factors), such as age, race, and gender, play a significant role in shaping the transference as well as the sequence in which therapeutic issues emerge.

3–7. **Answer: B (1 and 3).** Reassignment of a therapist on the basis of gender is frequently recommended. It is often thought to mobilize a stalemated situation. Unless there has been a sexual interaction with a prior therapist, however, it is rare that gender itself is the significant variable in the majority of therapies that are not successful. Reassignment to another therapist based on gender may be a way of avoiding responsibility for dealing with the embarrassment of a negative outcome. Erotic transference is a common development in psychotherapy and is not an indication to transfer the patient to a therapist of a different gender.

3–8. **Answer: A (1, 2, and 3).** Data are accumulating that suggest gender is a major factor in how group members respond to the leader. In female-led groups, men describe experiencing a sense of loss of control because they feel their ability to function as males is hindered. They often express relief and a return to normalcy when they are able to join male-led groups. Women who refuse to relinquish their assertive roles have been the targets of anger from both male and female members. Men are more likely to respond negatively to female leaders while positively reinforcing and reassuring male leaders who say the same things. Researchers have also noted that the more women talk in group situations, the more they tend to be ignored.

3–9. **Answer: 4.** The early view that the major determinant of gender development is the discovery of anatomical genital differences is no longer considered valid. The most important influence is how the parents relate to the infant regarding male and female roles. Even chromosomal factors can be overridden to some extent by parental assumptions about the gender of the child and relating to the child based on those gender assumptions. Boys and girls have different developmental experiences, with the differences largely related to cultural expectations of males and females.

3–10. **Answer: 2.** *Gender identity* is one's internalized sense of maleness or femaleness as well as a knowledge of one's biological sex, including the associated psychological attributes. Gender identity begins to evolve in early childhood and appears to be firmly established by about age 18 months. It derives from many influences, including identifications with parents and their attitudes, expectations, and behaviors, as well as biological and cultural factors. *Gender role* is a cultural construct referring to the expectations, attitudes, and behaviors that are considered to be appropriate for each gender in a particular culture.

3–11. **Answer: 3.** The process of diagnosis itself may be influenced by sex role stereotypes and gender bias. Agoraphobia is more commonly diagnosed in women and clearly relates to conflicts about autonomy, independence, and vulnerability to loss, issues all associated with female sexual stereotypes. Depression and borderline personality disorder (BPD) are also more commonly diagnosed in women than in men. Male patients who have the characteristics of BPD may be diagnosed as having narcissistic or antisocial personality disorder instead. Conversely, some women whose condition fulfills the criteria for antisocial personality disorder are diagnosed with BPD.

3–12. **Answer: 3.** Menopause is a marker of the life cycle that does not occur for men. Stereotyped expectations about women's life cycle and the attribution of midlife symptoms to menopause have resulted in the confusion of the experiences of this time of life, such as concerns about aging, family changes, shifts in expectations, and retirement, with the physiological event of cessation of menses. There is no evidence to support the notion that menopause causes depression. Those women who become depressed in midlife are generally those who have had depressions at other times in their lives. Estrogen replacement therapy does not address emotional or psychological problems, and responses to menopause are strongly influenced by cultural expectations.

CHAPTER 4

Cross-Cultural Issues in Psychiatric Treatment

DIRECTIONS: For questions 4–1 through 4–4, select the single best answer.

4–1. Which of the following terms is defined by "a set of meanings, behavioral norms, and values utilized by members of a particular society as they construct their unique view of the world"?

1. Ethnicity
2. Culture
3. Race
4. Values

4–2. Modern psychotherapy, which emerged from turn-of-the-century Western Europe, has questionable cross-cultural validity for all of the following reasons **except**

1. Modern psychotherapy espouses a predominantly psychological view of subjective experience, in which at times somatic expressions of distress are seen as more primitive.
2. Modern psychotherapy endorses independence and autonomous function at the expense of interdependence and belonging to a larger social unit.
3. Modern psychotherapy focuses to a great extent on ethnic origins of the patient.
4. Modern psychotherapy fails to see the individual's position in his or her family, society, and culture as an important determinant of the clinical presentation.

4–3. The term *emic* refers to

1. The conceptually narrow view by people in a given culture of a phenomenon occurring within that culture.
2. A presumed universal approach to the viewing of problems.
3. The imposition of a particular cultural perspective on observation about a different culture.
4. The biopsychosocial etiology of mental illness.

4-4. The concept of "locus of control" is defined as

1. A paranoid tendency to feel controlled by outside malevolent forces.

2. The extent to which a person believes that reinforcements in life are contingent upon his or her own efforts or determined by outside forces such as luck, chance, or fate.

3. The experience of one's actions, feelings, and expectations being controlled by other cultures.

4. None of the above.

■ DIRECTIONS: For statements 4–5 through 4–8, indicate whether the statement is true or false.

4-5. _____ The overwhelming majority of Asian, African, and Central and South American peoples actually experience distress somatically, so psychological interpretations of suffering may not be helpful.

4-6. _____ The category *black* refers to a group of individuals who share the same cultural values.

4-7. _____ Chinese and Chinese-American patients may view mental disorder as a sign of social and even supernatural disharmony that leads to a loss of face for individual and family alike.

4-8. _____ The syndrome known as *ataque de nervios* is a culturally determined somatically based syndrome found in Native American populations.

■ DIRECTIONS: For questions 4–9 through 4–12, indicate

A if answers 1, 2, and 3 are correct.

B if answers 1 and 3 are correct.

C if answers 2 and 4 are correct.

D if only answer 4 is correct.

E if all are correct.

4-9. In DSM-IV, the code V62.89 is to be used when a religious or spiritual problem is the principal focus of attention. This code would include which of the following situations?

1. Purely religious or spiritual problems

2. Mental disorders with a religious or spiritual content

3. Psychoreligious or psychospiritual problems not attributable to mental disorders

4. Delusions with religious content growing out of psychotic disorders

4-10. Nontraditional healing practices include which of the following?

1. *Espiritismo*

2. *Santería*

3. *Umbanda*

4. *Zar*

4–11. Which of the following is an outcome of acculturation when an individual migrates into the United States?

1. Individualism

2. Integration

3. Substantiation

4. Marginalization

4–12. In comparison to Caucasians and African-Americans, a much larger percentage of Asians are said to be "fast acetylators." This trait has an impact on the metabolism of which of the following drugs?

1. Clonazepam

2. Fluoxetine

3. Phenelzine

4. Haloperidol

■ **ANSWERS:**

4–1.   **Answer: 2.** Culture is defined as a set of behavioral norms, meanings, and values that are reference points and include social relationships, language, nonverbal expression of thoughts and emotions, religious beliefs, moral thought, technology, and financial philosophy. Culture is not a static notion, but one that changes as it is taught by one generation to the next.

4–2.   **Answer: 3.** Modern psychotherapy has *not* focused on the ethnic origins of the patient. The predominant models used in psychotherapeutic practice are oriented toward an intrapsychic view of subjective experience in which somatic expressions of emotional distress are seen as more primitive. Independence tends to be overvalued, and little emphasis is placed on the role of the larger social unit or the individual's position in the family, society, and culture.

4–3.   **Answer: 1.** As used in cross-cultural psychiatry, the term *emic* refers to the conceptually narrow view by people in a given culture of a phenomenon occurring within that culture. In some cultures, for example, an emic explanation of a severe stomachache may suggest that the cause of the abdominal discomfort is derived from the mixing of foods of different temperatures in the stomach. The term *etic* refers to a presumed universal approach to the viewing of such problems. When observers from one culture impose their own cultural perspective on observations about another culture, the result is a *pseudoetic* or "imposed etic" view.

4–4.   **Answer: 2.** Locus of control is a concept related to the issue of autonomy versus interdependence in cross-cultural studies. It is generally defined as the extent to which a person believes that reinforcements in life are contingent upon his or her own efforts (internal control) or are determined by outside forces such as luck, chance, fate, or powerful others (external control). In Asian culture, for example, a view of the individual as subject to situational forces beyond his or her control promotes the perception of an external locus of control. This culturally derived perception can be reinforced by the traumatizing experience of migration to a society in which one perceives others as oppressive and harsh.

4–5. **True** Many peoples around the world do not share the "psychologically minded" Western European and North American view of emotional distress. Asian, African, and Central and South American peoples not only express subjective distress in somatic terms but may experience this distress somatically. As a result, psychological interpretations may not be helpful.

4–6. **False** The category *black* has been used in many studies with the fallacious assumption that people in this category share the same cultural values. In fact, blacks may come from Jamaica, the United States, Great Britain, Haiti, or Africa, all of which have vastly different cultural values.

4–7. **True** It is difficult for many Chinese and Chinese-American patients to seek help for psychiatric illness because of the loss of face associated for both the individual and the family.

4–8. **False** The syndrome known as *ataque de nervios* is indeed a culturally determined somatically based syndrome used to express personal distress, but it is found in Puerto Rican populations, not in Native Americans.

4–9. **Answer: A (1, 2, and 3).** It has long been felt that psychiatry has been insensitive to the religious and spiritual issues that patients bring into treatment. The new code in DSM-IV is designed to include situations of purely religious or spiritual problems, mental disorders with religious or spiritual content, and psychoreligious or psychospiritual problems not attributable to a mental disorder.

4–10. **Answer: E (All).** *Espiritismo* is a culturally sanctioned practice of philosophy in Puerto Rico and other Hispanic Caribbean settings. It concerns the belief that many of life's misfortunes and conflicts can be helped by contact with the world of spirits that is said to surround the material world. *Santería* is a belief system native to Cuba that has been born of a syncretism between the religion of African slaves and the Catholic beliefs of their Spanish masters. *Umbanda* is a cult in Brazil that also involves syncretism between the African Yoruba beliefs and the Catholic credo. The *Zar* cult of the Northern Sudan is a healing movement practiced by women for the benefit of women.

4–11. **Answer: C (2 and 4).** Berry and Kim studied the outcome of acculturation and postulated four possible outcomes of the acculturative process. *Integration* is when an individual establishes positive relations with the dominant society without losing touch with his or her own culture of origin. An individual that neither feels strongly tied to his or her culture of origin nor feels well disposed to obtain support from the dominant culture has acquired a stance of *marginalization*. A stance of *separation* is adopted by individuals who feel tied to and supported by their culture of origin to the point where they see no benefit in associating with members of the dominant society. The stance of *assimilation* is said to be the outcome of those individuals who decide to embrace the dominant culture while partially or completely discounting the importance of their own culture of origin.

4–12. **Answer: B (1 and 3).** Polymorphisms of aldehyde dehydrogenase and alcohol dehydrogenase are more common in Asians than in Caucasians or African Americans. The result is that Asians are more likely to be "fast acetylators." This chemical difference has an impact on the metabolism of drugs such as clonazepam, caffeine, and phenelzine.

Disorders Usually First Diagnosed in Infancy, Childhood, or Adolescence

CHAPTER 5

Psychiatric Disorders in Mentally Retarded Persons

■ **DIRECTIONS: For questions 5–1 through 5–3, select the single best answer.**

5–1. Treatment modalities that are efficacious for persons with mental retardation include all the following **except**

1. Family therapy.
2. Insight/expressive long-term individual psychotherapy.
3. Pharmacological intervention.
4. Behavior modification.

5–2. Which of the following are sexual stereotypes of mentally retarded individuals?

1. They are sexually inhibited or have no sexual desires.
2. They are sexually immature and never develop sexual interests.
3. They are indiscriminate in their sexual behavior.
4. All of the above.

5–3. Which of the following are **not** adaptations of psychotherapeutic techniques necessary when working with developmentally handicapped persons?

1. Matching the technique to the person's intellectual development
2. Taking an indirect, nonconfrontive supportive style
3. Maintaining flexibility in the choice of treatment methods
4. Providing assistance in acknowledging the extent of the handicap

■ **DIRECTIONS: For questions 5–4 through 5–10, indicate**

A if answers 1, 2, and 3 are correct.

B if answers 1 and 3 are correct.

C if answers 2 and 4 are correct.

D if only answer 4 is correct.

E if all are correct.

5-4. Which persons will benefit most from psychotherapy?

    1. Those who have the capacity to recognize the similarity of their current life situations to previous situations

    2. Those who have experienced traumatic psychosocial experiences

    3. Those who have maladaptive personality functioning

    4. Those with moderate-to-mild mental retardation

5-5. Attachment theory is pertinent to which of the following aspects of psychotherapy for mentally retarded persons?

    1. The provision of a secure base in the therapeutic relationship

    2. The discovery of greater-than-anticipated communication handicaps

    3. The establishment of autobiographical competence

    4. The importance of establishing genital sexuality

5-6. The goal of behavior therapy is not only to reduce undesirable behaviors but to promote appropriate behaviors and responses to environmental stimuli. Of the following behaviors, which are most amenable to behavior modification?

    1. Stereotypic behaviors

    2. Destructive behaviors

    3. Noncompliance

    4. Inappropriate social interactions

5-7. Which of the following statements are **true** regarding the use of neuroleptics in mentally retarded persons?

    1. The prevalence rate of tardive dyskinesia in individuals with mental retardation on neuroleptics is as high as 30%, and persons with mental retardation are at increased risk for tardive dyskinesia.

    2. Risperidone, a combined serotonin-dopamine antagonist, is not efficacious in treating individuals with persistent behavioral disturbances.

    3. Young adults who are treated with thioridazine for behavioral dyscontrol may experience increased symptoms when the drug is withdrawn.

    4. Haloperidol is effective in the treatment of hyperactivity, self-injury, and assaultive behavior in children and adults with mental retardation.

5-8. What factors must be considered when deciding whether to prescribe antidepressants to mentally retarded persons?

    1. Individuals with mental retardation do not experience affective disorders.

    2. Antidepressant medications are effective in persons with mental retardation.

    3. Informed consent cannot be given by mentally retarded individuals.

    4. An increase in behavioral disturbances may occur.

5-9. Which of the following statements are **true** regarding group therapy for mentally retarded individuals?

    1. There is an opportunity to directly practice social skills.

    2. Adults, adolescents, and children all benefit equally from group therapy.

3. The therapist actively provides structure and facilitates communication.

4. Participants feel less comfortable discussing topics with others who have similar disabilities.

5–10. Which of the following statements are **false** regarding the treatment of mentally retarded individuals?

1. The family must be excluded to promote the development of transference in the therapy.

2. Confidentiality is imperative, and information should not be shared with caretakers.

3. Play therapy is inappropriate because it will only facilitate a regression in the patient.

4. Because thinking is characteristically disordered, psychotherapy is inadvisable.

■ **ANSWERS:**

5–1. **Answer: 2.** Although mildly retarded individuals (IQ 50–70) may greatly benefit from supportive and some insight-oriented psychotherapy, an intensive course of in-depth exploratory insight/expressive long-term individual psychotherapy is not the treatment of choice.

Family therapy is crucial in the treatment of individuals with mental retardation. The goals of family therapy include 1) allowing the mentally retarded individual to develop autonomy and self-reliance in a family system that may overprotect the patient, 2) addressing jealousy and other feelings of the unaffected siblings who may perceive that the patient receives more parental attention (or the feelings of the patient whose development lags behind the siblings), and 3) facilitating parental grieving over the child's developmental delays. Because mental retardation is a process that spans the life cycle, family therapy is valuable even for those persons who are chronologically adults, especially those individuals who require assistance with daily living skills.

Behavior modification techniques are central to the treatment of stereotypic behaviors, psychophysiological symptoms, noncompliance (65%–75% success rate), and destructive behaviors (45%–65% success rate). The goal of behavior therapy is not only to reduce undesirable behavior but also to promote appropriate behavior. Behavior modification techniques are particularly important when working with individuals with more severe mental retardation (IQ < 45), because the techniques do not require the use of language or conscious motivation. These interventions are less successful in establishing new social skills and in generalizing behaviors to other settings.

Pharmacological management has been used to address aggressive and impulsive behaviors, as well as affective and psychotic symptoms. Medication is not the first or the only treatment for difficult-to-manage behaviors. Consideration must be given to physical health, recent changes in everyday routines, and environmental and psychosocial adjustments. Neuroleptics such as haloperidol, chlorpromazine, and thioridazine are the most commonly prescribed agents for control of behavioral and psychotic symptoms. Lithium has also been used to manage aggression, with variable results. Psychostimulants such as methylphenidate, dextroamphetamine, and pemoline are generally considered drugs of choice in the pharmacological treatment of attention-deficit/hyperactivity disorder in children of normal intelligence. These medications may be safe and effective for hyperactive children with mild-to-moderate mental retardation (IQ 35–70). When antidepressants are used to treat major depression in mentally retarded persons, they were found to be as efficacious as in the treatment of non–mentally retarded individuals. Anticonvulsants may also be effective in treating behavioral dyscontrol in mentally retarded persons; however, the benefits must be carefully weighed against the side effects of blood dyscrasias and cognitive blunting.

5–2. **Answer: 4.** Based on stereotypes about inhibited, absent, or indiscriminate sexual activity in mentally retarded persons, sterilization was routinely practiced in the past. One treatment issue especially prominent in the older population of mentally retarded persons may be the loss of procreativity through sterilization and the effects of forced surgical treatment. Sexual interest generally corresponds to mental rather than chronological age; therefore, those individuals with severe or profound mental retardation may not achieve genital sexual interest. Mildly retarded individuals (IQ 50–70) may have limited access to social experiences with peers because of an overstructuring of their school or home environments, which may leave them with little opportunity to develop appropriate interpersonal skills and experiences with their peers. Family members may be reluctant to discuss sexual matters such as contraception, venereal disease, and basic sexual anatomy with their mentally retarded children or adolescents. Providing basic information may be addressed in individual therapy. Alternatively, the therapist may assist a parent or other family member in providing this information. Encouragement of relationships and teaching of appropriate social skills are prerequisites to facilitate the development of normal sexual identification.

5–3. **Answer: 2.** The following adaptations are recommended when working with handicapped persons. A directive approach is needed to maintain the focus of the therapy. Firm and clear limits should be established for aggressive, destructive, or excessive age-inappropriate affectionate behavior. The therapist must recommend alternative ways of coping with stressors. When specific questions are posed, the therapist should consider answering directly rather than exploring for unconscious fantasies. Providing feedback for effective behavior and offering reassurance when successes are reported are imperative. The therapist must be cognizant of any language or communication handicap and match his or her language with the patient's developmental level. Using sign language or communication boards may be critical. Syntactically simple language geared to the level of development is also essential. Immediately relevant and concrete examples must be provided to illustrate various points. Flexibility in therapeutic techniques is important. Play therapy may be used even with persons whose chronological age is well past childhood. The length and frequency of therapy sessions should be based on the individual's ability to tolerate the session; shorter and more frequent sessions may be necessary. The family and caretaking staff must be utilized to provide information, function as co-therapists, and provide support. Family members and caretaking staff also need support in working with handicapped persons. Confidentiality must be maintained, and the patient must be made to feel that he or she is an important provider of information. The patient's preferences must be respected and heeded as realistically as is possible. As with every therapy, the therapist must recognize the contributions of his or her own interpersonal distortions and prejudices. In addition, the desire to overprotect the patient must also be addressed. Finally, the impact of the disability and the chronicity must be reviewed with the patient.

5–4. **Answer: E (All).** The capacity for self-reflection and self-understanding is important in the person's ability to utilize verbal therapy. The individual must be able to anticipate the intentions of others and to act based on these anticipations. This capacity is linked to the cognitive stage of development that may be achieved by those with moderate-to-mild mental retardation. Persons with traumatic psychosocial experiences that have resulted in internalized conflict and persons with maladaptive personality functioning may be most amenable to psychotherapeutic interventions.

5–5. **Answer: B (1 and 3).** One purpose of psychotherapy with handicapped individuals is to allow them to achieve increased autonomy, which may be accomplished by providing a secure base in the therapeutic relationship. Similarly, the establishment of autobiographical competence is critical in developing the ability to transfer experiences and knowledge from one environment to a new setting. The discovery of communication handicaps that are far greater than anticipated, although not unusual, is not part of attachment theory. Providing information about sexual anatomy, sexually transmitted diseases, and contraception is important, but the development of genital sexuality is in part dependent on cognitive development and cannot be facilitated by therapy.

5–6. **Answer: A (1, 2, and 3).** Stereotypic behaviors, destructive behaviors, noncompliance, and psychophysiological symptoms are the most responsive to behavioral treatment (65%–75% success rate). Destructive behaviors are fairly responsive (45%–65% success rate). Inappropriate social interactions are the least responsive.

5–7. **Answer: B (1 and 3).** The typical prevalence rate of tardive dyskinesia in individuals with mental retardation on neuroleptics is as high as 30%; however, the risk factors are higher for being female, being older, and longer use of the neuroleptic. Persons with mental retardation are not at increased risk for tardive dyskinesia. Young adults treated with thioridazine for inappropriate behaviors may experience a small but significant increase in symptoms if the medication is withdrawn. Risperidone is efficacious in treating individuals for behavioral dyscontrol. Haloperidol has been shown to have highly variable results for treatment of hyperactivity, self-injury, and assaultive behavior in children. Even less compelling is the use of haloperidol for adults. Stereotyped behaviors may respond to haloperidol in adults and children.

5–8. **Answer: C (2 and 4).** Individuals with mental retardation may experience but have difficulty expressing symptoms of affective disorders because of limitations in cognitive development or communication. However, individuals with moderate-to-mild mental retardation may experience and be able to express their symptoms of affective disorders. Informed consent may be given by mentally retarded individuals, but family and caretakers should be involved in the decision. Antidepressant medications are effective in persons with mental retardation, but an increase in behavioral disturbances may occur, especially in individuals with severe or profound mental retardation.

5–9. **Answer: B (1 and 3).** Group therapy is generally most effective with adults and adolescents. Children may not have the attention span and verbal capacity to participate adequately. Discussing disabilities and social experiences may be facilitated by the group's including others with the same or similar difficulties. As with individual therapy, the therapist actively participates by maintaining structure and facilitating interactions between group members. Group therapy provides an opportunity to directly practice social skills and learn how to develop supportive extrafamilial relationships.

5–10. **Answer: E (All).** The family and caretakers should be included in treatment, and confidentiality must simultaneously be respected. Family members and caretakers may function as co-therapists and provide crucial additional support for the patient. The appropriateness of play therapy depends not on the chronological age but on the mental age of the individual and the degree of the impairment in communication. Thinking in persons with mental retardation is not characteristically disordered. Individual, group, and family therapy are all efficacious in the treatment of individuals with mental retardation.

CHAPTER 6

Learning Disorders

■ **DIRECTIONS: For statements 6–1 through 6–10, indicate whether the statement is true or false.**

6–1. _____ In the treatment of learning disorders, pharmacotherapy plays a primary role.

6–2. _____ The most frequent comorbid disorder in children with learning disorders is depression.

6–3. _____ Learning disorders are chronic, lifelong disabilities.

6–4. _____ Girls and boys are equally likely to be diagnosed with learning disorders.

6–5. _____ Children in private and parochial schools are not eligible for special services within the public school system.

6–6. _____ Through the Education for All Handicapped Children Act (Public Law 94-142), children are guaranteed an individualized education program.

6–7. _____ School principals must act within 30 working days if they receive a verbal request for a learning disorder screening from parents.

6–8. _____ If a screening process reveals a learning disorder, then the school system is obligated to provide services.

6–9. _____ With appropriate interventions, learning disorders can be cured.

6–10. _____ Learning disorders affect only a child's academic performance.

■ **ANSWERS:**

6–1. **False** There are no effective pharmacological interventions for children with learning disorders. Pharmacotherapy may be used to treat comorbid disorders such as attention-deficit/hyperactivity disorder (ADHD) or major depression. Learning disorders are most appropriately treated through an educational approach.

6–2. **False** The most commonly diagnosed comorbid disorder is ADHD.

6–3. **True** Although the way in which the learning disorder manifests itself varies over the life cycle, the underlying disability is persistent. Most learning disorders are diagnosed during the school years as a result of the child's inability to meet specific academic demands. Learning disorders may interfere with how the person performs on the job or interacts in relationships.

6–4. **False** Boys are diagnosed more frequently because of their behavioral disruption in the classroom; however, it is unclear if the actual incidence is higher in boys.

6–5. **False** Children in public, private, and parochial schools are all eligible for special services within the public school system.

6–6. **True** Through the Education for All Handicapped Children Act (PL 94-142) and its later revisions, students with disabilities are guaranteed all of the following:

1. That a free public education will be provided for all individuals between the ages of 3 and 21.

2. That for each person an *individualized education program* (IEP) will be developed. The IEP must be written; must be jointly developed by the school, teacher, and parent; and must include an analysis of the student's present achievement level, difficulties, and goals. Specific services that are to be provided must be identified. Specific ways of assessing progress must be noted.

3. That children with disabilities and without disabilities will be educated together to the fullest extent it is appropriate. That is, students with disabilities must be educated in the "least restrictive environment" that will allow for necessary services. The level of services need not mean that education is provided in the regular classroom. For some students, the least restrictive environment might be the most restrictive environment.

4. That tests and other evaluation materials used will be prepared and administered in such a way that they are not racially or culturally discriminatory. They must be presented, when needed, in the child's native language.

5. That these rights and guarantees apply to these children in private as well as public schools. That is, students in private schools are entitled to receive the same services from the public school as students in the public school.

6–7. **False** The 30-day time limit for a school principal to act on a request from parents for a learning disorder screening applies *only* when the request is made *in writing*.

6–8. **False** Individual school systems are allowed to set their own standards for learning disorders, including norms and "cut-off" scores.

6–9. **False** Appropriate interventions, including tutoring, specific styles of teaching, and career guidance, will all help the child manage the disability, but there is no cure.

6–10. **False** Learning disorders affect a child's or an adult's performance at school and at work and how he or she interacts in social relationships.

CHAPTER 7

Pervasive Developmental Disorders

■ **DIRECTIONS: For questions 7–1 through 7–11, indicate**

A if answers 1, 2, and 3 are correct.

B if answers 1 and 3 are correct.

C if answers 2 and 4 are correct.

D if only answer 4 is correct.

E if all are correct.

7–1. Autism is a chronic and pervasive disorder; therefore, it is important to set realistic short-term and long-term goals. Which of the following statements are **true** about the treatment objectives?

1. Behavioral symptoms should be decreased, but attention to continued development is not critical.
2. Pharmacotherapy may be the sole treatment for temper tantrums, aggression, hyperactivity, and stereotypies.
3. Modification of the child's environment produces no lasting effects.
4. Treatment should also take into account the needs of the family.

7–2. Medical and graduate student education has increasingly emphasized specialization as the amount of technical information has burgeoned. A drawback to specialization is that professionals tend to be interested in or accountable for solely their own discrete area of specialization. Other features associated with this model are

1. Everyone takes responsibility for the child.
2. The parents receive inconsistent or contradictory information on diagnosis and treatment.
3. The child is enrolled in the latest studies.
4. It is difficult for anyone to take responsibility for all of the child's needs.

7–3. The generalist model has been implemented in the TEACCH Program. This widely used program that crosses language and cultural barriers includes knowledge in which of the following areas?

1. Communication and normal speech development
2. Characteristics of pervasive developmental disorders (PDDs), including autism

      3. Behavior management

      4. Pharmacological treatment

7–4. Classrooms that have served children with autism have been developed with clear structure, expectations, and consequences. Which of the following have been important advances in classroom teaching of children with autism?

      1. The use of visual structure

      2. Emphasis on mild negative reinforcement and punishment

      3. Focus on "functional skills" such as self-care, basic work skills, and community functioning

      4. Emphasis on auditory learning

7–5. Communication is a major barrier in the treatment and prognosis of children with PDDs, including autism. Indeed, prognosis is significantly worse if the child does not develop useful interactive communication by age 5 years. Which of the following statements are **false** regarding communication and children with autism or another PDD?

      1. Facilitated communication is dictated by the client.

      2. Children may respond better to communication that is a predictable part of a set routine.

      3. Bodily gestures and motions are readily understood and are quite distinctive.

      4. Teaching spontaneous communication is efficacious.

7–6. Self-mutilation and self-injurious behaviors are common in children with autism. Which of the following techniques may be useful in decreasing these disturbing and potentially harmful behaviors?

      1. Pharmacotherapy

      2. Time-out, as in removing the child from a desirable social interaction

      3. Electric skin shock

      4. Positive reinforcement of socially acceptable replacement behaviors

7–7. Pharmacotherapy should never be the sole treatment of children with autism or another PDD. However, medication may improve specific target symptoms. For which of the following might pharmacotherapy be appropriate?

      1. Self-injurious behaviors

      2. Temper tantrums

      3. Hyperactivity

      4. Poor cognitive processing

7–8. Which of the following statements are **true** regarding the use of neuroleptics in the treatment of children with autism?

      1. Neuroleptics are the medications that have been most extensively studied in the treatment of autism.

      2. Higher IQ and greater severity of illness are associated with greater improvement.

      3. Older children respond more favorably than younger children.

      4. Dyskinesias are easily differentiated from stereotypies.

7–9. Which of the following statements are **true** regarding fenfluramine and its use in the treatment of children with autism?

    1. It is efficacious.

    2. Therapeutic gains are maintained.

    3. Effects on social interaction and hyperactivity are pronounced.

    4. Reduction of serotonin levels in the blood is associated with the administration of this medication.

7–10. Which of the following statements are **true** regarding clomipramine and its use in the treatment of children with autism?

    1. It is superior to placebo in reducing stereotypies, compulsive behaviors, and hyperactivity and in improving social interactions.

    2. Electrocardiogram changes include prolongation of the PR and QRS intervals.

    3. Seizures are not a concern.

    4. Constipation and urinary retention are particularly troublesome in this population.

7–11. Social deficits underlying the syndrome of autism are considered one of the most debilitating aspects of the disorder. Groups that involve social skills training share which of the following properties?

    1. They are conducted in a confrontive environment.

    2. Activities do not require in-depth understanding or production of complex language.

    3. The physical and temporal structure of the group revolves around conforming to social norms.

    4. Cooperation and attention to others are encouraged.

■ **DIRECTIONS: For questions 7–12 and 7–13, choose all answers that apply to each question.**

7–12. Which of the following statements are **true** regarding agents used in the treatment of autism and PDDs?

    1. Methylphenidate may produce a worsening of preexisting stereotypies.

    2. Hypotension may limit the use of beta-blockers and clonidine.

    3. Buspirone may be effective in reducing hyperactivity.

    4. Clonidine may produce long-lasting decreases in hyperactivity.

    5. Fluoxetine is a potent inhibitor of serotonin reuptake.

    6. Megavitamin therapy is efficacious.

    7. Sedation is a limiting factor in the use of clonidine.

    8. Buspirone has mixed dopaminergic and serotonergic properties.

7–13. Which of the following statements are **true** regarding individual therapy for individuals with autism?

    1. Therapy should emphasize real-life problems.

2. A therapeutic relationship may assist with identifying subtleties of interpersonal relationships.

3. These individuals will not form strong therapeutic relationships and may be treated by various therapists on rotation.

4. Confidentiality in therapy precludes having any contact with the family.

■ ANSWERS:

7–1. **Answer: D (Only 4).** Decreasing behavioral symptoms such as temper tantrums, aggression, motoric overarousal, and stereotypies is critical and is brought about by the use of medications, alterations in the child's environment, behavior modification techniques, and support of the parents in new procedures. Medication should never be the sole treatment. Indeed, the only lasting effects of drug therapy are believed to be indirect and secondary to modification of the patient's interaction with the environment. Assisting the child and family toward continued development is essential in the treatment of children with any PDD. The treatment needs of the family, with the family viewed both as a unit and as individuals, should be addressed and reassessed regularly, because this will facilitate the child's treatment. The importance of parent-professional collaboration cannot be overstated in developing a treatment plan for children with PDDs.

7–2. **Answer: C (2 and 4).** The trend toward specialization and subspecialization actually isolates the child and the family from receiving comprehensive and up-to-date care. Families are subjected to multiple opinions and views, which may further confuse the overall care of the child. In the model of specialization, no one person or team assumes full responsibility for the child.

7–3. **Answer: A (1, 2, and 3).** There are eight areas of general knowledge that should be mastered in the TEACCH Program: 1) characteristics of autism and other PDDs, 2) formal and informal diagnostic assessment, 3) structured teaching and reduction in behavior problems, 4) collaboration with families to expedite patient adaptation, 5) communication issues, 6) independence and vocational training, 7) social and leisure skills training, and 8) behavior management. This program uses a team approach, embracing professionals and family, to the long-term care of children and adults with autism and other PDDs. This method was developed by Schopler and has been implemented in the United States, Europe, and Japan.

7–4. **Answer: B (1 and 3).** Children with autism and other PDDs tend to be weak in auditory processing, in memory unrelated to their idiosyncratic interests, and in organization of their thoughts. They are relatively strong in visuospatial skills and visual processing. Cognitive approaches that incorporate visual processing and emphasize strategies for learning global skills have a greater long-term impact. Positive reinforcement and the above changes in curriculum produce better results than negative reinforcement or punishment.

7–5. **Answer: B (1 and 3).** More than 24 studies have shown that facilitated communication is dictated by the facilitator and not the client. Alphabet communication has been of varying usefulness with a wide range of children with communication difficulties. Pictures or picture rings may be particularly useful in children with autism or other PDDs, given the relative strengths that the children have in visual processing. Bodily gestures and motions may be valuable; however, they are not distinctive across a spectrum of children. Teaching spontaneous communication, especially in the context of a set or daily routine, can be the most productive way of promoting verbal skills.

7–6. **Answer: E (All).** Intense conflict concerning the use of only rewards and no aversive procedures, regardless of the behavior, exists among both parents and professionals. A consensus panel convened by the National Institutes of Health (1990) to address this issue, after considerable discussion and debate, recommended that emphasis be placed on behavior enhancement with rewards and that aversive procedures be used with destructive behaviors "only if the clinical situation require[s] short-term use of such restrictive interventions and *only* after appropriate review and consent are obtained." Some behaviors may be life-threatening, and the use of aversive procedures, such as a *mild* electric shock, may be lifesaving. Pharmacotherapy may be helpful in decreasing behaviors and the intense anxiety that some autistic individuals appear to relieve through certain behaviors, which frequently are damaging. There is a continued trend toward integrating behavioral and cognitive approaches.

7–7. **Answer: A (1, 2, and 3).** Target symptoms such as hyperactivity, temper tantrums, self-injurious or aggressive behaviors, and irritability may respond to medications. Approximately 70% of children with autism or another PDD function at the mentally retarded range, and medications will not improve their cognitive processing. Medications may allow the child to fully utilize inherent capabilities by modulating the behaviors that interfere with learning.

7–8. **Answer: A (1, 2, and 3).** Dyskinesias occur in 26.9%–29.27% of children treated with haloperidol and are generally reversible. The differentiation of drug-related dyskinesia from stereotypies is particularly difficult. Older children, children with higher IQs, and those with more severe behavioral symptoms all respond better than younger children, those with severe or profound mental retardation, or those with mild-to-moderate behavioral symptoms. This class of medications has been most extensively studied in autism.

7–9. **Answer: D (Only 4).** Fenfluramine is associated with a decrease in blood serotonin levels; however, it is neither safe nor efficacious. Therapeutic gains are lost after 6 months. The most pronounced effects of fenfluramine are on social interaction and hyperactivity, but these effects are quite variable.

7–10. **Answer: C (2 and 4).** Desipramine and clomipramine, potent inhibitors of serotonin reuptake, were both found to be efficacious in reducing stereotypies, compulsive behaviors, and hyperactivity, but not in improving social interactions. Clomipramine, amoxapine, and bupropion are all antidepressants associated with drug-induced seizures and may lower seizure threshold. Constipation and urinary retention are particularly troublesome in young children and in a population who have poor communication skills. Chronic constipation may lead to impaction that requires surgical intervention. Urinary retention predisposes the individual to urinary tract infections, requiring treatment with yet another medication. Like other heterocyclic antidepressants, clomipramine has a quinidine-type effect of prolonging conduction, including PR, QRS, and QT intervals, and producing a resting tachycardia.

7–11. **Answer: C (2 and 4).** Groups that involve social skills training are conducted in a positive, supportive environment that emphasizes the needs of individuals with autism. Social norms are addressed within the group context, but the physical and temporal structure of the group revolves around the needs of the group members. Activities that emphasize cooperation and attention to others are stressed. These activities are designed to use simple language geared to the group's level of functioning.

7–12. **Answer: 1, 2, 3, 4, 5, 7, and 8.** Methylphenidate has been noted to worsen preexisting stereotypies; however, in some studies, a decrease in motoric over-arousal was noted. No definite conclusions can be made about the usefulness of methylphenidate in the treatment of children with autism. Clonidine is a centrally acting alpha-adrenergic receptor partial agonist and an antihypertensive agent. Most recently, it has been used to treat motoric overarousal and poor attention associated with attention-deficit/hyperactivity disorder. It is also used to treat Tourette's syndrome. It may be effective in reducing hyperactivity and irritability. The most common side effect is sedation. Hypotension may limit the use of clonidine and beta-blockers. The efficacy of beta-blockers has not been established, although there are some reports of a decrease in self-injurious behaviors. Fluoxetine is a potent inhibitor of serotonin reuptake and may decrease self-injurious behaviors. Side effects include hyperactivity, agitation, restlessness, insomnia, and decreased appetite. Buspirone, an anxiolytic medication with mixed dopaminergic and serotonergic effects, may be useful in decreasing hyperactivity. Megavitamin therapy has not been proven to be efficacious in autism.

7–13. **Answer: 1 and 2.** Individual therapy can be efficacious in treating a verbal individual with autism or another PDD. These individuals can depend on the regularity and familiarity of weekly sessions and can utilize this feature as a bridge to understanding the external world by using the therapist to work on subtleties of interpersonal relationships and to solve problems of daily living. Although these individuals may be slow to form a therapeutic alliance, once it is created, the relationships tend to be strong and enduring. Autistic individuals are not good candidates for clinics, where there is a high turnover rate of therapists. From the initiation of the therapy, a relationship with the patient's support network must be established.

CHAPTER 8

Attention-Deficit/Hyperactivity Disorder: Pharmacotherapy

DIRECTIONS: For questions 8–1 through 8–15, match the pharmacological agent with the associated property (properties), mechanism(s) of action, or side effect(s). Each response may be used once, more than once, or not at all.

8–1.	Desipramine	a.	Typical starting dose 18.75–37.5 mg
8–2.	D-Amphetamine	b.	Sudden death
8–3.	Propranolol	c.	Increases tricyclic antidepressant (TCA) levels
8–4.	Sertraline	d.	Toxic psychosis
8–5.	Imipramine	e.	Anorexia
8–6.	Nortriptyline	f.	Tic disorders
8–7.	Bupropion	g.	Tertiary amine
8–8.	Deprenyl	h.	Hypotension
8–9.	Magnesium pemoline	i.	Half-life 10–17 hours
8–10.	Fluoxetine	j.	Increases heart rate and blood pressure
8–11.	Paroxetine	k.	Electrocardiogram (ECG) necessary
8–12.	Clonidine	l.	Secondary amine
8–13.	Methylphenidate	m.	Associated with seizures
8–14.	Phenelzine	n.	Quinidine-like effect
8–15.	Amitriptyline	o.	Dietary regimen must be followed
		p.	Associated with weight gain
		q.	Liver toxicity
		r.	Tooth decay
		s.	Indirect dopamine agonist
		t.	Rebound hypertension
		u.	Lethal in overdose
		v.	Depressive symptoms

w. Plasma levels used clinically

x. Priapism

y. Sudden withdrawal associated with flulike symptoms

z. Total daily dose 0.3–3 mg/kg/day

■ **DIRECTIONS: For questions 8–16 and 8–17, choose all answers that apply.**

8–16. Which of the following statements are **false** regarding attention-deficit/hyperactivity disorder (ADHD)?

1. Pharmacotherapy is curative.

2. Children will outgrow their ADHD.

3. At least 30% of children with ADHD have concomitant learning disorders.

4. There is a genetic origin for ADHD.

5. Behavioral interventions have long-lasting effects.

6. Psychosocial interventions can be generalized to untrained situations.

8–17. Which of the following are **true** statements regarding the pharmacological management of ADHD?

1. Stimulants are the mainstay of treatment for children and adolescents, but not for adults, with ADHD.

2. Magnesium pemoline, methylphenidate, and D-amphetamine are short-acting compounds that must be given every 4 hours.

3. The mechanism of action of stimulants is to block the reuptake of catecholamines.

4. Paroxetine, fluoxetine, and sertraline are associated with increased TCA levels.

5. ADHD symptoms improve in 90% of children treated with L-deprenyl.

6. Studies have shown that 70% of individuals with ADHD respond to stimulant medication alone.

7. Propranolol is a selective beta-adrenergic antagonist.

8. Response to stimulant medication may be inhibited in children who are highly anxious or depressed.

■ **DIRECTIONS: For questions 8–18 through 8–22, indicate**

A if answers 1, 2, and 3 are correct.

B if answers 1 and 3 are correct.

C if answers 2 and 4 are correct.

D if only answer 4 is correct.

E if all are correct.

8–18. Which of the following statements are **false** regarding the treatment of ADHD?

   1. The patient may be seen monthly during the initiation of medication.
   2. Thirty percent of patients treated with stimulants may have an insufficient response.
   3. There are no extraordinary risks when stimulant medication is used in the treatment of children with conduct disorder and ADHD.
   4. Desipramine may be safely administered to children.

8–19. Which of the following statements regarding ECGs and the pediatric population are valid?

   1. Heart rates of 100–130 beats per minute are not necessarily considered to be abnormal or to have major hemodynamic significance.
   2. An incomplete right bundle branch block (RBBB; QRS 100–120 msec) may be found in 10% of the pediatric population.
   3. A complete RBBB (QRS > 120 msec) does not necessarily imply impaired cardiac function.
   4. Atrioventricular block (A-V block; PR ≥ 200 msec) is a frequent finding in the pediatric population.

8–20. Which of the following medications may be used to treat the signs and symptoms of both ADHD and tic disorders?

   1. Clonidine
   2. Pimozide
   3. Methylphenidate and nortriptyline
   4. Haloperidol

8–21. Which of the following medications will have little to no effect on the use of stimulant medication?

   1. Isocarboxazid
   2. Paroxetine
   3. Pseudoephedrine
   4. Diphenhydramine

8–22. Which of the following comorbid disorders are found in at least 15% of children with ADHD?

   1. Learning disorders
   2. Mood disorders
   3. Anxiety disorders
   4. Conduct disorders

■ **ANSWERS:**

8–1. Desipramine: **b, i, j, k, l, n, r, u, w, y**

8–2. D-Amphetamine: **d, e, j, v, z**

8–3. Propranolol: **h, k, t**

8–4. Sertraline: **e**

8–5. Imipramine: **g, i, j, k, n, r, u, w, y**

8–6. Nortriptyline: **i, j, k, l, n, r, u, w, y**

8–7. Bupropion: **m, s**

8–8. Deprenyl: **c, h**

8–9. Magnesium pemoline: **a, d, j, q, r, v, z**

8–10. Fluoxetine: **c, e**

8–11. Paroxetine: **e**

8–12. Clonidine: **h, k, t**

8–13. Methylphenidate: **d, e, f, j, v, z**

8–14. Phenelzine: **c, h, o**

8–15. Amitriptyline: **g, i, j, k, n, r, u, w, y**

8–16. **Answer: 1, 2, 4, 5, and 6.** ADHD is a chronic disorder persisting throughout the life cycle. The precise etiology of ADHD is unknown, although twin and adoption studies suggest that a genetic component appears to account for some forms of the disorder. Other etiologies are also likely, such as psychological traumas and perinatal insults. Approximately 3%–5% of all school-age children meet the criteria for the diagnosis, and 2% of adults also have ADHD. In those children diagnosed with ADHD, 10%–60% have symptoms as adults. This disorder may be a relatively common adult disorder that may be underdiagnosed. Although pharmacotherapy can greatly ameliorate the behavioral and attentional components of this disorder, it is not curative. Behavioral and psychosocial interventions can be helpful, but they have not proven to be long-lasting and generalizable in untrained situations. Learning disorders are one of the most common comorbid disorders found in ADHD children, with 30% of the children meeting the criteria for diagnosis of at least one learning disorder.

8–17. **Answer: 3, 5, 6, and 8.** Stimulant medication continues to be the mainstay of pharmacological management of children, adolescents, and adults with ADHD. There have been more than 100 controlled studies that have documented the efficacy and safety of stimulants. Overall, there is a 70% response rate to stimulant medication alone. The mechanism of action for stimulants is to prevent the reuptake of all catecholamines into presynaptic nerve endings, preventing degradation of the catecholamines by monoamine oxidase. Methylphenidate and D-amphetamine are both short-acting compounds with peak onset between 1 and 3 hours of administration. They must be given approximately every 4 hours. Magnesium pemoline is a long-acting preparation that is given in a single daily dose. Fluoxetine, but not paroxetine and sertraline, strongly inhibits hepatic enzymes such as P450, thereby increasing the blood levels of TCAs. L-Deprenyl, a selective monoamine oxidase–B inhibitor that does not require strict dietary restrictions, was found to be effective in reducing ADHD symptoms in 90% of the children studied. Propranolol is a central- and peripheral-acting nonselective beta-adrenergic receptor antagonist that may exacerbate asthma and mask hypoglycemia in individuals with diabetes mellitus. The impact of comorbidity on treatment response is not well studied. There is some evidence that children with ADHD who are also depressed or overly anxious may not respond optimally to stimulant medication. These children have been shown to respond to desipramine.

8–18. **Answer: B (1 and 3).** Weekly contact with the ADHD patient and family is necessary during the initial phase of treatment. Stimulant medications are highly prized contraband in the delinquent subculture and therefore should be avoided in children with comorbid conduct disorder who are not receiving careful supervision. As many as 30% of individuals with ADHD may have no or an inadequate response to stimulant medication. These patients may respond to a TCA, selective serotonin reuptake inhibitor (SSRI), or clonidine, or they may require multiple medications to manage their symptoms. The investigation by a task force from the Work Group on Research from the American Academy of Child and Adolescent Psychiatry showed that despite markedly increased exposure to desipramine, the number of fatalities from sudden death associated with desipramine did not increase. A careful evaluation of the risks and benefits must be undertaken before using desipramine, but this medication has been shown to be clinically safe and efficacious.

8–19. **Answer: A (1, 2, and 3).** In the first decade of life, sinus tachycardia is found at baseline in 20% of children. An incomplete RBBB is considered a normal variant in the pediatric population. A complete RBBB in the absence of cardiac disease does not imply impaired cardiac function. RBBB may impede electro-mechanical function of the right ventricle; therefore, a noninvasive study of the quality of myocardial contraction (ejection fraction and cardiac output) is warranted. A-V block is found in only 0.5% of children at baseline and is not a normal variant. The presence of an A-V block at baseline warrants a complete cardiac workup.

8–20. **Answer: B (1 and 3).** Approximately 10% of all children with ADHD have an associated tic disorder, and 50% of patients with Tourette's syndrome may have comorbid ADHD. In the pediatric population, clonidine alone may suffice for the treatment of ADHD and tic disorders. Clonidine may also be combined with a stimulant or a TCA. The use of stimulants alone may actually decrease the frequency of the tics, or it may exacerbate the tics. Stimulants may be combined with a TCA in the treatment of ADHD and tics. Neuroleptics, pimozide, and haloperidol are not effective in the treatment of ADHD.

8–21. **Answer: C (2 and 4).** Isocarboxazid is a monoamine oxidase inhibitor and will have synergistic reactions with stimulants. Pseudoephedrine is a synthetic catecholamine found in many over-the-counter cold preparations, including those given to children, and may potentiate the effect of stimulant medication. Diphenhydramine is an antihistamine and will not generally have a clinically discernible effect on stimulants. Paroxetine, sertraline, and fluoxetine are all SSRIs. Fluoxetine, but not paroxetine and sertraline, increases the blood levels of TCAs. To date, there is no known interaction between stimulants and the SSRIs.

8–22. **Answer: E (All).** Thirty percent of children with ADHD have a concomitant learning disorder, 15%–75% will experience an affective disorder at some time, 25% will have an anxiety disorder (including posttraumatic stress disorder), and 30%–50% will meet the diagnostic criteria for conduct disorder. In addition, 10% of children with ADHD will also have a tic disorder.

CHAPTER 9

Conduct Disorder

■ **DIRECTIONS: For questions 9–1 through 9–6, choose all answers that apply.**

9–1. Disruptive behavior disorder is the most stable of all childhood disorders. The gender-specific rates are 9% for males and 2% for females. What other statements are **valid** regarding disruptive behavior disorder?

1. Punishment increases disruptive behaviors in a child with disruptive behavior disorder.

2. Antisocial parents are more likely than nonantisocial parents to produce a child with disruptive behavior disorder.

3. Parents of children with disruptive behavior disorder frequently request and follow through with treatment.

4. Approval and encouragement are sufficient rewards for the child with disruptive behavior disorder.

9–2. What countertransference factors may elicit a menacing or assaultive response in children with conduct disorders?

1. Fear of the child

2. Anger at the child or parents

3. Judgmental attitudes regarding the patient's behavior or belief system

4. Anxiety

9–3. Medication should not ordinarily be used to control behavior. Children and adolescents with disruptive disorders need to assume a developmentally appropriate level of responsibility for their actions. Medication is indicated for which of the following conditions?

1. The behaviors are escalating to the point of destroying a previously adequate placement.

2. The child has no desire to change or work on his or her difficulties.

3. There is an underlying condition such as ADHD or psychosis.

4. There is an underlying paranoid ideational component.

9–4. What medications are the most commonly used to control aggressive outbursts?

1. Haloperidol

2. Lithium

     3. Carbamazepine

     4. Chlorpromazine

9–5. Parent management training is based on social learning theory and is part of the cognitive-behavioral techniques used in the treatment of youths with disruptive behavior disorder. Which of the following are critical aspects of this technique regarding the parents' role?

     1. Providing social rewards for the child

     2. Developing a tolerance for their child's behaviors

     3. Establishing age-appropriate rules

     4. Negotiating compromises

9–6. What type of family therapy is the most appropriate for families with a child with disruptive behavior disorder?

     1. Client-centered family therapy

     2. Psychodynamic family therapy

     3. Functional family therapy

     4. No type is successful

■ **DIRECTIONS: For questions 9–7 through 9–9, indicate**

     A if answers 1, 2, and 3 are correct.

     B if answers 1 and 3 are correct.

     C if answers 2 and 4 are correct.

     D if only answer 4 is correct.

     E if all are correct.

9–7. Cognitive problem-solving skills are based on the early work of Luria, who observed that children would first comment out loud on the tasks to be performed and talk themselves through the task. Problem-solving therapy in children with disruptive behavior disorder is focused on which of the following goals?

     1. Establishment of an internal dialogue

     2. Appraisal of situations and anticipation of their impact on others

     3. Constructive management of anger

     4. Development of external guides for self-evaluation

9–8. Which of the following are common reasons that treatment programs for youths with disruptive behavior disorder fail?

     1. The parents overtly or covertly support the child's behavior.

     2. The child's ego development is not sufficient to manage the particular program.

     3. The child has been "written off" by parents and others.

     4. The parents receive too little social support.

9–9. To create a workable home-based treatment program for youths with disruptive behavior disorder, what services must the children and their parents have?

1. Probation officers

2. Court-ordered treatment

3. After-school groups

4. Individual psychotherapy

■ ANSWERS:

9–1. **Answer: 1 and 2.** Unlike for healthy children, for whom punishment decreases a behavior, for the child with disruptive behavior disorder, punishment only serves to increase the problematic behavior. Antisocial behaviors tend to run in families. Adoption studies show a fairly strong genetic loading for criminal behavior; however, antisocial parents can also produce children with disruptive behavior disorder through deficiencies in the family environment. Indeed, parental discord is the strongest predictor of delinquency, and parental response (whether exaggerated or minimal) to delinquent behaviors is the strongest prognostic indicator. Parents of children with disruptive behavior disorder and the children themselves rarely request treatment. Treatment is frequently court ordered. Children with disruptive behavior disorder have little regard for praise or encouragement and respond best to concrete rewards.

9–2. **Answer: 1, 2, 3, and 4.** A high level of any expressed emotion may elicit an assaultive or menacing response from the child. A firm, clear, supportive, and patient response is the optimal approach to these children. The physician and other treaters must avoid overreacting or minimizing antisocial behaviors, remembering that it is the patient who must regain self-control.

9–3. **Answer: 1, 3, and 4.** Maintaining a placement may become critical in today's environment of limited funding. Long-term hospital treatment had proven useful in the past for youths with disruptive behavior disorder. However, there are now few adequate hospital or residential settings. Medications on a time-limited basis may help control the child's behavior as well as help maintain the child in the placement. If the youth has no desire to change, then medication may simply become yet another power struggle. However, if the youth is in an appropriate environment in which supportive structure is provided, and if the child is motivated to change but is unable to do so because of emotional lability, impulsivity, or paranoid ideation, then medication may be used. The diagnosis of disruptive behavior disorder is based on a collection of behaviors and does not address dynamic or etiological factors. Comorbid diagnoses of bipolar disorder, schizophrenia, learning disorders, attention-deficit/hyperactivity disorder, posttraumatic stress disorder, and major depression must be carefully addressed and appropriately treated.

9–4. **Answer: 1 and 4.** Haloperidol and chlorpromazine remain the most commonly prescribed medications to control aggressive outbursts. Short-term side effects of excessive sedation and acute dystonia are frequent with haloperidol. Furthermore, haloperidol has a significant negative impact on cognition. Both medications reduce aggression, explosiveness, and temper tantrums. Lithium is as effective as haloperidol and does not have a negative impact on cognition;

however, it can be lethal in an overdose and requires thyroid and serum level monitoring (range 0.5–1.5 mEq/L). Carbamazepine has antiaggressive effects that are independent of electroencephalographic (EEG) abnormalities, yet a review of the studies has yielded equivocal results with regard to its efficacy in the treatment of aggression.

9-5. **Answer: 3 and 4.** Children with disruptive behavior disorder do not respond to social rewards but will respond to nonsocial, concrete reinforcers. Families of youths with disruptive behavior disorder frequently overrespond and underrespond to their child's behavior. Teaching parents how to respond to antisocial behavior in a firm and concrete manner is important in family therapy work.

9-6. **Answer: 3.** Family therapy can be successful with even moderately motivated families of children with disruptive behavior disorder. Just as they do with their children, these families may become more volatile when intense emotional issues and relationships are explored along the lines of psychodynamic family therapy. Client-centered family therapy does not work well with these families because they have difficulty processing information and then constructively acting on the given information. Functional family therapy, like the cognitive problem-solving skills techniques used with the children, emphasizes problem-solving techniques and communication.

9-7. **Answer: A (1, 2, and 3).** The goal for this therapy is to have the youth develop an internal dialogue for self-evaluation. This therapy first involves having the youth talk his or her way through a task and then learn to anticipate the impact of his or her actions on others and plan ahead. Constructive anger management is also an important aspect of this therapy.

9-8. **Answer: E (All)** Parents whose child has disruptive behavior disorder may themselves have antisocial personalities, substance abuse, somatization disorders, major depression, or other affective disorders that render them unable to discern their child's behavior as age appropriate, socially acceptable, or even criminal. Parents who have struggled for many years with their child may be emotionally, physically, and fiscally drained and unable to support yet another attempt at treatment. The child and his or her parents may be too fragile to manage a given program because the low level of ego development or overwhelming environmental pressures exerted on both the child and parents render a placement untenable.

9-9. **Answer: B (1 and 3).** For a home placement to succeed, it need not be court ordered, but the parents must be solidly committed to following through with treatment, including use of the legal system when it is warranted. Probation officers who are trained to work with adolescents and children are critical to long-term home placement. Within the educational system, social workers who work with the children and their families, as well as specialized classrooms that can adequately contain the children, are necessary. Because the children need nearly round-the-clock supervision, day treatment and after-school groups are also necessary. Traditional outpatient psychotherapy works well with the child who has a high level of ego integration, experiences guilt, is capable of empathy, and forms meaningful relationships. Individual psychotherapy is not necessarily a critical component in the treatment of most youths with disruptive behavior disorder. If the child cannot be maintained in the home, then group or residential programs are the next step.

CHAPTER 10

Tic Disorders

■ **DIRECTIONS: For question 10–1, choose all answers that apply.**

10–1. Which of the following statements are **true** regarding tic disorders?

1. The genetics of Tourette's syndrome (TS) and obsessive-compulsive disorder (OCD) are unrelated.

2. Intrapsychic conflicts may be more disabling than the actual tics.

3. Impairment correlates best with the magnitude and duration of the tics and the circumstances at the peak levels of severity.

4. The relationship between the child and the family has no correlation with prognosis.

5. Approximately 50% of children with tic disorders may meet the criteria for attention-deficit/hyperactivity disorder (ADHD).

6. The male-to-female ratio is 4:1.

7. The lifetime prevalence may be as high as 10%.

■ **DIRECTIONS: For questions 10–2 through 10–11, select the single best answer.**

10–2. Children with TS will frequently have learning difficulties. Which of the following is the most common learning disorder in children with TS?

1. Spelling
2. Handwriting
3. Reading
4. Arithmetic

10–3. The goal of treatment in children and adults with tic disorders is

1. To reduce symptoms.
2. To further research into the etiology of tic disorders.
3. To facilitate overall development.
4. To have the patient accept his or her symptoms.

10–4. What is the mainstay of treatment for TS?

    1. Education

    2. Pharmacotherapy

    3. Psychodynamic family therapy

    4. A specialized classroom setting

10–5. Which one of the following medications or combinations is used in the treatment of tic disorder but not in the treatment of ADHD and tic disorders?

    1. Deprenyl and clonidine

    2. Clonazepam

    3. Desipramine and pimozide

    4. Methylphenidate and haloperidol

10–6. What area of the brain is thought to be involved in TS?

    1. Frontal cortex

    2. Cerebellum

    3. Thalamus

    4. Basal ganglia

10–7. Which of the following therapeutic modalities may be useful in reducing depression or anxiety and may facilitate understanding of how TS may interact with other tic disorders and ADHD?

    1. Client-centered individual therapy

    2. Supportive individual therapy

    3. Interpersonal individual therapy

    4. Brief time-limited individual therapy

10–8. Which of the following is **not** part of a behavioral program for TS?

    1. Clear expectations

    2. Separate programs for home and school

    3. Predictability

    4. Appropriate and timely rewards

10–9. Which of the following medications has the fewest side effects and has proven efficacy in the treatment of TS?

    1. Haloperidol

    2. Clonidine

    3. Pimozide

    4. Propranolol

10–10. Which of the following medications is the first choice in individuals with co-morbid ADHD and TS?

    1. Clonidine

    2. Magnesium pemoline

    3. Nortriptyline

    4. Pimozide

10–11. Self-injurious behaviors are the most dangerous of all the symptoms of TS. What is the first line of treatment?

    1. Dopaminergic blocking agents

    2. Behavior therapy

    3. Family therapy

    4. Individual psychotherapy

■ **ANSWERS:**

10–1. **Answer: 2, 3, and 5.** There is a strong genetic link between TS and OCD. As many as 40% of patients who have TS for 10 years will have OCD. Intrapsychic conflicts are frequently more disabling than the actual tics. Impairment in tic disorders correlates with magnitude and duration of the tics and the circumstances at the peak levels of severity rather than the mean number of tics. Videotapes may provide more accurate accounting of subtle tics and frequency than verbal reports by the patient or the family. As with any chronic illness, there is a pronounced mutual influence between the child's symptoms and the family relationships. Approximately 50% of children with TS meet the criteria for ADHD, and 10% of children with ADHD meet the criteria for TS. The male-to-female ratio is 1.6:1 to 3:1. The lifetime prevalence for tic disorders may actually be as high as 20%.

10–2. **Answer: 4.** Several studies have suggested deficits in mathematical skills. Children with both ADHD and TS may have more global deficits in visual-motor integration. Treatment of the arithmetic disorder should follow the same guidelines as those used in the treatment of any learning disorder.

10–3. **Answer: 3.** The goal of treatment for tic disorders is to facilitate developmental progress and adaptation. Symptom reduction is an ancillary objective. In the process of treatment, the patient may come to work with the disorder and accept it as a somatic reality, but the goal of treatment is not to prod the patient into passive acceptance. Patients and their families may wish to enroll in various studies concerning the treatment and pathogenesis of tic disorders; however, the goal of treatment is not to uncover a specific etiology.

10–4. **Answer: 1.** Educating the patient, the family, and the school system about the etiology and natural history of the disorder can reduce anxiety, place symptom severity in perspective, and lay the groundwork for later treatment. Educating teachers and school nurses about TS can be the first step in the care of an individual patient. Pharmacotherapy can be useful in reducing symptoms. Medications must always be prescribed in the context of a therapeutic relationship in which the patient understands the target symptoms and side effects. TS can place burdens on family members and close relationships. Initially providing a format of education and understanding may diffuse stress and blaming. In general, children with TS should receive whatever educational placement is most appropriate, which does not necessarily mean placement in a specialized classroom setting.

10–5. **Answer: 2.** Clonazepam is a benzodiazepine that is conventionally used as an anticonvulsant for petit mal, minor motor, and infantile spasm seizure disorders.

It has proven useful in a group of TS patients. It has relatively few side effects (sedation and dizziness are the most common) and is safe for long-term administration. Deprenyl is a selective monoamine oxidase–B inhibitor that does not require the dietary restrictions of the other monoamine oxidase inhibitors and has proven efficacious in the treatment of ADHD. Methylphenidate is a short-acting psychostimulant and is a mainstay in the treatment of ADHD. Nortriptyline is a secondary amine tricyclic antidepressant with fewer cardiac effects and a therapeutic window of 50–150 ng/mL. Desipramine is a secondary amine tricyclic antidepressant that has been extensively studied. Both nortriptyline and desipramine have proven efficacious in the treatment of ADHD without exacerbating tics. Clonidine is a centrally and peripherally acting alpha2-noradrenergic receptor partial agonist that has proven effective in the treatment of tics and ADHD.

10–6. **Answer: 4.** Medications that reduce tic symptomatology work on far-reaching areas of the central and peripheral nervous system. Recent work has linked cortico-striato-thalamo-cortical pathways to the basal ganglia, and magnetic resonance imaging (MRI) scanning data suggest changes in the basal ganglia in individuals with TS.

10–7. **Answer: 3.** Because TS is a chronic disorder that may initially manifest in childhood, brief time-limited therapy will not sufficiently address intrapsychic conflicts and developmental issues. Supportive therapy will not explore the intrapsychic conflicts of self-esteem, identifications, and self-perceptions that may powerfully influence the tic disorder. Interpersonal and cognitive therapies have proven particularly effective in the treatment of depression, and interpersonal therapy will allow for resolution of internal conflicts.

10–8. **Answer: 2.** Many of the strategies that are useful in school will also be useful in the home environment. Creating an integrated program will provide the child with a consistent, predictable system with clear expectations and appropriate and timely rewards. Such behavioral systems foster communication between parents and the school system and lower the level of anxiety while promoting appropriate development.

10–9. **Answer: 2.** Although 80% of patients will respond to haloperidol or pimozide, as many as 50% of patients will develop side effects. The long-term risk of tardive dyskinesia must also be weighed when considering using a neuroleptic. Propranolol is not generally used to treat TS. Clonidine has a slow onset of action, requiring 12 weeks for a clinical trial, and fewer individuals may respond. Clonidine, however, has no known long-term side effects and the fewest short-term side effects.

10–10. **Answer: 1.** Clonidine is the only medication with documented efficacy in the treatment of ADHD and TS without exacerbating the tic disorder. Magnesium pemoline is the longest-acting psychostimulant and is efficacious in treating ADHD; however, as with the other stimulants, it may exacerbate tic symptoms. In addition, magnesium pemoline is associated with hepatic toxicity. Nortriptyline is a tricyclic antidepressant that is efficacious in the treatment of ADHD but not in the treatment of TS. Pimozide is an antipsychotic that is efficacious in the treatment of TS but not in the treatment of ADHD. If there is no response to clonidine alone, then the addition of dopaminergic blocking agents is warranted.

10–11. **Answer: 1.** Because self-injurious behaviors may be life-threatening, dopaminergic blocking agents may be the first line because they are more likely than other agents to work and they act more rapidly. Behavioral, family, and individual therapies are all adjunctive treatments. Clonidine may be used if side effects to dopaminergic agents arise. Selective serotonin reuptake inhibitors may also be tried if the patient has a personal or family history of OCD. Repetitive self-injurious behaviors may be a manifestation of a compulsion or a complex tic.

CHAPTER 11

Elimination Disorders

■ DIRECTIONS: For questions 11–1 and 11–2,
choose all answers that apply.

11–1. Which of the following statements apply to enuresis?

1. There is rarely evidence of functional urinary tract abnormalities.
2. There is a relationship with disorders of sleep and sleep architecture.
3. There may be a history of developmental delays.
4. The disorder may have a familial aggregation.
5. There are specific psychiatric disorders associated with the disorder.
6. Constipation may be a concomitant problem.
7. Children who are not "dry" by age 3 years are at risk.

11–2. Which of the following statements apply to encopresis?

1. Fecal retention occurring before age 1 year can predict later encopresis.
2. The anus is anteriorly displaced.
3. Stressful events may be associated with the onset.
4. The disorder is associated with neglectful toilet training.
5. Constipation may have a familial aggregation.
6. Other psychiatric disorders are commonly associated with the disorder.

■ DIRECTIONS: For questions 11–3 through 11–9, indicate

A if answers 1, 2, and 3 are correct.
B if answers 1 and 3 are correct.
C if answers 2 and 4 are correct.
D if only answer 4 is correct.
E if all are correct.

11–3. Cindy is a 6-year-old girl who has frequent urinary tract infections and wets her pants both during the day and at night. Her toilet training began at 15 months of age. She walked at 10 months and spoke simple sentences at 26 months. She is currently doing well in first grade. Her mother considers her daughter's behavior "normal" and is not concerned. Which of the following statements apply to this case?

1. Given the mother's normalization of this behavior, there is reason to inquire about a family history of bed-wetting or daytime enuresis.
2. Fluid restriction before bed will be an effective long-term treatment.
3. Imipramine will be an ineffective treatment in this child.
4. It is likely that Cindy's enuresis is caused by the frequent urinary tract infections.

11–4. Which of the following statements apply to the alarm method of behavior therapy for enuresis?

1. It is most successful for combined day and night enuresis.
2. Significant relapse occurs in one-third of children despite an adequate 12-week course of treatment.
3. It is as efficacious in the treatment of children who have additional psychiatric disorders as it is in the treatment of those who have only enuresis.
4. A cure is defined as 14 consecutive dry nights and is usually achieved in the second month of treatment.

11–5. Daytime wetting is best conceptualized as a disorder of toileting. What treatments may be useful for this disorder?

1. Oxybutynin chloride, belladonna, and imipramine
2. A regular schedule of anticipatory reinforced toileting
3. Intranasal desamino-D-arginine vasopressin (DDAVP)
4. A careful exploration for urinary tract abnormalities

11–6. Bobby is a 5-year-old boy who has had hard stools since 2 years of age but had no overt problems with encopresis until he moved with his parents to a new state 6 months ago. Since the move, Bobby soils his pants at least once a month, and he wets his bed nightly and occasionally wets his pants. Bobby walked at 26 months (normal range 10 to 18 months), and toilet training started at that time. At present, Bobby only knows three colors and does not recognize any letters or numbers. Which of the following statements apply to this case?

1. Enuresis occurs in approximately one-third of children with encopresis.
2. Bobby's developmental delay and the enuresis are probably associated.
3. There was a significant stressor in this child's life.
4. The constipation that has been evident since age 2 years may be genetically determined.

11–7. In the aforementioned case involving Bobby, what forms of treatment would be advisable?

1. A bowel clean-out involving suppositories and enemas
2. Maintenance therapy using mineral oil or milk of magnesia
3. Behavior therapy with a bed alarm
4. Imipramine at a dose of 1.0 to 2.5 mg/kg

11–8. The mechanism of action of desamino-D-arginine vasopressin (DDAVP) is thought to involve a reduction of nocturnal urine flow. What are other aspects of DDAVP?

1. It has a higher success rate than imipramine.

2. Hyponatremia may occur.

3. Nasal congestion and conjunctivitis may occur.

4. Most children do not relapse once treatment is stopped.

11–9. Behavioral-educational treatment of encopresis comprises

1. Reinforcing consistent toilet usage.

2. Providing a system of positive reinforcements.

3. Educating both the child and parents about the disorder.

4. Requiring the child to clean his or her clothes after soiling.

■ ANSWERS:

11–1. **Answer: 3, 4, and 6.** There is evidence of increased functional urinary tract abnormalities in enuretic patients, including reduced bladder volume. In the history of the enuretic child, there may be evidence of developmental delays, minor neurological abnormalities, low intelligence, delayed initiation of toilet training beyond 18 months, and a history of constipation. This disorder may have a genetic component. Many families appear to believe that bed-wetting in particular is "just part of growing up." There is no evidence of association with a specific psychiatric disorder. Children who are not "dry" by age 4 years are at increased risk for enuresis. There is no evidence that enuresis is associated with abnormal sleep or sleep architecture.

11–2. **Answer: 2, 3, and 5.** Fecal retention occurring between ages 1 and 2 years can predict later encopresis. Neglectful or punitive toilet training previously was thought to play a major role in the development of encopresis. Although it may be part of the etiology in some cases, it certainly is not frequently a contributing factor. Less than one-third of children are completely toilet-trained by age 2. Bowel continence is established in the majority of children by age 5 years. Anal fissures, anal irritation, or an anteriorly displaced anus may all contribute to encopresis. Genetic factors are recognized in constipation. Stressful events were associated with the onset of encopresis in 25% of cases in one study. As with enuresis, there is no specific association of encopresis with other psychiatric disorders.

11–3. **Answer: B (1 and 3).** Enuresis is equally common in males and females until age 5 years. By age 11 years, the male-to-female ratio is 2:1. Diurnal enuresis occurs in about 3% of children age 5 to 7 years. Daytime wetting occurs more commonly in girls and is associated with higher rates of psychiatric disturbance, urinary tract anomalies, and urinary tract infections. Daytime and nighttime enuresis may actually spawn the urinary tract infections, rather than the other way around. Fluid restriction and forced nighttime toileting are commonsense measures that occasionally work for brief periods. Imipramine at 1.0 to 2.5 mg/kg given at bedtime reduces symptoms in up to 85% of children with nighttime enuresis but is not effective in the treatment of daytime enuresis. The mother's normalization of the problem should prompt an investigation into parental knowledge concerning child development as well as a family history of enuresis. Cindy's development appears on target for her age.

11–4.   **Answer: C (2 and 4).** The alarm method of behavior therapy is most successful for nighttime enuresis. A cure is defined as 14 consecutive dry nights. A prolonged course of treatment of at least 12 weeks is necessary, and a cure, if such takes place, is most likely achieved in the second month of treatment. Approximately one-third of children will relapse despite adequate treatment. The alarm method is less successful with children who are mentally retarded or institutionalized and with those who have diabetes mellitus.

11–5.   **Answer: C (2 and 4).** Anticholinergic medications that increase functional bladder capacity and delay the desire to void, such as belladonna, oxybutynin chloride, and terodiline, may be beneficial in the treatment of daytime enuresis. Imipramine is not efficacious in the treatment of daytime enuresis and may exacerbate the condition by producing constipation that may even further decrease the functional bladder capacity. Intranasal DDAVP is successful in as many as 50% of the children with *nighttime* enuresis, but it is not useful in the treatment of daytime enuresis. A regular schedule of anticipatory toileting and forcing fluids to increase the number of toileting responses is the most frequently used mode of therapy. Daytime enuresis is more frequently associated with disorders of the urinary tract, and a careful investigation should be conducted.

11–6.   **Answer: E (All).** Bobby has motoric and cognitive developmental delays, which are associated with enuresis. Significant life stressors are frequently present in children with enuresis or encopresis. For a 5-year-old child, a move is a significant life event. Enuresis occurs in approximately one-third of children with encopresis. There is a body of evidence indicating that constipation—and especially early-onset constipation—has a genetic component.

11–7.   **Answer: A (1, 2, and 3).** Constipation is associated with most, but not all, children who present with encopresis. Behavior therapy alone is usually not sufficient to curtail the symptoms. A physical exam including a rectal exam is critical to determine if the child has fissures or an anteriorly displaced anus. Regimens of laxative therapy and regular toileting are the mainstay of treatment. The initial phase consists of bowel clean-out involving suppositories and enemas to remove the underlying impaction. Following the removal of the impaction, maintenance therapy should include using mineral oil and milk of magnesia, increasing fiber in the diet, and using bowel motility-enhancing agents. Because this child also experiences diurnal enuresis, a bedtime and possibly a day alarm system may provide some symptom relief. Imipramine has not proven useful in children with both day and night enuresis.

11–8.   **Answer: A (1, 2, and 3).** DDAVP is associated with a higher success rate (50%) than is imipramine (30%) in the treatment of nocturnal enuresis in children; however, *both* medications are associated with high relapse rates when the medication is discontinued. Hyponatremia is a rare complication that may be prevented by ensuring appropriate fluid intake. Nasal pain and congestion, rhinitis, and conjunctivitis are common side effects.

11–9.   **Answer: E (All).** The first step in the behavioral-educational treatment of encopresis is educating the child and parents about the disorder and its relationship to regular bowel action. Consistent toilet usage, generally immediately following a meal to take advantage of the gastrocolic reflex, is a strong component in this system. Positive reinforcements for appropriate toileting, as well as mild punishment (such as requiring older children to clean their soiled clothes), are also elements of this system.

CHAPTER 12

Anxiety and Anxiety Disorders

DIRECTIONS: For questions 12–1 through 12–4, select the single best answer.

12–1. What is the longest period of time between physical examinations acceptable for an evaluation of a child with a suspected anxiety disorder?

    1. 6 months

    2. 24 months

    3. 12 months

    4. 18 months

12–2. What proportion of children with an anxiety disorder will meet the criteria for a second anxiety disorder?

    1. 1/4

    2. 1/3

    3. 1/2

    4. 3/4

12–3. What proportion of children with an anxiety disorder will have comorbid major depression?

    1. 1/4

    2. 1/3

    3. 1/2

    4. All

12–4. Which anxiety disorder is likely to be the most disabling in school-age children?

    1. Social phobia

    2. Generalized anxiety disorder

    3. Agoraphobia

    4. Separation anxiety with school refusal

■ **DIRECTIONS: For questions 12–5 through 12–20, indicate**

    A if answers 1, 2, and 3 are correct.
    B if answers 1 and 3 are correct.
    C if answers 2 and 4 are correct.
    D if only answer 4 is correct.
    E if all are correct.

12–5.   Before initiating pharmacotherapy, which of the following should be ordered?

1. Electroencephalogram
2. Electrocardiogram
3. Computed cerebral tomography
4. Renal and hepatic screens

12–6.   According to DSM-IV nomenclature, which of the following anxiety disorders are classified as usually diagnosed during infancy, childhood, or adolescence?

1. Generalized anxiety disorder
2. Overanxious disorder of childhood
3. Panic disorder
4. Separation anxiety disorder

12–7.   Children and their parents may report different signs and symptoms. Of the following, which are most likely to be accurately reported by the child?

1. Feelings of impending doom
2. Suicide ideation
3. Cardiac palpitations and tachypnea
4. The number of times the child has refused to go to school

12–8.   Clonidine may be useful for reducing autonomic overarousal, catastrophic undifferentiated anxiety, or excessive psychophysiological reactiveness. What are the most important adverse effects of this medication?

1. Sedation
2. Irritability
3. Hypotension
4. Skin rash

12–9.   Which of the following need special consideration when one is diagnosing or treating anxiety disorders?

1. Prescription medications
2. Consumption of carbonated beverages
3. Sexual activity
4. Athletic activities

12–10.   Disorders that preclude the use of propranolol include

1. Asthma.
2. Heart failure.

3. Diabetes mellitus.

4. Allergic rhinitis.

12–11. In most cases, the child and family voluntarily seek evaluation and treatment. This is not likely to occur when the child has which of the following disorders?

1. Separation anxiety disorder

2. Social phobia

3. Somatization disorder

4. Generalized anxiety disorder

12–12. Which of the following should guide treatment decisions?

1. The diagnosis

2. The case formulation

3. The severity of symptoms

4. The existence of comorbid diagnosis or symptoms

12–13. Which of the following neurotransmitters are closely associated with obsessive-compulsive disorder (OCD)?

1. Gamma-aminobutyric acid

2. Dopamine

3. Norepinephrine

4. Serotonin

12–14. Which of the following unconscious conflicts are commonly found in anxious children and adolescents?

1. Identity and self-concept

2. Autonomy

3. Aggression

4. Abandonment

12–15. Anxious children often have anxious or otherwise affectively disturbed family members. Even when a child's parents do not have a psychiatric disorder, the child's symptoms frequently evoke strong reactions from family members. Which of the following statements apply to dealing with families who have an anxious child?

1. The clinician should express confidently to the anxious child that he or she is able to manage a situation despite his or her anxiety.

2. The clinician should assure the family that anxiety is not contagious.

3. The clinician should give the parents a realistically reassuring prognosis.

4. The child's excessive power is not a contributing factor in creating or maintaining anxiety in a child.

12–16. The use of benzodiazepines in children and adolescents with anxiety disorders is still under investigation. The results from several studies are equivocal; yet, the use of a benzodiazepine may be efficacious for an individual patient. Concerning the use of benzodiazepines in children, which of the following statements are **false**?

1. Behavioral disinhibition is seen with equal frequency in adults and in children.

    2. Three to four doses per day of lorazepam are frequently necessary.

    3. Short-acting benzodiazepines are particularly likely to accumulate in the body.

    4. Long-acting benzodiazepines may minimize symptom breakthrough.

12–17. Which defense mechanisms are viewed as contributing to pathology in children with anxiety disorders?

    1. Displacement

    2. Projective identification

    3. Repression

    4. Sublimation

12–18. The choice of a tricyclic or heterocyclic medication is usually based on the clinician's experiences and the tolerance to, or even desirability of, side effects such as sedation. Which of the following are part of the workup necessary before initiation of this type of medication?

    1. Electrocardiogram

    2. Pulse

    3. Blood pressure

    4. Complete cell count

12–19. In children with generalized anxiety disorder or posttraumatic stress disorder, autonomic activity may be continuously excessive. Which of the following medications are more effective for treating the overarousal?

    1. Imipramine

    2. Buspirone

    3. Fluoxetine

    4. Clonazepam

12–20. Which of the following neuroleptics appear to induce separation anxiety in some patients?

    1. Pimozide

    2. Thioridazine

    3. Haloperidol

    4. Thiothixene

■ **DIRECTIONS: For questions 12–21 through 12–28, match the treatment modality or method with the appropriate statement(s). Each statement may be used once, more than once, or not at all.**

12–21. Gradual desensitization   a. This method is behavioral.

12–22. Relaxation training   b. This method deals with unconscious conflicts.

12–23.	Prolonged exposure	c.	A fixed ratio of rewards may be used.
12–24.	Modeling	d.	This method is completed in 10 to 20 sessions.
12–25.	Positive reinforcement	e.	Symptoms result from inaccurate self-talk.
12–26.	Negative reinforcement	f.	This method is used empirically.
12–27.	Cognitive-behavior therapy	g.	Problems are identified, listed, and prioritized.
12–28.	Psychodynamic therapy	h.	The only major disadvantage to this method is that it is relatively slow to work.
		i.	This method is not useful if the primary gain (the reduction of psychological distress) is driving the behavior.
		j.	This method involves withholding a reinforcer.
		k.	This method is associated with a soothing, monotonous voice.
		l.	Puppets may be used.
		m.	Does not work well with oppositional children.
		n.	The relationship with a neutral therapist is seen as a model for important relationships with parents.
		o.	This method may be painful and not well tolerated.
		p.	Sessions may be daily to weekly.
		q.	Adaptive behaviors are rewarded.
		r.	This method replaces unworkable defenses with better ones.
		s.	Homework is a key component.
		t.	Prepared scripts are available.

■ **DIRECTIONS: For statements 12–29 through 12–36, indicate whether the statement is true or false.**

12–29. _____ The most serious adverse side effect associated with buspirone is psychosis.

12–30. _____ Primary reinforcers must be exchanged for something of value.

12–31. _____ Medications should be used as the sole treatment modality.

12–32. _____ The most powerful schedule for increasing the frequency of a given behavior is the variable ratio schedule.

12–33. _____ For an interpretation to be effective—that is, for it to elicit an "Aha!" response—the child, at the very least, must acknowledge it as being correct.

12–34. _____ In modeling therapy, the model need not be similar in age, cultural background, or gender.

12–35. _____ Oppositional behavior is frequently seen in anxious children.

12–36. _____ Children with generalized anxiety disorder respond better to intensive psychoanalytically based treatment than to weekly psychodynamic therapy.

■ ANSWERS:

12–1. **Answer: 3.** A principal component of the evaluation of a child with a suspected anxiety disorder is a timely physical examination. If an examination has not been performed within the past 6 to 12 months, the child should be referred for a thorough physical. If the clinical history is suggestive of a physical disorder, then appropriate referral should, of course, be obtained. At the very least, vital signs should be checked in the psychiatrist's office.

12–2. **Answer: 2.** Approximately one-third of children with an anxiety disorder will meet the criteria for a second anxiety disorder.

12–3. **Answer: 3.** At least approximately one-half of children with an anxiety disorder will meet the criteria for major depression.

12–4. **Answer: 4.** Frank disability is relatively uncommon in young people with primary anxiety disorders. There is some debate concerning the chronicity of anxiety disorders in children. In a child with an anxiety disorder who has a parent with a mood disorder, the anxiety disorder may become chronic. Separation anxiety with school refusal is the disorder that will cause the most disability in school-age children.

12–5. **Answer: C (2 and 4).** An electrocardiogram, renal and hepatic screens, and, for menstruating females, a pregnancy test are all indicated before initiating pharmacological management. If the initial history and physical examination so indicate, then thyroid studies, urine drug screening, endocrine studies, anemia screening, electroencephalograms, or computed tomography may be ordered.

12–6. **Answer: D (Only 4).** Only one anxiety disorder—separation anxiety disorder—is classified as "usually diagnosed in infancy, childhood, or adolescence." The diagnosis of overanxious disorder of childhood has been deleted from the nosology. If a child previously met the criteria for overanxious disorder, the diagnosis now would be generalized anxiety disorder.

12–7. **Answer: A (1, 2, and 3).** Several studies have shown that children are better reporters of internal feeling states associated not only with anxiety but with any affective disorder than their parents. Even a child of age 4 or 5 years may accurately describe feelings of disappearing or vanishing, quick breathing, pounding heart, or thoughts of self-harm. Parents are far better at recording and categorizing overt behaviors, such as school refusal.

12–8. **Answer: E (All).** Sedation is frequently observed in the first 2 weeks of treatment with clonidine. Irritability may be dose related, and lowering the dose may decrease this symptom without mitigating the effectiveness of the medication for overarousal. The original use of clonidine was as an antihypertensive medication, so hypotension may be a side effect when given to normotensive individuals. Approximately 3%–5% of children who are treated with the transdermal (patch) system of clonidine develop a skin rash.

12–9. **Answer: A (1, 2, and 3).** Over-the-counter cold preparations may contain sympathomimetics, such as pseudoephedrine. Even with correct administration, these medications may induce a syndrome analogous to a panic attack or elements of generalized anxiety in a particularly vulnerable population. Adolescents may use over-the-counter medications as substances of abuse in an attempt to "get high," producing tachycardia, palpitations, nausea, diaphoresis, headaches, and breathlessness. Carbonated beverages contain variable amounts of caffeine. Children may surreptitiously consume several containers of these beverages, or their parents may not be aware of the amount of caffeine in these beverages, leaving the children at risk for caffeinism. Sexual activity should be discussed to ascertain any history of abuse, fear of exposure of sexual activity that is not sanctioned by the parents, fear of pregnancy, or sexually transmitted diseases. Athletic activities in general are anxiolytic, unless children are pressured into performing beyond their capacity.

12–10. **Answer: E (All).** Propranolol is a nonselective beta-adrenergic receptor antagonist that may exacerbate asthma and allergic rhinitis and contribute to heart failure. In persons with diabetes, the use of propranolol may mask the presence of hypoglycemia.

12–11. **Answer: B (1 and 3).** Separation anxiety disorder is frequently accompanied by school refusal, and the parents overtly or covertly accept the behavior. If the child has missed too much school, authorities may insist on an evaluation. Children whose anxiety is manifested solely through somatic symptoms may be subjected to numerous medical procedures before being referred for psychiatric evaluation by their primary care physicians or a pediatric specialist.

12–12. **Answer: E (All).** A case formulation consisting of psychodynamic issues (intrapsychic and interpersonal), family system functions, family history, environmental variables, and biological variables, in addition to the actual diagnosis and severity of symptoms, should guide treatment planning. The existence of comorbid disorders may affect treatment. For example, a child with dysthymic disorder with symptoms that have their onset after the onset of panic disorder may be best served by having the anxiety disorder treated first. The depressive symptoms may remit with treatment of the underlying anxiety disorder.

12–13. **Answer: D (Only 4).** Currently, the exact physiology of anxiety is not well understood. Gamma-aminobutyric acid, serotonin, and norepinephrine may all be involved in different manifestations of anxiety. OCD symptoms are associated primarily with serotonin.

12–14. **Answer: E (All).** Several areas of unconscious conflict come up repeatedly in the treatment of anxious children and adolescents: reexperiencing frightening events, separation, and abandonment and experiencing confusion and conflict over identity, self-concept, social acceptance, aggressive urges, autonomy, control, sexual urges, and family roles. These conflicts may be evident in specific statements or implicit in play themes. Repetitive behaviors or responses to environmental stimuli may also be clues to the underlying unconscious conflicts.

12–15. **Answer: B (1 and 3).** Families with an ill child need realistic reassurance concerning prognosis and what may be expected from the child given the overall level of cognitive, physical, and emotional development. Frequently, there is a tendency to "rescue" and provide comfort to an anxious child. This action may give these children the indication that there is a "real" danger or that they are indeed too ill to accomplish a particular task. Children with an anxiety disorder may respond best to a low level of expressed emotion, to a consistent nurturing environment with developmentally appropriate expectations, and to parents who function as authority figures. Children who are "in charge" can become overwhelmed by the power, and this may then increase their anxiety and oppositional behaviors. When serious difficulties in family functioning are noted, formal family therapy is indicated.

12–16. **Answer: B (1 and 3).** The frequency of behavioral disinhibition with benzodiazepines is not known, but it does occur more frequently with children than with adults. Long-acting, not short-acting, benzodiazepines are more likely to accumulate.

12–17. **Answer: B (1 and 3).** Displacement, repression, and somatization are the classic defense mechanisms utilized by individuals with an anxiety disorder. One goal of treatment is to replace these with the more reliable and mature defense mechanisms of humor, sublimation, suppression, altruistic behavior, and anticipation. Projective identification is more characteristic of individuals with personality disorders such as borderline personality disorder.

12–18. **Answer: A (1, 2, and 3).** Baseline and periodic electrocardiograms are essential with heterocyclic or tricyclic antidepressant use. Baseline and periodic evaluations of pulse and blood pressure are also required. A small but statistically relevant increase in pulse is noted in children who are placed on tricyclics and heterocyclics. A complete cell count is frequently obtained but is not critical.

12–19. **Answer: C (2 and 4).** Benzodiazepines such as diazepam (Valium), lorazepam (Ativan), clonazepam (Klonopin), clorazepate dipotassium (Tranxène), and the nonbenzodiazepine anxiolytic buspirone (BuSpar) may be used to address excessive autonomic activity. Imipramine (Tofranil) is a tricyclic antidepressant that may be used to treat a comorbid depressive disorder, panic symptoms, or excessive psychophysiological reactiveness. Clonidine (Catapres), a partial alpha2-receptor agonist, may also decrease autonomic overarousal. Fluoxetine (Prozac) belongs to the class of antidepressants known as selective serotonin reuptake inhibitors (SSRIs). SSRIs may be used to treat obsessions or ruminations.

12–20. **Answer: B (1 and 3).** Pimozide and haloperidol appear to induce separation anxiety in some patients.

12–21. Gradual desensitization: **a, h**

12–22. Relaxation training: **a, k, p, t**

12–23. Prolonged exposure: **a, o**

12–24. Modeling: **a, l, m**

12–25. Positive reinforcement: **a, c, f, q**

12–26. Negative reinforcement: **a, c, i, j**

12–27. Cognitive-behavior therapy: **d, e, g, s**

12–28. Psychodynamic therapy: **b, l, n, p, r**

12–29. **True**

12–30. **True**

12–31. **False**

12–32. **True**

12–33. **False**

12–34. **False**

12–35. **True**

12–36. **True**

CHAPTER 13

Mood Disorders and Suicidal Behavior

DIRECTIONS: For questions 13–1 through 13–11, select the single best answer.

13–1. Which of the following modalities have proven efficacy greater than that of placebo?

1. Tricyclic antidepressants (TCAs)
2. Selective serotonin reuptake inhibitors (SSRIs)
3. Interpersonal psychotherapy
4. None of the above

13–2. Short-term studies have indicated a high level of chronicity for depression in children and adolescents. How many months elapse before most children (80%–90%) recover?

1. 36 months
2. 12 months
3. 6 months
4. 48 months

13–3. Which of the following psychotherapeutic techniques have demonstrated efficacy in the treatment of affective disorders in children and adolescents?

1. Psychoanalysis
2. Individual psychotherapy
3. Behavior therapy
4. Brief supportive psychotherapy

13–4. What is the most common place for youth to commit suicide?

1. School
2. Place of employment
3. Home
4. A relatively unknown place

13–5. Tricyclic antidepressants may be particularly helpful to children who have which of the following disorders in addition to depression?

    1. Asthma

    2. Diabetes

    3. Obesity

    4. Migraine headaches

13–6. Of the following medication side effects, which would be the most commonly reported in children and adolescents on a TCA?

    1. Agitation

    2. Diarrhea

    3. Blurred vision

    4. Increased salivation

13–7. In a previously well-functioning adolescent with an acute psychotic depression and psychomotor retardation, what is the likelihood of a subsequent manic episode?

    1. < 5%

    2. 10%–20%

    3. 20%–30%

    4. 30%–40%

13–8. Which of the following methods for suicide is the least common?

    1. Gunshot

    2. Household poisons

    3. Hanging

    4. Overdose

13–9. Which of the following is not an element of the Coping With Depression Course for Depressed Adolescents?

    1. Group therapy process

    2. Parallel parent process

    3. Social skills training

    4. Behavior modification

13–10. Which of the following medications has Food and Drug Administration (FDA) approval for the treatment of depression in children and adolescents?

    1. Imipramine

    2. Paroxetine (Paxil)

    3. Nortriptyline (Pamelor)

    4. None of the above

13–11. What is the goal of psychodynamic psychotherapy in the treatment of children and adolescents with a mood disorder?

    1. To effect complete resolution of all symptoms

    2. To change the personality

3. To reestablish the normal developmental path

4. To determine who is responsible for creating the child's depression

■ **DIRECTIONS: For questions 13–12 through 13–23, indicate**

A if answers 1, 2, and 3 are correct.

B if answers 1 and 3 are correct.

C if answers 2 and 4 are correct.

D if only answer 4 is correct.

E if all are correct.

13–12. Which of the following should be regarded as basic pieces of information when one is formulating a treatment plan for a child or adolescent with a mood disorder?

1. Intelligence of the child

2. Prior drug history

3. History of psychiatric treatment

4. Weight

13–13. Which of the following electrocardiogram (ECG) changes in a child would call for a reduction or discontinuation of a TCA?

1. QRS of greater than 0.12 seconds

2. Resting heart rate of greater than 100 beats per minute in an 8-year-old

3. P-R interval of greater than 0.20 seconds in a 12-year-old

4. Increase in QRS interval to 40% above baseline

13–14. The goal of the time-limited approach in cognitive therapy is to provide relief from depressive symptoms and prevent future depressive episodes by changing cognitions. Which of the following statements are **true** regarding negative cognitive patterns?

1. They are negative thoughts only about oneself and one's future.

2. Cognitive errors serve to maintain negative beliefs.

3. Negative thoughts are reinforced by the environment.

4. They are negative schemas involved in processing information.

13–15. Which of the following are justification for the use of plasma levels for TCAs?

1. To assess compliance

2. To improve the likelihood of therapeutic response

3. To avoid toxicity

4. For medicolegal documentation

13–16. Which of the following psychotherapeutic techniques are commonly used with young children?

1. Playing with puppets

2. Interpreting dreams

3. Drawing

4. Discussing issues directly

13–17. Which of the following statements are **true** regarding the use of tricyclic medications in children and adolescents?

1. The medication is started at 1–2 mg/kg at bedtime.

2. A rhythm strip is obtained at 5 mg/kg.

3. An incomplete right bundle branch block (RBBB) (0.10- to 0.12-second QRS) does not contraindicate the use of tricyclic medication.

4. The dose is increased every 3 days.

13–18. Interpersonal psychotherapy (IPT) is based on the assumption that depression evolves in a social context and that, consequently, the onset and outcome of depression are influenced by interpersonal relationships. What are the major goals of IPT?

1. To decrease depressive symptoms

2. To enhance communication

3. To improve interpersonal relationships

4. To change an individual's negative schemas

13–19. What group of children is most suitable for IPT?

1. Children who are actively suicidal

2. Children with normal intellectual functioning

3. Children aged 5 to 18 years

4. Children who have major depression without comorbid disorders

13–20. Group therapy is the most extensively examined psychosocial approach to treating depression in youth. What are the major drawbacks to the group therapy studies?

1. School samples were used.

2. The children were all severely depressed.

3. The children did not have to meet the criteria for major depression.

4. Comorbid diagnoses were not examined.

13–21. In which of the following situations is hospitalization essential?

1. The parents no longer want the adolescent in their household because of the adolescent's behaviors.

2. The child's paranoia and subsequent blaming behaviors are assumed to be part of an externalizing behavior disorder.

3. The child's threatening suicide has become a lifestyle.

4. The family covertly gives the child messages that he or she should end his or her life by making lethal means available despite requests to rid their household of these items.

13–22. Which of the following have proven efficacy as environmental deterrents to suicide in adolescents?

1. Therapists

2. Caring friends

      3. Adequate supervision

      4. Public education

13–23. Which of the following are interventions in the self-control model of depression?

      1. Learning skills for self-monitoring

      2. Setting less perfectionistic standards

      3. Setting realistic subgoals

      4. Thinking positive thoughts

■ **DIRECTIONS: For questions 13–24 through 13–38, match the medication with the applicable response(s). Each response may be used once, more than once, or not at all.**

13–24.	Imipramine	a.	Is tricyclic or heterocyclic in nature.
13–25.	Fluoxetine	b.	Induces enzymatic degradation of itself.
13–26.	Bupropion	c.	Mozzarella cheese cannot be consumed.
13–27.	Desipramine	d.	Blood level should be 3–11 mg/L.
13–28.	Paroxetine	e.	May cause agitation or excitation.
13–29.	Tranylcypromine	f.	Orthostatic hypotension can be a problem.
13–30.	Carbamazepine	g.	Priapism can occur.
13–31.	Amoxapine	h.	Therapeutic range is 0.7–1.4 mEq/L.
13–32.	Nortriptyline	i.	Inhibits degradation of neurotransmitters.
13–33.	Phenelzine	j.	Average dose range is 3–5 mg/kg.
13–34.	Lithium	k.	Is used for rapid-cycling bipolar disorder.
13–35.	Sertraline	l.	Nonsteroidal anti-inflammatory agents increase levels.
13–36.	Valproic acid	m.	Hepatotoxicity may be fatal.
13–37.	Trazodone	n.	Constipation is a side effect.
13–38.	Clomipramine	o.	Overdose is lethal.
		p.	Plasma level should be 60–100 ng/mL.
		q.	Is an SSRI.
		r.	Level may be checked via saliva.
		s.	Hypotension is a side effect.
		t.	Periodic TSH, T4, and T3 levels are necessary.
		u.	May cause the Stevens-Johnson syndrome.
		v.	Increases norepinephrine, serotonin, and dopamine levels.
		w.	Can cause bone marrow suppression.
		x.	Causes weight gain.
		y.	Causes sedation.
		z.	Baseline ECG is needed.
		aa.	Dose-related seizures can occur.
		bb.	Is used as an anticonvulsant.

■ **ANSWERS:**

13–1. **Answer: 4.** Tricyclic antidepressants are the most well-studied group experimentally. There have been a few open and double-blind trials of fluoxetine (Prozac) and paroxetine (Paxil) in adolescents. With respect to psychotherapy outcome studies, the data are even more limited. The most striking feature is that none of these treatments were more efficacious than placebo.

13–2. **Answer: 2.** For 80%–90% of youth, recovery from depression takes 12 months. The relapse rate is high: one-third to two-thirds will relapse within 3 years.

13–3. **Answer: 1.** Psychoanalytic treatment for affective disorders in children and adolescents has been demonstrated to be efficacious and superior to other psychotherapies.

13–4. **Answer: 3.** The most common place for suicide to be committed is in the home.

13–5. **Answer: 4.** TCAs and monoamine oxidase inhibitors (MAOIs) have a tendency to produce weight gain, so they would not be a first choice in obese children. MAOIs, but not TCAs, interact adversely with bronchodilators. There is no evidence that TCAs are particularly helpful to children with asthma. The interaction of antidepressants with exogenous insulin or hypoglycemics in children is not well studied. TCAs are helpful in the treatment of migraine headaches and pain syndromes.

13–6. **Answer: 3.** The most commonly reported side effects from TCAs are sedative (drowsiness, lethargy, feeling drugged) or anticholinergic (dry mouth, constipation, blurred vision, dizziness, nausea). Agitation is one of the most common side effects of SSRIs.

13–7. **Answer: 3.** The treatment of depression, particularly in adolescents, is complicated by the possibility that the presenting depression is actually a component of a bipolar disorder. A careful historical search for the possibility of a previous hypomanic episode must be obtained in every adolescent who presents with a major depression. A family history of bipolar disorder also strengthens the possibility that the depression is part of a bipolar disorder. Even without a positive personal or family history, 20%–30% of adolescents who present with an acute psychotic depression and psychomotor retardation will go on to develop a bipolar disorder.

13–8. **Answer: 2.** Gunshot is the most common way to *complete* suicide, and overdose is the most common way to *attempt* suicide. Males attempt to hang themselves more often than do females. Although household cleaning solutions and other poisons are the most common means of inadvertent poisoning in young children, it is rare for a child or adolescent to use these substances as a means of suicide.

13–9. **Answer: 4.** The Coping With Depression Course for Depressed Adolescents is a group therapy process designed for 4 to 10 adolescents. The course involves 16 2-hour sessions over an 8-week period with individualized booster sessions at 4-month intervals in the first two posttreatment years. This process has a parental component and also includes social skills training, anxiety management with relaxation techniques, cognitive training, and increasingly pleasant activities. Communication training is also taught, with an emphasis on skills such as actively responding, maintaining good eye contact, and reducing putdowns, interruptions, and accusations.

13–10. **Answer: 4.** No antidepressants have been approved by the FDA for treatment of depression in children and adolescents.

13–11. **Answer: 3.** Complete resolution of all symptoms is not the goal of pharmacotherapeutic or psychodynamic treatment. Alleviating symptoms is a more reasonable goal. The child's personality may or may not be the focus of the therapeutic process. Establishing blame is neither productive nor reasonable. The goal of psychodynamic interventions is to return the child to a normal developmental pathway through improving his or her ability to deal with unconscious thoughts and feelings that have been linked to maladaptive behaviors.

13–12. **Answer: E (All).** Basic information necessary when one is creating a treatment program for a child or adolescent with a mood disorder includes intelligence, age, weight, and prior drug history (including compliance history, hypersensitivity, hyposensitivity, and allergic responses). Particularly in young children, medications are administered based on the child's weight. Intelligence and overall development are important in determining psychological interventions as well as the level of family involvement. In cases of mentally retarded adolescents, the primary caretaker may continue in a parenting role despite the chronological age of the child. The past history of a psychiatric disorder is relevant for assessing past treatment responses, for evaluating comorbidity, and for determining whether the current process is the beginning of a chronic illness.

13–13. **Answer: B (1 and 3).** The following criteria are used for reduction or discontinuation of a TCA: 1) a QRS interval greater than 0.12 seconds or increased to 50% above baseline; 2) a P-R interval of greater than 0.18 seconds in a child age 10 years or younger, or a P-R interval of 0.20 seconds in a child older than age 10 years; and 3) a resting heart rate of greater than 110 beats per minute in children age 10 years or younger, or a resting heart rate of greater than 100 beats per minute in children older than age 10 years.

13–14. **Answer: C (2 and 4).** The cognitive triad consists of negative thoughts about the self, world, and future. Cognitive errors serve to maintain negative beliefs despite the presence of contradictory information from the environment.

13–15. **Answer: E (All).** There is a great deal of variability in the dose in milligrams per kilogram and the subsequent plasma level for an individual child. If a child is taking more than 3 mg/kg and is not experiencing deleterious or beneficial effects from the medication, then a plasma level should be drawn. If the level is at the upper limits, the child probably will not respond to this particular medication. Desipramine has been implicated in several sudden deaths of children, so documentation of plasma levels for TCAs has medicolegal justification.

13–16. **Answer: A (1, 2, and 3).** Helping the child to understand and master internalized conflicts is a major goal of individual therapy. Playing with puppets or other toys that lend themselves to exploration of the child's inner world, interpreting dreams, and drawing are all commonly used techniques in play therapy with the young child. Discussing issues and conflicts directly is usually reserved for the more cognitively developed older child or adolescent.

13–17. **Answer: B (1 and 3).** Tricyclic medication can be initiated at bedtime at 1–2 mg/kg and should be increased every 4 to 5 days by 10 mg–25 mg to a maximum dose of 5 mg/kg. A minimum of 2 hours should separate the doses.

A repeat rhythm strip should be obtained at 3 mg/kg. An incomplete RBBB is found in approximately 10% of the pediatric population and is considered a normal variant.

13–18. **Answer: A (1, 2, and 3).** The goals of IPT are to decrease depressive symptoms and to improve interpersonal relationships through enhanced communication. Altering negative schemas is part of cognitive therapy.

13–19. **Answer: C (2 and 4).** IPT is conceptualized as a treatment for children ages 12 to 18 years who have normal intelligence, who have a major depressive disorder without comorbid disorders (e.g., substance abuse, anxiety disorders, conduct disorders, bipolar disorders, or psychosis), and who are not suicidal. The outcome research on IPT is complicated by the nearly 50% placebo response rate observed in depressed youth, regardless of treatment type.

13–20. **Answer: B (1 and 3).** The majority of studies on group therapy used school samples and did not require that children meet the criteria for major depression, thus raising questions about the generalizability of findings to clinical samples.

13–21. **Answer: C (2 and 4).** Children whose behavior is "out of control" may be hospitalized because of lack of other options, but in general, these children may be placed in group homes, respite foster homes, or residential treatment facilities or may enter the juvenile court system. Family therapy and individual processes used in conjunction with pharmacological management may enable some of these children to remain in their homes. Likewise, youths who chronically threaten suicide may not always be best served by repeated hospitalizations and, instead, may require intensive individual and/or family therapy or an out-of-home placement. Children who are functioning in the midst of a thought disorder require hospitalization to prevent them from harming themselves and others. This is especially true if their behaviors are viewed as an externalizing behavior disorder under their full control. Unfortunately, there are families who covertly give their suicidal child the message that he or she should end his or her life by continuing to provide access to weapons, pills, and car keys. These children must be removed from this life-threatening situation.

13–22. **Answer: A (1, 2, and 3).** Public education has not proven efficacious in reducing suicidal behaviors in youth. There is some evidence that copycat suicides occur if there is media sensationalism of the event, especially if the child or adolescent was a popular figure in the school or community. Adequate supervision of suicidal children and adults is imperative. If adequate supervision cannot be obtained, then hospitalization may be necessary. Therapists and caring significant relationships can reduce the frequency of suicide attempts.

13–23. **Answer: E (All).** The self-control model of depression emphasizes links between depression and deficits in self-monitoring, self-evaluation, and self-reinforcement. Interventions focus on self-monitoring (i.e., attend to good things that happen, things one enjoys doing, positive thoughts, and delayed as well as immediate gratification), self-consequences (i.e., reward oneself rather than punish), self-evaluation (i.e., set less perfectionistic standards), and goal setting (i.e., set realistic and obtainable subgoals and goals).

13–24. Imipramine: **a, f, j, n, o, v, x, z**

13–25. Fluoxetine: **e, q**

13–26. Bupropion: **aa**

13–27. Desipramine: **a, f, j, n, o, v, x, z**

13–28. Paroxetine: **q**

13–29. Tranylcypromine: **c, e, i, o, s, v, x**

13–30. Carbamazepine: **b, d, k, u, w, bb**

13–31. Amoxapine: **a, f, n, o, t, v, x, aa**

13–32. Nortriptyline: **a, f, n, o, p, v, x, z**

13–33. Phenelzine: **c, i, o, s, v, x, y**

13–34. Lithium: **h, l, o, r, t, z**

13–35. Sertraline: **q**

13–36. Valproic acid: **k, m, w, bb**

13–37. Trazodone: **g, y**

13–38. Clomipramine: **a, f, j, n, o, x, z**

CHAPTER 14

Childhood Posttraumatic Stress Disorder

■ **DIRECTIONS: For questions 14–1 through 14–10, select the single best answer.**

14–1. What treatment modality is the most frequently prescribed in the treatment of childhood posttraumatic stress disorder (PTSD)?

1. Pharmacological management, because this modality addresses the autonomic overarousal.
2. Group therapy, because this modality alleviates the sense of isolation.
3. Individual psychotherapy, because this modality is capable of modifying the internal world.
4. Family therapy, because children live within the context of their family environment and only by modifying this environment can they have new experiences.

14–2. Which of the following statements are **true** regarding the use of artwork or play therapy in the treatment of children with PTSD?

1. Art and play therapy are counterproductive. The child, no matter how young, should be encouraged to use only verbal conversation.
2. Play therapy should be reserved for the very young child.
3. Posttraumatic play in children with PTSD dwindles off as adolescence approaches.
4. Art and play therapy should be allowed and encouraged, especially during the early course of psychotherapy.

14–3. Some children who have been repeatedly traumatized may exhibit the compulsive need to masturbate, proposition adults and children for sexual activity, or repeat their traumatic experiences in sexually inappropriate behaviors. Which medication may alleviate some of these behaviors when combined with psychotherapy?

1. Buspirone
2. Haloperidol
3. Clomipramine
4. Clonazepam

14–4. What is the objective to be met by the end of the middle phase of therapy with a child with PTSD?

1. The child's trauma-specific fears should be resolved.
2. Most posttraumatic play should receive "corrective denouements."
3. The child should be able to give a full traumatic narrative.
4. The child should realize what future problems may relate to past traumatic experiences.

14–5. What may be helpful for the therapist to directly tell the child?

1. The therapist who has experienced a personal trauma should reveal the experience to the child.
2. The therapist should tell the child what the therapist has been told by the child's parents or other authority figures.
3. The therapist should explain to the child the child's part in creating the traumatic experience.
4. The therapist should explain that there is a pattern to traumatic events so that the child is better able to anticipate and cope with those events.

14–6. In children who demonstrate frequent self-mutilation, trichotillomania, or compulsive eating disturbances, which medication is the most useful?

1. Desipramine
2. Diazepam
3. Clonidine
4. Carbamazepine

14–7. What type of psychotherapeutic approaches are helpful to the child with PTSD?

1. Using behavior modification with in vitro and in vivo desensitization
2. Relating accounts of other children and how they dealt with their traumatic events
3. Facilitating "lucid dreaming"
4. All of the above

14–8. Which medication is useful when given approximately 40 minutes before the child's meeting a potential source of trauma or facing an event that evokes a reexperiencing of the trauma?

1. Propranolol
2. Imipramine
3. Lorazepam
4. Clonidine

14–9. Group therapy is a potentially strong treatment for traumatized children. What is the purpose of group therapy with this population?

1. To help the children express their individual stories
2. To have the children explain in detail their traumatic experiences
3. To help the children recognize maladaptive personality patterns
4. None of the above

14–10. Which of the following statements is **true** regarding working with a child who is being maintained in an abusive home?

    1. Work with the parent who is the perpetrator should be avoided.

    2. Involvement with the legal system should be avoided.

    3. Most abusive parents will never fully admit the abuse.

    4. Termination of parental rights should not be recommended.

■ ANSWERS:

14–1. **Answer: 3.** All of these modalities—pharmacological management, group therapy, individual psychotherapy, and family therapy—can be helpful in the treatment of children with PTSD. Traumatized children may have abandoned all trust in individuals and institutions. Individual psychotherapy allows these children to create, at their own pace, a trusting relationship with a well-trained adult who will not cringe from the unfolding narrative of the traumatic experiences the children relate.

14–2. **Answer: 4.** Early in therapy, the therapist encourages the child to use whatever medium is the most comfortable for the child (e.g., artwork, poetry, music, dramatic scenarios, conversations), no matter what the age of the child. Unlike the typical pretend play of childhood, posttraumatic play does not diminish as the child approaches adolescence.

14–3. **Answer: 3.** Clomipramine (Anafranil) is approved for the treatment of obsessive-compulsive disorder (OCD) and may be efficacious in the treatment of children with PTSD who manifest compulsive behaviors. Haloperidol (Haldol) is an antipsychotic medication and should be reserved for the treatment of psychosis. Buspirone (BuSpar) is a novel antianxiety medication not related to the benzodiazepine class of medications that may relieve anxiety in children with PTSD. Clonazepam (Klonopin) is a long-acting benzodiazepine that may be useful in alleviating anxiety in children with PTSD.

14–4. **Answer: 1.** During the first four to six sessions of therapy, the child should be encouraged to tell in words or by whatever means possible how he or she understands the traumatic events. During the middle phase of therapy, the child is helped to discover new modes of control over what previously had been uncontrollable. By the end of the middle phase, the child's trauma-specific fears should be resolved. In the last phase of therapy, most posttraumatic play should receive "corrective denouements," allowing the child to develop new endings to traumatic experiences. By the end of therapy, the child should realize what future problems may relate to past trauma.

14–5. **Answer: 2.** The therapist should *not* reveal any personal trauma experience to the child. Sharing traumatic memories with these children will add to their fears, may cause them to assume responsibility for protecting the therapist from their narrative or from perceived outside forces, and may inhibit their development. The therapist must carefully indicate to these children that they are *not* responsible for the traumatic events and that traumatic events occur at *random*. Toward the completion of therapy, it is important for these children to understand how their past may influence their reactions to future events, but not to predict future trauma.

14–6.   **Answer: 4.** Carbamazepine (Tegretol) is an anticonvulsant that is recognized as a standard medication used to treat seizure disorders in children and adults. In situations such as self-mutilation, trichotillomania, and compulsive eating disturbances, carbamazepine may be efficacious. Diazepam (Valium) may be useful to initiate sleep or to relieve anxiety in children with PTSD. Desipramine (Norpramin) is a tricyclic antidepressant. This class of medication has not been well studied in children with PTSD. Clonidine (an alpha2-receptor agonist) may be useful in decreasing motoric and autonomic overarousal.

14–7.   **Answer: 4.** In behavior modification, the child is gradually exposed to the traumatic event, initially through conversations and play, and then by careful exposure to the actual circumstances. For example, a child who was in a near-drowning incident may first discuss the event, then draw pictures and play with a water table (i.e., a miniature pond set up in a table), and finally make a trip to the place of the near-drowning. This same child may also be enrolled in swimming classes to facilitate mastery of the event. Hearing distant accounts or watching videos of how other children managed their own traumatic experiences may lessen the sense of isolation and facilitate problem-solving skills. *Lucid dreaming* is a technique used to decrease nightmares. The child relates a nightmare and, with the therapist's assistance, fashions a new ending to the dream. The child then decides to dream the dream again, except with the new ending.

14–8.   **Answer: 1.** Propranolol is a nonspecific beta-blocking agent that may be used approximately 40 minutes before exposure to an anxiety-producing stimulus. This medication may also be used in divided doses throughout the day to alleviate autonomic overarousal. Imipramine is a tricyclic antidepressant. The use of tricyclic medications in PTSD in children has not been well studied. Lorazepam (Ativan) is a short-acting benzodiazepine that may be quite useful as a sleeping agent in children whose anxiety prevents them from falling asleep. Clonidine is an alpha2 presynaptic agonist that may be given throughout the day in divided doses to increase the child's sense of well-being as well as to decrease any motoric overarousal.

14–9.   **Answer: 3.** There are two serious risks in creating a group therapy process for traumatized children: contagion and worsening of the child's traumatic condition. Trauma is one of the most contagious of psychiatric disorders. To this end, the amount of detail divulged in the group therapy process should be minimized, with the children using an individual therapy process for relating the majority of the details as well as their overall narrative. Group therapy can help these children to share creative expressions of trauma, to recognize maladaptive personality patterns, and to explore the transference of personal problems onto the group members at large.

14–10. **Answer: 3.** The child's therapist should maintain close involvement with the child's parents, both the abusing and the nonabusing parent. The parents may attend the child's therapy sessions either regularly or as deemed advisable. *Filial therapy,* as developed by Erna Furman, is a treatment in which the therapist offers interpretations to the parents, who then impart these interpretations to their child. This approach may be used to bring the parent into the therapeutic process, which may enable the parents to alter their potential for abuse or may stop their forcing the child into silence about the trauma. Involvement with the legal and welfare systems is part of working with traumatized children.

If parents do not move positively in the direction of caring for and protecting their child, then termination of parental rights may be suggested by the child's therapist. Most abusive parents will never fully admit the abuse. Small changes in attitude and behaviors, in addition to regular pediatric evaluations and monitoring by the legal and social welfare systems, may be used to assess any changes in the parents' attitude and behavior toward their child.

CHAPTER 15

■

Obsessive-Compulsive Disorder

■ **DIRECTIONS: For questions 15–1 through 15–10, indicate**

    A if answers 1, 2, and 3 are correct.

    B if answers 1 and 3 are correct.

    C if answers 2 and 4 are correct.

    D if only answer 4 is correct.

    E if all are correct.

15–1. Which diagnoses are frequently found in conjunction with obsessive-compulsive disorder (OCD) in children?

    1. Tic disorders

    2. Major depression

    3. Simple phobia

    4. Posttraumatic stress disorder

15–2. Treatment planning for children with OCD must encompass which of the following?

    1. The child's developmental level

    2. The child's age

    3. Comorbidity

    4. Family dynamics

15–3. Which of the following modalities are the most beneficial in the treatment of OCD in children?

    1. Pharmacotherapy

    2. Behavior therapy

    3. Cognitive therapy

    4. Psychoanalysis

15–4. Which of the following serotonin reuptake inhibitors has a Food and Drug Administration (FDA)–approved indication for its use in children and adolescents (10 years and older) for the treatment of OCD?

    1. Paroxetine

    2. Fluoxetine

    3. Sertraline

    4. Clomipramine

15–5. Which of the following features are particularly responsive to exposure and response prevention?

    1. Repetitive handwashing

    2. Obsessional thoughts of death and dying

    3. Circling the chair exactly 10 times before sitting down

    4. Obsessional slowness

15–6. The role of the family is critical in the behavioral management of children with OCD. What is the rationale behind this statement?

    1. Depending on their ego strengths and developmental (i.e., emotional, chronological, physical, cognitive, and psychological) level, children with OCD may view and report their behaviors differently than their parents.

    2. Parents may participate as cotherapists.

    3. Parents may overtly or covertly participate in their child's rituals.

    4. Parents may overreact to their child's behavior.

15–7. Which of the following statements are **false**?

    1. Intense flooding does not disrupt treatment in children with compulsions or obsessions.

    2. Children with obsessions are good candidates for flooding.

    3. Postpharmacotherapy relapse rates are low.

    4. Booster therapy may be useful.

15–8. Which of the following medications lower the seizure threshold?

    1. Fluoxetine

    2. Clomipramine

    3. Sertraline

    4. Bupropion

15–9. What is the role of psychotherapy in the treatment of OCD in children?

    1. Improves peer relationships.

    2. Teaches coping skills.

    3. Allows family relationship issues to be worked through.

    4. Treats primary obsessive-compulsive symptoms.

15–10. The relationship of obsessional defenses, obsessive-compulsive personality disorder, and perfectionism is not well understood. What type of treatment best addresses these difficulties?

    1. Pharmacotherapy

    2. Family therapy

    3. Behavior therapy

    4. Insight-oriented psychotherapy

■ ANSWERS:

15–1. **Answer: A (1, 2, and 3).** The following comorbid diagnoses are found (listed in descending order of frequency): tic disorders (30%), major depression (26%), specific developmental delay (24%), simple phobia (17%), overanxious disorder (16%), adjustment disorder with depressed mood (13%), oppositional defiant disorder (11%), attention-deficit disorder (10%), conduct disorder (disruptive behavior disorder) (7%), and separation anxiety disorder (7%). Posttraumatic stress disorder is not usually found in children with OCD.

15–2. **Answer: E (All).** When a comprehensive treatment program is being planned, psychosocial factors such as the child's chronological age, developmental level (i.e., emotional, cognitive, social, physical, and psychological), and family dynamics (a parent with OCD or another psychiatric disorder) must be considered. Any comorbid diagnosis must also be treated. An example is the use of a serotonin reuptake inhibitor, which may increase the anxiety level of an already overanxious child but will decrease the OCD symptoms. One solution may be the use of an anxiolytic in conjunction with a serotonin reuptake inhibitor.

15–3. **Answer: A (1, 2, and 3).** Although OCD is one of the psychiatric disorders that most closely follow the classical analytic model of pathogenesis, it is highly resistant to psychoanalytic interventions. Pharmacotherapy, used in conjunction with cognitive and behavior therapies, provides the greatest relief from symptoms.

15–4. **Answer: D (Only 4).** Clomipramine (Anafranil), a tricyclic, is a potent serotonin reuptake inhibitor. It is the first and most thoroughly studied pharmacological agent in the treatment of OCD in children and adults. It is the only medication that has FDA approval in the treatment of childhood OCD.

15–5. **Answer: B (1 and 3).** Exposure and response prevention appear to be more successful with compulsions and repetitive behaviors than with obsessions, repetitive thoughts, or obsessional slowness. This approach is also the behavioral treatment of choice for children with OCD.

15–6. **Answer: E (All).** Because parents necessarily spend time with their child and have strong emotional attachments to their child, both affirmative and negative ones, parents are an essential part of the child's therapy. Young children may or may not report their obsessions as disturbing, whereas the concerned parent may find these thoughts most distressing. Children, especially those with ego or other developmental deficits, frequently are not as good at reporting their behavioral symptoms as are their parents. In a concerted effort to maintain the family, or in conjunction with parental psychopathology, parents may collude with their child in the symptoms.

15–7. **Answer: A (1, 2, and 3).** Flooding (prolonged exposure to the most anxiety-provoking stimuli) has proven efficacy in adolescents with compulsions but not in children with compulsions or obsessions. Intense flooding may exacerbate anxiety and disrupt the treatment process. Once pharmacotherapy is discontinued, relapse rates may be high and booster behavior therapy may prevent a complete relapse.

15–8. **Answer: C (2 and 4).** Clomipramine (Anafranil), bupropion (Wellbutrin), and amoxapine (Asendin) are all antidepressants that are associated with dose-related seizures and lowered seizure threshold. Fluoxetine (Prozac) and sertraline (Zoloft) are selective serotonin reuptake inhibitor antidepressants and are *not* associated with seizures.

15–9. **Answer: A (1, 2, and 3).** Individual psychotherapy may be used with children with OCD to address comorbid diagnosis, family issues, and interpersonal issues. This therapeutic intervention may improve coping skills. Treatment of the primary obsessive-compulsive symptoms is not usually the thrust of individual therapy.

15–10. **Answer: D (Only 4).** Insight-oriented psychotherapy is the treatment best suited for obsessional defenses, obsessive-compulsive personality disorder, and debilitating perfectionism. The other therapies may be used in conjunction with insight-oriented psychotherapy.

CHAPTER 16

Substance Abuse and Substance Use Disorders

■ **DIRECTIONS: For questions 16–1 through 16–6, indicate**

    A if answers 1, 2, and 3 are correct.

    B if answers 1 and 3 are correct.

    C if answers 2 and 4 are correct.

    D if only answer 4 is correct.

    E if all are correct.

16–1. What pretreatment factors argue for a more favorable treatment outcome in childhood substance abuse?

    1. Being female

    2. Absence of academic problems

    3. Later age at onset of drug use

    4. Voluntary entrance into treatment

16–2. What information should be gained from an interview for assessment of substance abuse?

    1. Route of administration

    2. Beliefs about benefits of drug use

    3. Duration of use

    4. Age at initial use

16–3. Appropriate referral is important to a successful treatment outcome. Which signs and symptoms would direct the clinician to make a referral for inpatient or residential treatment?

    1. Impaired function in educational, social, or vocational areas

    2. Antisocial behavior

    3. Compulsive or addictive drug use

    4. Complicating psychopathology

16–4. Which of the following scenarios represent the highest risk for relapse for the adolescent patient?

1. Enrollment in a 7-day-a-week partial hospitalization program
2. Provision of 4 months of aftercare
3. An ongoing commitment to a 12-step recovery program
4. Discharge to the home environment

16–5. Pharmacotherapy may be important in the initial treatment of substance abuse in adolescents. Which features being present would support the use of medications?

1. Major depression
2. Prolonged agitation
3. Psychosis
4. Craving

16–6. At present, there are few data on the temporal relationship between psychoactive substance abuse patterns and specific psychiatric syndromes. The disorders frequently associated with substance abuse are

1. Conduct disorder.
2. Anxiety disorders.
3. Attention-deficit disorder.
4. Bipolar disorder.

■ **DIRECTIONS: For statements 16–7 through 16–11, indicate whether the statement is true or false.**

16–7. _____ Parents are often unaware of their children's substance use.

16–8. _____ Withdrawal symptoms are common in the adolescent population.

16–9. _____ If adolescent substance abuse does not appear to be maladaptive, then it may be sufficient for the clinician to warn the adolescent about the negative consequences of drug experimentation.

16–10. _____ Relapse rates for adolescents and adults are roughly the same.

16–11. _____ Adolescents are interested in the long-term consequences of their substance abuse.

■ **ANSWERS:**

16–1. **Answer: A (1, 2, and 3).** Pretreatment factors, including female gender, Caucasian race, higher educational level, later age at onset of drug use, lack of criminal activity, younger age at admission, and lack of comorbid psychiatric disorders, are all associated with a favorable treatment outcome. Treatment factors associated with a favorable treatment outcome include voluntary entrance into the program, greater length of treatment (for residential only), favorable perceptions of the experience, parental involvement, and special services (educational, recreational, and vocational).

16–2. **Answer: E (All).** Questions in the assessment of substance abuse should focus on the identification of the drug or drugs used, the route of administration, the duration and frequency of use, the setting of drug use, and the age at initial use. Belief systems about the physical (such as steroid abuse by athletes), psychological (mind-expanding), and social benefits of drug use should be queried. The amount of time an adolescent spends getting, using, and thinking about the drug is important information.

16–3. **Answer: E (All).** Referral for inpatient or residential treatment should occur if there is 1) compulsive or addictive drug use; 2) persistent antisocial behavior; 3) impaired function in educational, social, legal, or vocational areas; 4) psychopathology requiring behavioral and/or pharmacological management; 5) imminent danger posed by the physical or mental health of the child; 6) failure of outpatient treatment; and 7) behavior that presents a danger to self or others that requires containment.

16–4. **Answer: C (2 and 4 correct).** Adolescents discharged to the home environment are at the highest risk for relapse. A minimum of 6 months of aftercare is critical for the treatment of adolescents.

16–5. **Answer: A (1, 2, and 3).** Detoxification/withdrawal, major depression, active psychosis, prolonged agitation or combative behaviors, and bipolar disorder all require prompt medical management. Craving is a less well-defined entity in the adolescent population and does not require medical management.

16–6. **Answer: E (All).** Several disorders are associated with psychoactive substance abuse, including conduct disorder (disruptive behavior disorder), antisocial personality disorder, anxiety disorders, attention-deficit disorder, bipolar disorder, and other mood disorders.

16–7. **True** Parents are often unaware of their children's substance use. Separate interviews for the child and for the parents should be undertaken. In addition, the child may be unaware of the extent of their parents' substance abuse or use history.

16–8. **False** Withdrawal symptoms are relatively uncommon in the adolescent population because of the choice of drug, the relatively brief duration of use, or intermittent use.

16–9. **True** Those adolescents who are in the experimental stage of substance abuse may heed the advice and warnings of a trusted adult.

16–10. **True** Relapse rates for adolescents range between 35% and 85%. The relapse rate for adults is approximately 66%.

16–11. **False** Adolescents who have moved into the stage of substance abuse or dependence are not extremely concerned about the long-term consequences of substance abuse. These youth are most concerned about the here-and-now effects of substance use.

CHAPTER 17

Childhood-Onset Schizophrenia

■ **DIRECTIONS: For questions 17–1 through 17–10, indicate**

A if answers 1, 2, and 3 are correct.

B if answers 1 and 3 are correct.

C if answers 2 and 4 are correct.

D if only answer 4 is correct.

E if all are correct.

17–1. Which of the following are critical components in the treatment of childhood-onset schizophrenia?

1. Family therapy or parental guidance

2. Social skills training

3. Special education

4. Pharmacotherapy

17–2. Which of the following statements are **true** regarding the use of neuroleptic medications in children and adolescents with schizophrenia?

1. More than 100 controlled studies have documented the efficacy of neuroleptics in children and adolescents.

2. Children and adults have the same response rate to neuroleptics.

3. Children and adolescents experience few side effects.

4. As with adults, neuroleptics have greater impact on positive symptoms in children and adolescents.

17–3. In a youth presenting with an initial episode of psychosis, which of the following should be considered as part of the workup?

1. Electroencephalogram

2. Toxicology screen

3. Physical examination

4. Neuroimaging

17–4. Clozapine was the first of the atypical antipsychotic medications introduced in the United States. What are the risks associated with its use?

1. 1% to 2% incidence of potentially irreversible agranulocytosis

    2. Lenticular deposits

    3. Seizures

    4. 2% to 3% incidence of obstructive hepatitis

17–5. Which of the following are critical factors in the differential diagnosis of schizophrenia in children and adolescents?

    1. Developmental level of the child

    2. Severe abuse and neglect

    3. Affective disorders

    4. Asperger's syndrome

17–6. What are the most common side effects in children and adolescents on clozapine?

    1. Seizures

    2. Drooling

    3. Agitation

    4. Sedation

17–7. Which of the following statements are **true** regarding risperidone?

    1. It has a lower incidence of extrapyramidal symptoms than haloperidol.

    2. It is not convincingly superior to standard neuroleptics in treatment-resistant cases.

    3. It is not less likely to produce tardive dyskinesia.

    4. It is associated with aplastic anemia.

17–8. The educational handicaps of children with schizophrenia include which of the following?

    1. Poor attention

    2. Cognitive impairment

    3. Increased vulnerability to stress

    4. Specific learning disorders

17–9. Which of the following statements are **true** regarding psychotherapy for children and adolescents with schizophrenia?

    1. Psychotherapy may enhance coping skills.

    2. Psychotherapy may assist with here-and-now issues.

    3. Psychotherapy may assist with monitoring suicidality.

    4. Psychotherapy is not indicated for children and adolescents with schizophrenia.

17–10. Family therapy is an important component in the treatment of children and adolescents with schizophrenia. Which of the following statements are **false** regarding family therapy?

    1. Family therapy should always be conducted with every member of the family present.

    2. Family therapy lowers the relapse rate.

    3. Open and frank discussion with family members about the diagnosis is too overwhelming for them.

    4. A critical issue is allowing developmentally appropriate independence.

■ ANSWERS:

17–1. **Answer: E (All).** Although pharmacotherapy is a critical component in the treatment of childhood-onset schizophrenia, it is not sufficient by itself. Attention must be directed to reestablishment of as normal a developmental path as possible. Family therapy and parental guidance are critical to maintaining a chronically ill child in the home. Social skills training can be employed to teach these children how to approach and play with their peers. Special education in small, nurturing, and highly structured classrooms provides the best opportunity for these children to succeed academically.

17–2. **Answer: D (Only 4).** There are only two controlled studies documenting the use of neuroleptics in children and adolescents. The physiological development of children may influence the metabolism of neuroleptics, and schizophrenia in children may differ from that in adults. Children and adolescents are at least as vulnerable to extrapyramidal effects and sedation, with one study reporting that 75% experienced untoward effects. The primary impact of medications is on positive symptoms; medications are less effective with negative symptoms.

17–3. **Answer: E (All).** A comprehensive personal and family history is necessarily required for a youth presenting with an initial episode of psychosis. Even in those children and adolescents who deny substance use, a urine drug screen should be obtained. Young children may be coerced into using substances by older peers, siblings, or other family members. In a first episode of psychosis, careful consideration should be given to obtaining an electroencephalogram (EEG), particularly if there is any history suggestive of temporal lobe or other epileptic type of activity, as well as a neuroimaging study.

17–4. **Answer: B (1 and 3).** The major side effects of clozapine include a 1% to 2% incidence of potentially irreversible agranulocytosis and a dosage-related risk, ranging from 1% to 5%, of the induction of seizures. Chlorpromazine can cause pigmentation deposits in the eye, chiefly in the back of the cornea and the front of the lens. Retinal pigmentation occurs only with thioridazine. A form of allergic obstructive hepatitis is associated with high doses of chlorpromazine.

17–5. **Answer: E (All).** The developmental level of the child is critical in the differential diagnosis of schizophrenia. For example, a vivid fantasy life of a preschooler may be misconstrued as perceptual disturbances. Concrete and at times illogical thinking may be developmentally appropriate and may not indicate a formal thought disorder in young children. A history of severe abuse and neglect in the presence of auditory hallucinations and poor thought processing should alert the clinician to the possibility of multiple personality or other dissociative disorders. Distinguishing between bipolar disorder, major depression with psychotic features, and the first psychotic episode of schizophrenia may be clinically impossible in an acute setting. Affective disorders are always considered in the differential diagnosis. Many clinicians will use a mood-stabilizing agent such as lithium, carbamazepine, or valproic acid with an antidepressant and/or a benzodiazepine in an effort to avoid the use of neuroleptics in children and adolescents. There is a preponderance of evidence that establishes schizophrenia and autism as separate disorders. Asperger's syndrome is a variant of pervasive developmental disorder that has the distinguishing feature of no impairment in cognitive development. A minority of children with schizophrenia may have symptoms that overlap with those of children who have one of the pervasive developmental disorders.

17–6. **Answer: C (2 and 4).** The most common side effects of clozapine in children and adolescents are sedation, dizziness, tachycardia, orthostatic hypotension, and drooling. In one study, 55% of the children and adolescents showed sharp biphasic EEG waves during treatment compared with 30% before treatment. Seizures were not a common side effect. Agitation is not a usual side effect.

17–7. **Answer: A (1, 2, and 3).** Risperidone has a lower incidence of extrapyramidal symptoms than haloperidol. Unlike clozapine, it is not associated with aplastic anemia and is not convincingly superior to standard neuroleptics in treatment-resistant cases. To date, there is no evidence that risperidone is less likely to produce tardive dyskinesia.

17–8. **Answer: E (All).** Children with schizophrenia have numerous educational difficulties, including specific learning disorders, which may be difficult to ascertain in the midst of poor attention; thought disorders; cognitive impairments; behavioral disturbances; and social impairments. These children may have additional cognitive impairments that further complicate their ability to learn.

17–9. **Answer: A (1, 2, and 3).** Supportive psychotherapy that emphasizes coping and problem-solving skills, monitors medication compliance, educates the patient about the illness, and monitors suicide risk may be essential in the treatment of children and adolescents with schizophrenia.

17–10. **Answer: B (1 and 3).** Depending on the child's development and the acuity of the illness, the child may or may not be present for each therapy session. Empathic, open, and frank discussions of the diagnosis and basic epidemiological data with an emphasis on discussion of "myths" about schizophrenia actually reduce the family members' anxiety. At least with adult patients, family therapy lowers the relapse rate. Issues such as developmentally appropriate limit setting and allowing independence are critical when working with a family with a chronically ill child.

CHAPTER 18

Sleep Disorders

■ **DIRECTIONS: For questions 18–1 through 18–7, select the single best answer.**

18–1. What percentage of 1-year-olds who have previously slept through the night experience night waking?

    1. 20%

    2. 30%

    3. 50%

    4. 75%

18–2. A sleep apnea event is an interruption of breathing during sleep that lasts what length of time?

    1. 1 second

    2. 5 seconds

    3. 8 seconds

    4. 10 seconds

18–3. Secretion of which hormone may be severely impaired in childhood obstructive sleep apnea?

    1. Growth hormone

    2. Thyroid

    3. Testosterone

    4. Estrogen

18–4. Nightmares usually begin between what ages?

    1. 1 and 2 years

    2. 3 and 6 years

    3. 7 and 12 years

    4. After puberty

18–5. Which of the following is characteristic of a night terror?

    1. The child leaves the home to rendezvous with peers.

    2. The child is able to fully recount the dream in the morning.

3. The child appears awake and is terrified but recalls nothing.

4. The child walks out of the bedroom and does not respond when his or her name is called out.

18–6. What percentage of healthy 9-month-old infants will exhibit disturbances of sleep-wake transitions, such as head banging, head turning, or rocking?

1. 10%

2. 30%

3. 60%

4. 100%

18–7. What percentage of adolescents report falling asleep in school?

1. 10%

2. 20%

3. 30%

4. 50%

■ **DIRECTIONS: For questions 18–8 through 18–17, indicate**

A if answers 1, 2, and 3 are correct.

B if answers 1 and 3 are correct.

C if answers 2 and 4 are correct.

D if only answer 4 is correct.

E if all are correct.

18–8. Which of the following are part of the treatment for sleep terrors?

1. Lorazepam

2. A 30- to 60-minute afternoon nap

3. Trazodone

4. Parental reassurance

18–9. Which of the following statements are **true** regarding delayed sleep phase syndrome?

1. This syndrome is more common in adolescents than in young children.

2. The disorder is characterized by the child's being unable to fall asleep at a socially normative time.

3. The treatment of the disorder involves delaying both sleep times and rise times by 1 to 2 hours each day.

4. Once a bedtime and wake time are established, there is little risk of the disorder returning.

18–10. What factors are related to the development of a dyssomnia in a child?

1. Maternal personality

2. Physical discomfort

3. Maternal psychopathology

4. Temperament

18–11. Which physicians are the most likely to prescribe hypnotics to the pediatric population to treat sleep disturbances?

1. Child psychiatrists
2. Pediatricians
3. Pediatric neurologists
4. Family practitioners

18–12. Which of the following are behavioral approaches used to treat night waking in children?

1. Tolerating the child's crying
2. Practicing conjoint sleeping
3. Awakening the child before the usual waking time
4. Having a consistent ritual of rocking the child to sleep

18–13. How many apnea or hypopnea events must occur per hour of sleep before a diagnosis of obstructive sleep apnea disorder can be made?

1. 5 apnea events
2. 10 apnea events
3. 10 apnea/hypopnea events
4. 15 apnea/hypopnea events

18–14. What information is obtained from a standard polysomnographic recording?

1. Oxygen saturation
2. Cardiac rhythm
3. Amount of sleep fragmentation
4. Determination of daytime sleepiness

18–15. What types of surgical interventions may be necessary for the treatment of obstructive sleep apnea?

1. Uvulopalatopharyngoplasty
2. Tonsillectomy and adenoidectomy
3. Mandibular and maxillary advancement
4. Tracheostomy

18–16. In patients with narcolepsy, human leukocyte antigen (HLA) is essentially 100% positive for which of the following HLA haplotypes?

1. HLA-DR2
2. HLA-DR3
3. HLA-DQw1
4. HLA-DQw2

18–17. What will provoke cataplexy in patients with narcolepsy?

1. Laughing
2. Sexual excitement
3. Anger
4. Contentment

■ **DIRECTIONS: For statements 18–18 through 18–23, indicate whether the statement is true or false.**

18–18. _____ In the treatment of delayed sleep phase syndrome, phase advancement and phase delay are carried out at the same rate.

18–19. _____ Delayed sleep phase syndrome is easily treated in adolescents.

18–20. _____ There are strong clinical data supporting the use of sedative hypnotics for the treatment of sleep disturbances in children.

18–21. _____ The presenting signs and symptoms of sleep disorders in children may mimic those of attention-deficit/hyperactivity disorder.

18–22. _____ Parents frequently recognize the "stopped" breathing during sleep in children with obstructive sleep apnea.

18–23. _____ Parasomnias are found with equal frequency in boys and girls.

■ **ANSWERS:**

18–1. **Answer: 3.** Approximately half of all 1-year-olds who have previously accomplished sleeping throughout the night experience some night waking.

18–2. **Answer: 4.** A sleep apnea event is an interruption of breathing that lasts at least 10 seconds.

18–3. **Answer: 1.** The multiple awakenings of obstructive sleep apnea may disrupt the secretion of growth hormone. Children with obstructive sleep apnea may present with mild growth retardation or failure to thrive.

18–4. **Answer: 2.** Nightmares usually start between the ages of 3 and 6 years.

18–5. **Answer: 3.** Night terrors occur in stage 3 and stage 4 sleep. The child is amnestic for the event, despite appearing terrified. Children (most often adolescents) who leave home to rendezvous with peers or to perform other highly complex activities in the night do not have a pure sleep disturbance. Unlike children with night terrors, children who have nightmares are fully oriented and are frequently able to recount their dreams. Somnambulism (sleep walking) is a disorder of stage 3 and stage 4 sleep in which the child walks about in a trancelike state.

18–6. **Answer: 3.** Approximately 60% of healthy 9-month-old infants will exhibit some type of repetitive movement in the sleep-wake transition periods. These disorders are usually outgrown.

18–7. **Answer: 3.** Approximately 30% of adolescents report falling asleep in class, and many more complain of being tired.

18–8. **Answer: C (2 and 4).** Late-afternoon or early-evening naps of 30 to 60 minutes will reduce the amount of stage 4 sleep and may decrease the frequency of the night terrors. Most children will outgrow their night terrors, and parental education and reassurance may be sufficient.

18–9. **Answer: A (1, 2, and 3).** Delayed sleep phase syndrome is more common in adolescents than in younger children, who have less control over their bedtimes and fewer social, economic, and academic demands imposed on them. The disorder is characterized by the child's being unable to fall asleep at a socially normative time and then being unable to wake up in the morning. One form of treatment (phase delay) is to have the child delay sleep and waking times by 1 to 2 hours each night until a bedtime of 10:00 or 11:00 P.M. is achieved. Once the schedule is achieved, the sleep and wake times must be rigidly adhered to or the delayed sleep phase syndrome will return.

18–10. **Answer: E (All).** Intrinsic factors such as temperament and extrinsic factors such as physical discomfort, nutritional states, parental conflict, maternal personality, and maternal psychopathology have been linked to dyssomnias in young children.

18–11. **Answer: C (2 and 4).** Pediatricians and family practitioners are more likely to prescribe hypnotics to children with sleep disorders.

18–12. **Answer: A (1, 2, and 3).** Tolerating the child's crying or crying out is difficult for many parents, but this approach may extinguish the behavior. Conjoint sleeping is practiced in many cultures and provides the child with a sense of security. Scheduling awakenings before the time expected decreases the reward associated with crying out. A consistent ritual that is not associated with rocking or feeding may decrease the child's separation anxiety.

18–13. **Answer: B (1 and 3).** Sleep apnea syndromes, such as obstructive sleep apnea, are characterized by 5 apnea events or 10 apnea/hypopnea combinations per hour of sleep.

18–14. **Answer: A (1, 2, and 3).** Only polysomnography (PSG) provides an accurate recording of the type of apnea episode and its association with the sleep stage. Oxygen saturation and cardiac rhythm are obtained in PSG. The multiple sleep latency test (MSLT) is a daytime polysomnographic procedure that elicits daytime naps at regular intervals to determine daytime sleepiness or accumulated sleep debt.

18–15. **Answer: E (All).** Uvulopalatopharyngoplasty, tonsillectomy, adenoidectomy, mandibular and maxillary advancement, and tracheostomy are all surgical procedures that may alleviate obstructive sleep apnea. In the past, removal of tonsils and adenoids was a common pediatric procedure, and fewer cases of obstructive sleep apnea were diagnosed.

18–16. **Answer: B (1 and 3).** HLA testing is essentially 100% positive for HLA-DR2 and HLA-DQw1 in patients with narcolepsy.

18–17. **Answer: A (1, 2, and 3).** Strong affects such as intense joy, sexual excitement, and anger will induce cataplexy in patients with narcolepsy.

18–18. **False** Phase advancement, requiring the child to go to bed early by 15 to 30 minutes each night, is a more gradual process than phase delay.

18–19. **False** Treatment of delayed sleep phase syndrome requires a highly motivated adolescent and a cooperative family.

18–20. **False** There are few data supporting the use of sedative-hypnotics in the treatment of sleep disturbances in children.

18–21. **True** Children with obstructive sleep apnea may present with irritability, declining school performance, and difficulty with attending in the classroom.

18–22. **True** Parents are particularly good observers of "stopped" breathing in their children.

18–23. **False** Parasomnias are more common in males than in females.

Delirium, Dementia, and Amnestic and Other Cognitive Disorders

CHAPTER 19

■

Delirium Due to a General Medical Condition, Delirium Due to Multiple Etiologies, and Delirium Not Otherwise Specified

■ DIRECTIONS: For questions 19–1 through 19–7, select the single best answer.

19–1. Delirium is a sign of impending death in what percentage of cases?

1. 15%
2. 25%
3. 35%
4. 45%

19–2. All of the following patient groups are at high risk for delirium **except**

1. Elderly patients.
2. Patients with extensive burns.
3. Children postcardiotomy.
4. Patients with human immunodeficiency virus (HIV) infection.

19–3. Delirium is the most commonly diagnosed brain disorder in patients with advanced acquired immunodeficiency syndrome (AIDS). What is the overall frequency of brain disorders in these patients?

1. 30%
2. 60%
3. 90%
4. 100%

19–4. Which of the following forms of delirium is indicative of the most severe cognitive disturbance?

1. Hyperactive delirium
2. Mixed delirium

3. Hypoactive delirium

4. None of the above

19–5. What is the only treatment that may reduce the incidence of postcardiotomy delirium?

1. Adequate hydration

2. Optimal management of any preoperative chronic medical condition

3. Psychiatric intervention

4. None of the above, because there is evidence that no treatment modality can effectively decrease the risk of postcardiotomy delirium

19–6. Which of the following is **not** part of the general treatment of patients with delirium?

1. Ensuring adequate oxygenation

2. Discontinuing all nonessential medications

3. Monitoring fluid input and output

4. Keeping the patient in a room with other patients with delirium that is as close as possible to the nursing station

19–7. Which of the following delirious patients will benefit from treatment with physostigmine?

1. A 23-year-old with ulcerative colitis who has overdosed on diphenhydramine

2. A 22-year-old who presents with acute phencyclidine (PCP) intoxication

3. A 20-year-old who has overdosed on amitriptyline

4. A 45-year-old with diabetes mellitus and sepsis secondary to a gangrenous foot

■ DIRECTIONS: For questions 19–8 through 19–15, indicate whether the statement is true or false.

19–8. _____ Patients who receive intravenous haloperidol have an increased incidence of extrapyramidal symptoms.

19–9. _____ Sensory deprivation alone is sufficient to cause delirium.

19–10. _____ Patients with borderline personality disorder are at high risk for delirium.

19–11. _____ Patients are frequently amnestic for the period of time that they were delirious.

19–12. _____ Patients with delirium are oriented to person but not to time or place.

19–13. _____ Auditory hallucinations are the most common perceptual disturbance in delirious patients.

19–14. _____ The delirious patient may develop a loosely knit paranoid delusional system.

19–15. _____ Intravenous haloperidol is efficacious in the treatment of delirium.

■ ANSWERS:

19–1. **Answer: 2.** The mortality associated with delirium is 25%.

19–2. **Answer: 3.** Adult patients who undergo cardiac surgery are at high risk for delirium, but children postcardiotomy do not appear to be at particularly high risk.

19–3. **Answer: 3.** The frequency of any type of organic mental disorders in patients with advanced AIDS is 90%.

19–4. **Answer: 3.** Hypoactive delirium, compared with the hyperactive and mixed types of delirium, is associated with the most severe cognitive disturbance. It may be mistaken as depression in a medically ill patient.

19–5. **Answer: 3.** Only preoperative psychiatric consultation has any effect on decreasing the risk of postcardiotomy delirium.

19–6. **Answer: 4.** The delirious patient should be moved as close as possible to the nursing station, and, if possible, a family member or close friend should remain with the patient. Keeping two delirious patients together will only exacerbate each patient's condition.

19–7. **Answer: 3.** A continuous infusion of physostigmine may be used to treat severe cases of anticholinergic toxicity. Contraindications for physostigmine are ulcerative colitis, asthma, diabetes mellitus, gangrene, mechanical obstruction of the urinary or gastrointestinal tracts, and cardiovascular disease.

19–8. **False** There is no increased incidence of extrapyramidal symptoms with intravenous haloperidol.

19–9. **False** Sensory deprivation may cause perceptual disturbances but not a full delirium.

19–10. **False** There is no evidence that patients with a personality disorder are at higher risk for delirium.

19–11. **True** Amnesia is part of delirium.

19–12. **True** Orientation to person is basic to being human and is the last orientation lost in delirium.

19–13. **False** Illusions and visual hallucinations are more common than auditory hallucinations.

19–14. **True** Paranoid delusions may be part of a delirium.

19–15. **True** Intravenous haloperidol has been shown to be effective in the treatment of delirium.

CHAPTER 20

━━━━━━━■━━━━━━━

Substance-Induced Delirium

■ **DIRECTIONS: For questions 20–1 through 20–41, match each substance to the appropriate statement(s). Each statement may be used once, more than once, or not at all.**

20–1.	Diazepam	a.	This is an anticholinergic agent.
20–2.	Aminophylline	b.	This is an over-the-counter medication that directly induces delirium.
20–3.	Amitriptyline	c.	This is an effective treatment for organo-phosphate poisoning.
20–4.	Meperidine	d.	This is an anticonvulsant agent.
20–5.	Lorazepam	e.	Hyperbaric oxygen is the treatment of choice for severe poisoning.
20–6.	Digoxin	f.	This is commonly used by farmers.
20–7.	L-Dopa	g.	As many as 50% of patients on this agent experience adverse neuropsychiatric events.
20–8.	Nortriptyline	h.	The action at the locus coeruleus may account for delirium.
20–9.	Propranolol	i.	Choreoathetoid movements may be associated with the delirious state.
20–10.	Clonidine hydrochloride	j.	Aseptic meningitis is associated with this agent.
20–11.	Phenobarbital	k.	This agent is used to treat asthma.
20–12.	Cyclosporine	l.	When this agent is freely available, it is preferred over food.
20–13.	Chlorpromazine	m.	This is an antiviral agent.
20–14.	Ethosuximide	n.	Hypothyroidism may increase the risk of drug-induced delirium with this agent.
20–15.	Fluoxetine	o.	This agent is used to treat hypertension.
20–16.	Trimethoprim/ sulfamethoxazole	p.	The nephrotoxic element of this drug may be part of the etiology of the substance-induced delirium state.

20–17. Amantadine   q. This agent is used in the treatment of HIV.

20–18. Cocaine   r. This agent is frequently used to treat urinary tract infections.

20–19. Ethanol   s. The binding of the beta-lactam ring to the gamma-aminobutyric acid (GABA) receptors may account for the neurotoxicity of the drug.

20–20. Morphine   t. This agent is a monoclonal antibody.

20–21. Prednisone   u. Hypokalemia increases the neurotoxicity of this agent.

20–22. OKT3   v. Enhanced activity in the adrenal medulla may be responsible for the neurotoxic effects of this agent.

20–23. Amoxicillin   w. Brain-stem spongiosis is a rare complication.

20–24. Didanosine   x. This agent disrupts folate metabolism.

20–25. Organophosphates   y. Worsening mentation within 2 hours after initiation of the medication may indicate the presence of neurotoxicity.

20–26. Paroxetine   z. Haloperidol may be used to treat the delirium.

20–27. Cimetidine   aa. Indomethacin use increases neurotoxicity.

20–28. Nifedipine   bb. Hypoglycemia may be so profound that delirium and coma may result.

20–29. Chlordiazepoxide   cc. This agent is an antiparkinson drug.

20–30. Amphotericin B   dd. Even topical application of this agent may be associated with delirium in susceptible patients.

20–31. Diphenhydramine   ee. This agent may produce EEG "silence."

20–32. Valproic acid   ff. Seizures often occur before the onset of the delirium.

20–33. Lidocaine   gg. This agent has muscarinic properties equivalent to those of imipramine.

20–34. Bromides   hh. This agent has potentially fatal interaction with monoamine oxidase inhibitors.

20–35. Metrizamide   ii. This agent may be used to treat delirium.

20–36. Dextromethorphan   jj. This medication is a tricyclic antidepressant.

20–37. Ibuprofen   kk. This agent is an immunosuppressant.

20–38. Lithium   ll. This agent is an H_2-receptor antagonist.

20–39. Interleukins (IKs)   mm. This is an antifungal agent.

20–40. Ciprofloxacin

20–41. Streptomycin

■ DIRECTIONS: Using the following clinical vignette, for questions 20–42 through 20–46, select the single best answer.

Mr. K. is a 43-year-old business executive who is 2 days status post–emergency exploratory laparotomy with drainage of two pancreatic pseudocysts. His transaminase levels are SGOT 1,200 (5–40 IU/L) and SGPT 1,000 (7–53 IU/L). His vital signs are BP 160/95, P 105 beats per minute, T 98.8°F. He adamantly denies drinking on "more than a social basis" and refuses to elaborate on how many drinks per day he consumes. A psychiatric consultation is sought to address his "seeing little green men who walk into his room" and his lack of cooperation with staying in bed. Mr. K. has been found repeatedly wandering the hallways oblivious to the pain that must have occurred when he ripped out intravenous lines.

20–42. What diagnosis would be the most likely explanation for Mr. K.'s psychiatric symptoms?

1. Alcohol withdrawal delirium
2. Anesthetic-induced delirium
3. Postoperative "psychosis"
4. Delirium due to sepsis

20–43. What percentage of general hospital inpatients abuse or are dependent on alcohol?

1. 20%
2. 30%
3. 40%
4. 50%

20–44. What is the medication of choice for the treatment of Mr. K.'s delirium?

1. Diazepam
2. Lorazepam
3. Chlordiazepoxide
4. Oxazepam

20–45. In addition to a benzodiazepine, what other medications should be administered?

1. Thiamine and chlorpromazine
2. Thiamine and haloperidol
3. Vitamin B_6 and haloperidol
4. No other treatment is necessary

20–46. Mr. K. is steadily improving with the combined efforts of the psychiatric, medical, and surgical services. One evening the resident receives a "stat" call to Mr. K.'s room, where they find him comatose. Pulse oximetry reveals an oxygen saturation of 85% on room air. His respirations are shallow, with a rate of 10 per minute. Vital signs are BP 100/60, P 68 beats minute, and T 97.5°F. Mr. K. had inadvertently received 10 times the ordered dose of benzodiazepine. What is the treatment of choice?

1. Immediate intubation
2. Flumazenil and O_2 by mask
3. Haloperidol and O_2 by mask
4. Forbidding the use of any benzodiazepines in this patient

■ **DIRECTIONS: For questions 20–47 through 20–49, select the single best answer.**

20–47. In which of the following conditions is the use of neuroleptics to treat the delirium contraindicated?

1. Nitrous oxide poisoning
2. Ifosfamide intoxication
3. Neuroleptic malignant syndrome
4. None of the above

20–48. Which of the following conditions is associated with ibuprofen overdose but not acetaminophen overdose?

1. Aseptic meningitis
2. Hepatic involvement
3. Comatose state
4. Death

20–49. Beta-blockers penetrate the central nervous system according to their lipophilicity. Which of the following beta-blockers is most often associated with mental status changes?

1. Atenolol
2. Propranolol
3. Clonidine hydrochloride
4. Nadolol

■ **DIRECTIONS: For questions 20–50 through 20–53, indicate**

A if answers 1, 2, and 3 are correct.
B if answers 1 and 3 are correct.
C if answers 2 and 4 are correct.
D if only answer 4 is correct.
E if all are correct.

20–50. Which of the following conditions may predispose an individual to delirium?

1. Hypoalbuminemia

2. Hyponatremia

3. Hypomagnesemia

4. Elevated transaminase levels

20–51. As many as 5% of patients taking corticosteroids will experience neuropsychiatric symptoms. What factors predispose a patient to these symptoms?

1. Receiving a total daily dosage of greater than 40 mg

2. Being elderly

3. Being female

4. Having had a prior or having a current psychiatric disorder

20–52. Which of the following drugs are associated with delirium in a state of intoxication and withdrawal?

1. Carbamazepine

2. Morphine

3. Lorazepam

4. Isoniazid

20–53. In the treatment of patients with Parkinson's disease who continue to be delirious even with a reduction in levodopa, which of the following medication strategies may be tried to treat the psychiatric symptoms?

1. Add thioridazine.

2. Add chlorpromazine.

3. Add clozapine.

4. Add haloperidol.

■ **ANSWERS:**

20–1. Diazepam: **z**

20–2. Aminophylline: **No answers**

20–3. Amitriptyline: **jj**

20–4. Meperidine: **z, hh**

20–5. Lorazepam: **d, ii**

20–6. Digoxin: **u, z**

20–7. L-Dopa: **cc**

20–8. Nortriptyline: **a, z, jj**

20–9. Propranolol: **o, z, dd**

20–10. Clonidine hydrochloride: **o, h**

20–11. Phenobarbital: **d**

20–12. Cyclosporine: **kk**

20–13. Chlorpromazine: **a**

20–14. Ethosuximide: **d**

20–15. Fluoxetine: **No answers**

20–16. Trimethoprim/sulfamethoxazole: **r, x, y**

20–17. Amantadine: **m, z, cc**

20–18. Cocaine: **l**

20–19. Ethanol: **z, ff**

20–20. Morphine: **z**

20–21. Prednisone: **z, kk**

20–22. OKT3: **kk**

20–23. Amoxicillin: **r, s, y**

20–24. Didanosine: **m, q**

20–25. Organophosphates: **f**

20–26. Paroxetine: **gg**

20–27. Cimetidine: **ll**

20–28. Nifedipine: **o**

20–29. Chlordiazepoxide: **z**

20–30. Amphotericin B: **mm**

20–31. Diphenhydramine: **a, z**

20–32. Valproic acid: **d, z**

20–33. Lidocaine: **g**

20–34. Bromides: **f, z**

20–35. Metrizamide: **z**

20–36. Dextromethorphan: **b, z**

20–37. Ibuprofen: **j**

20–38. Lithium: **n, aa**

20–39. Interleukins (IKs): **m, z**

20–40. Ciprofloxacin: **r, y**

20–41. Streptomycin: **w, y**

20–42. **Answer 1.** The most likely diagnosis to explain Mr. K.'s psychiatric symptoms is *alcohol withdrawal delirium.* Anesthetic-induced delirium usually occurs in the immediate postoperative period, and delirium due to sepsis occurs most frequently on postoperative days 5 to 7. The delirium described in this patient is a "hyperactive" delirium with motoric overarousal, visual hallucinations, and autonomic instability. There is no diagnostic category of postoperative "psychosis."

20–43. **Answer: 4.** In the general population, the incidence of alcohol abuse or dependence is approximately 7%. In general hospital inpatient populations, the incidence is approximately 50%.

20–44. **Answer: 2.** The patient has significantly elevated transaminase levels, indicating possible hepatic impairment. He has undergone a major abdominal procedure, necessitating the use of intramuscular or intravenous medications rather than an oral route of administration. Diazepam and chlordiazepoxide require hepatic oxidation before conjugation; both are poorly absorbed via intramuscular routes. Oxazepam does not undergo hepatic oxidation, but it is highly sedating and is not available in an injectable form. Lorazepam is the drug of choice because it does not undergo hepatic oxidation, it is intermediate acting (lessening the risk of accumulation of the drug), and it is well absorbed via the intramuscular route.

20–45. **Answer: 2.** Thiamine should be given for the first 3 days. Haloperidol is the neuroleptic of choice for treatment of severe perceptual disturbances.

20–46. **Answer: 2.** At present, Mr. K. is stable and does not require intubation. Flumazenil 2 mg intravenously should be attempted. This agent is a benzodiazepine antagonist that does not necessarily reverse benzodiazepine-induced respiratory depression.

20–47. **Answer: 3.** Neuroleptic malignant syndrome (NMS) is a rare, idiopathic, and potentially fatal reaction to central nervous system dopamine blockade. Delirium caused by NMS is one type of delirium for which treatment with neuroleptics is contraindicated. Ifosfamide is an alkylating agent used to treat certain types of cancer. The delirium associated with ifosfamide carries a particularly grave prognosis of irreversible encephalopathy followed by death. Nitrous oxide is an inhalation anesthetic that is occasionally associated with delirium in patients with advanced age or who are obese.

20–48. **Answer: 1.** The nonsteroidal anti-inflammatory agents (NSAIDs)—in particular, ibuprofen—are associated with aseptic meningitis. Hepatic involvement occurs in overdose situations with NSAIDs (hepatitis) and acetaminophen (hepatic necrosis). A hypoglycemic coma may result from acetaminophen overdose. In the case of NSAIDs, delirium progressing to a comatose state may occur. Death may result from overdose in both cases.

20–49. **Answer: 2.** Propranolol is the most lipophilic of the beta-blockers. Consequently, it is the medication most often implicated in mental status changes. Clonidine hydrochloride is not a beta-blocker.

20–50. **Answer: E (All).** Poor nutrition, liver disease, renal insufficiency, or chronic disease may lead to hypoalbuminemia, hyponatremia, hypomagnesemia, or elevated transaminase levels, all of which may predispose an individual to a toxic reaction or accumulation of even therapeutic doses of medications.

20–51. **Answer: A (1, 2, and 3).** Susceptibility to mental status changes induced by corticosteroids is increased by receiving a total daily dose of 30–40 mg, having an intercurrent illness, being elderly, and being female. A prior history of a psychiatric disorder does not necessarily predispose the patient to neuropsychiatric symptoms.

20–52. **Answer: B (1 and 3).** Anticonvulsants (carbamazepine), sedative-hypnotics (lorazepam), immunosuppressants, and anesthetic agents are all associated with delirium caused by intoxication or withdrawal. Opioids (morphine) and antineoplastics (isoniazid) are associated with delirium only during intoxication.

20–53. **Answer: A (1, 2, and 3).** A low-potency antipsychotic such as thioridazine or chlorpromazine, which has anticholinergic effects, or low-dose clozapine may reduce the delirium associated with dopaminergic agents. High-potency neuroleptics such as haloperidol may exacerbate parkinsonian symptoms.

CHAPTER 21

Alzheimer's Disease

■ **DIRECTIONS: For questions 21–1 through 21–9, indicate**

    A if answers 1, 2, and 3 are correct.

    B if answers 1 and 3 are correct.

    C if answers 2 and 4 are correct.

    D if only answer 4 is correct.

    E if all are correct.

21–1. Family members of patients with Alzheimer's disease (AD) provide most of the care for these patients. Which of the following statements regarding family caregivers of patients with AD are **true**?

    1. They have poorer overall physical health than do age-matched control subjects.

    2. They have less depressive symptomatology than do age-matched control subjects.

    3. They use more psychotropic medications than do age-matched control subjects.

    4. The majority of caregivers are the eldest sons in the family.

21–2. Modifications to the AD patient's home are essential in the behavioral management of wandering behaviors and to guard against other unsafe activities. Which of the following are part of ensuring a safe environment?

    1. Installing door alarms

    2. Making stoves and other appliances inoperable by the patient

    3. Installing outdoor fencing

    4. Having the patient wear a medical alert wrist bracelet

21–3. Patients with AD may develop incontinence. Which of the following statements regarding incontinence are **true**?

    1. It is an important factor in the family's decision to place the patient in an extended care facility.

    2. In patients with urinary incontinence, 30%–50% may episodically experience fecal incontinence.

3. Behavior therapy approaches are the treatment of choice for incontinence associated with AD.

4. Incontinence in AD patients is consistently due to their dementia.

21–4. In AD patients who develop a secondary seizure disorder, which medications are the treatment of choice?

1. Phenobarbital

2. Phenytoin

3. Ethosuximide

4. Carbamazepine

21–5. Behavioral disturbances can be disruptive to the AD patient's family and are highly resistant to pharmacological management. Which of the following are included in this category?

1. Repetitive questions

2. Apathy

3. Disinhibition

4. Verbal outbursts

21–6. Which of the following therapeutic modalities are efficacious in the treatment of AD patients?

1. Family therapy

2. Cognitive therapy

3. Behavior therapy

4. Insight-oriented therapy

21–7. Sleep disturbances are relatively common in AD patients. These disturbances may be treated with improved sleep hygiene and medications. Which of the following agents are associated with tolerance and withdrawal symptoms?

1. Trazodone

2. Temazepam

3. Thioridazine

4. Chloral hydrate

21–8. The most consistent neurotransmitter deficiency in AD patients is loss of basal forebrain cholinergic neurons that synthesize choline acetyl transferase (CAT). This feature has led to a great deal of research in augmentation of CAT or prevention of its degradation. Which of the following statements regarding these agents are **true**?

1. Administration of phosphatidylcholine increases cerebrospinal fluid (CSF) levels of CAT and improves cognitive functioning in AD patients.

2. 4-Aminopyridine increases acetylcholine release and improves cognitive functioning in AD patients.

3. Administration of choline increases CSF levels of CAT and improves cognitive functioning in AD patients.

4. Administration of tacrine retards the breakdown of CAT and improves cognitive functioning in AD patients.

21-9. Neuroleptic agents are the most commonly prescribed medications in nursing homes. Which of the following statements regarding their usage are **false**?

    1. Most AD patients will not experience extrapyramidal side effects when the dose is below 4 mg/day.

    2. Management of behavioral symptoms is usually accomplished with neuroleptic medication.

    3. No particular neuroleptic agent is therapeutically superior in the treatment of AD patients.

    4. Patients with Alzheimer's disease are fairly resistant to the various side effects of neuroleptics.

■ **ANSWERS:**

21-1. **Answer: B (1 and 3).** Family caregivers of AD patients are most frequently women, usually the spouse or an adult daughter. They have more depressive symptomatology, use more psychotropic medications, and have poorer overall physical health than do age-matched control subjects.

21-2. **Answer: E (All).** Modifications of the physical environment may be lifesaving to the AD patient. Such measures include installing door locks and alarms, making appliances inoperable by the patient, installing outdoor fencing, improving the lighting, and having the patient wear a medical alert bracelet.

21-3. **Answer: A (1, 2, and 3).** The etiology of incontinence should not presumptively be assigned to the patient's dementia. It may be secondary to infection, restricted mobility, urinary or fecal retention with overflow, atrophic vaginitis/urethritis, or medication side effects. The presence of incontinence strongly influences the family's decision to place the patient in an extended care facility. Approximately 30%–50% of patients with urinary incontinence will also experience fecal incontinence. Behavioral management such as scheduling toileting, increasing the visibility and availability of the facilities, and avoiding evening fluid intake are frequently helpful in managing the incontinence.

21-4. **Answer: C (2 and 4).** The relatively nonsedating properties of phenytoin (Dilantin) and carbamazepine (Tegretol) make these the drugs of choice for treatment of seizure disorders associated with Alzheimer's disease.

21-5. **Answer: E (All).** Wandering, verbal outbursts, hostility, repetitive questions, apathy, and disinhibition are behavioral disturbances that can be disruptive to the AD patient's family and particularly resistant to pharmacological interventions.

21-6. **Answer: E (All).** Early in the course of AD, insight-oriented therapy may be beneficial to a patient who is realizing the imminent loss of cognitive, emotional, and motoric capabilities. Family, cognitive, supportive, and behavior therapies are frequently key components in the treatment of AD patients.

21-7. **Answer: C (2 and 4).** Patients may develop tolerance and experience withdrawal symptoms from temazepam (a short-acting benzodiazepine) and chloral hydrate.

21–8. **Answer: D (only 4).** Choline and phosphatidylcholine both increase CSF levels of CAT, but there is no improvement in cognitive functioning. 4-Aminopyridine increases acetylcholine release but does not improve cognitive functioning in AD patients. At present, tacrine (THA) is the only medication approved by the FDA for treatment of cognitive deficits in patients with mild-to-moderate AD.

21–9. **Answer: C (2 and 4).** Management of behavior symptoms is rarely achieved through pharmacology. Patients with AD are highly sensitive to the side effects of neuroleptics.

CHAPTER 22

Vascular Dementia

Mr. Y. is a college-educated, 75-year-old business executive who smokes three packs of cigarettes per day. He has a history of hypertension, atrial fibrillation, and adult-onset diabetes mellitus. Last year he had a stroke that involved the left basal ganglia. Physical examination today reveals a blood pressure of 80/45.

22–1. Which of the following statements regarding poststroke mood disorders are **false**?

    1. Because his stroke was in the left basal ganglia, Mr. Y. is at low risk for depression.

    2. Electroconvulsive therapy (ECT) is efficacious in the treatment of poststroke depression.

    3. Antidepressants are not effective in the treatment of poststroke depression.

    4. Treatment of poststroke depression may alleviate some of the cognitive impairments.

22–2. Which risk factors for vascular dementia are missing in Mr. Y.?

    1. Hypertension

    2. Hypotension

    3. Atrial fibrillation

    4. Limited education

22–3. On clinical examination, Mr. Y. is alert, with no fluctuation in his sensorium. He is unable to interpret proverbs or understand similarities, and he appears confused and inarticulate about his business affairs. Which of the following may improve Mr. Y.'s cognitive functioning?

    1. Acetylsalicylic acid

    2. Dipyridamole

    3. Smoking cessation

    4. Buflomedil

22–4. If Mr. Y.'s cognitive impairments are not severe, which of the following treatments may be helpful?

    1. Ticlopidine

    2. Carotid endarterectomy

    3. Verapamil

    4. Estrogen replacement

■ ANSWERS:

22–1. **Answer: B (1 and 3).** Patients who have left-sided lesions, particularly left frontal or basal ganglia lesions, are at higher risk for depression than those who have right-sided lesions. Both ECT and antidepressants are effective treatments in poststroke depression. There is some evidence that treatment of poststroke depression may improve cognitive functioning.

22–2. **Answer: D (Only 4).** Hypertension is the single most influential risk factor for stroke and atherosclerosis, which themselves are risk factors for vascular dementia. Hypotension is also a risk factor for vascular dementia. Overly aggressive treatment of hypertension or other physiological states may create a hypotensive clinical picture in a high-risk patient. Atrial fibrillation, smoking, diabetes mellitus, a history of stroke, and limited education are also risk factors for vascular dementia.

22–3. **Answer: E (All).** Acetylsalicylic acid (ASA/aspirin) is a noncompetitive antiplatelet drug that is effective in the secondary prevention of stroke. Dipyridamole is also an antiplatelet drug that is effective in the secondary prevention of stroke. Buflomedil is a vasodilator drug that enhances red blood cell function; poor attention, cooperation, and impaired self-care are all positively affected by this medication. Smoking cessation, appropriate management of hypertension and diabetes mellitus, and potassium supplementation may decrease the risk of subsequent strokes.

22–4. **Answer: A (1, 2, and 3).** If carotid stenosis is between 20% and 99%, a carotid endarterectomy may be beneficial. Calcium channel blockers such as verapamil, and ticlopidine are useful agents. Estrogen replacement is indicated in postmenopausal women.

CHAPTER 23

■

Dementia Due to Other General Medical Conditions and Dementia Due to Multiple Etiologies

■ **DIRECTIONS: For questions 23–1 through 23–7, match each disease process to the corresponding item(s). Each item may be used once, more than once, or not at all.**

23–1.	Fahr's disease	a.	Autosomal dominant
23–2.	Huntington's disease	b.	Autosomal recessive
23–3.	Pick's disease	c.	Iron deposits in the substantia nigra
23–4.	Steele-Richardson-Olszewski syndrome	d.	Kayser-Fleischer rings
23–5.	Hallervorden-Spatz disease	e.	Obsessive-compulsive behaviors
23–6.	Wilson's disease	f.	Streptococcal infections
23–7.	Friedreich's ataxia	g.	Progressive supranuclear palsy
		h.	Diabetes mellitus
		i.	Klüver-Bucy syndrome
		j.	Chromosome 4
		k.	Wing-beating tremor
		l.	Pseudobulbar palsy
		m.	Basal ganglia calcification
		n.	Personality changes
		o.	D-Penicillamine
		p.	Zidovudine

■ **DIRECTIONS: For questions 23–8 through 23–18, indicate**

    A if answers 1, 2, and 3 are correct.

    B if answers 1 and 3 are correct.

    C if answers 2 and 4 are correct.

    D if only answer 4 is correct.

    E if all are correct.

23–8. Which of the following signs are seen in Parkinson's disease but not in pseudo-dementia?

    1. Mask facies

    2. Stooped posture

    3. Bradykinesia

    4. Tremor

23–9. Which of the following statements regarding psychiatric disorders in patients with Huntington's disease are **true**?

    1. Chronic depression occurs in 50% of patients.

    2. Intermittent explosive disorder occurs in 30% of patients.

    3. Hypomanic episodes occur in 20% of patients.

    4. Alcoholism occurs in 15% of patients.

23–10. Treatment of depression associated with Parkinson's disease includes which of the following modalities?

    1. Electroconvulsive therapy

    2. Paroxetine

    3. Bupropion

    4. Sertraline

23–11. Treatment of Huntington's disease involves which of the following medications?

    1. Amitriptyline

    2. Lithium

    3. Phenelzine

    4. Haloperidol

23–12. Sixty percent of patients with Parkinson's disease demonstrate improvement in which symptoms when treated with levodopa?

    1. Akinesia

    2. Tremor

    3. Cognitive impairment

    4. Depression

23–13. Treatment with physostigmine may result in improvement for which of the following disorders?

    1. Wilson's disease

    2. Olivopontocerebellar atrophies

3. Fahr's disease

4. Friedreich's ataxia

23–14. Twenty-four hours after undergoing resection of a parathyroid tumor, Mr. Z. is experiencing hallucinations and is worried that the nursing staff is secretly poisoning his food. Which of the following statements regarding this patient are **true**?

1. His psychosis is most likely self-limited.

2. If the tumor was removed within 5 years of the onset of symptoms, then considerable improvement in cognitive functioning is expected.

3. He may experience a fluctuating sensorium.

4. His present condition is secondary to hypercalcemia.

23–15. Which of the following may improve or decrease the likelihood of dialysis dementia?

1. Using peritoneal dialysis

2. Using clonazepam

3. Using deferoxamine

4. Reducing aluminum levels in dialysate

23–16. Replacement of which of the following vitamins will improve the associated dementia?

1. Cobalamin

2. Folic acid

3. Niacin

4. Ascorbic acid

23–17. The dementia associated with systemic lupus erythematosus may be treated by which of the following?

1. Corticosteroids

2. Placement of an intraventricular shunt

3. Electroconvulsive therapy

4. Propranolol

23–18. Surgical management may result in improvement of cognitive deficits for which of the following conditions?

1. Subdural hematomas

2. Hyperparathyroidism

3. Normal-pressure hydrocephalus

4. Hyperthyroidism

■ ANSWERS:

23–1. Fahr's disease: **a, m**

23–2. Huntington's disease: **a, j**

23–3. Pick's disease: **a, i, n**

23–4. Steele-Richardson-Olszewski syndrome: **e, g, l**

23–5. Halervorden-Spatz disease: **b, c**

23–6. Wilson's disease: **d, k, n, o**

23–7. Friedreich's ataxia: **b, h**

23–8. **Answer: D (Only 4).** Tremor is not a sign of pseudodementia. Decreased facial expression (mask facies), stooped posture, bradykinesia, and decreased cognitive skills are seen in both pseudodementia and Parkinson's disease.

23–9. **Answer: C (2 and 4).** Approximately 50% of patients with Huntington's disease will have an affective disorder, 20% will have a chronic depression, and 10% will experience hypomanic episodes. Intermittent explosive disorder is present in 30% of patients with Huntington's disease. Alcoholism occurs in 15% of patients with Huntington's disease.

23–10. **Answer: B (1 and 3).** Electroconvulsive therapy and bupropion are both effective treatments for depression associated with Parkinson's disease. Tricyclic antidepressants are also efficacious. The selective serotonin reuptake inhibitors paroxetine and sertraline indirectly inhibit dopaminergic neurons and may exacerbate the motor signs and symptoms of Parkinson's disease.

23–11. **Answer: E (All).** Tricyclic antidepressants (e.g., amitriptyline) and monoamine oxidase inhibitors (e.g., phenelzine) are effective in the treatment of depression seen in patients with Huntington's disease. Aggression and irritability seen in patients with Huntington's disease may decrease with the use of lithium. Neuroleptics (e.g., haloperidol) are effective in treating the choreic movement disorder associated with Huntington's disease.

23–12. **Answer: A (1, 2, and 3).** Depression in Parkinson's disease is probably an integral part of the basal ganglia disease and yet is unresponsive to treatment with levodopa. The motor symptoms associated with Parkinson's disease, including akinesia, tremor, and rigidity, all improve with levodopa. There is some improvement in cognitive functioning.

23–13. **Answer: D (Only 4).** Mild transient improvements are found in some patients with Friedreich's ataxia treated with physostigmine.

23–14. **Answer: B (1 and 3).** Postoperative hypocalcemia may result in a self-limited psychosis with impairment in consciousness. If the tumor is resected within 2 years, there is considerable improvement in the dementia.

23–15. **Answer: E (All).** Peritoneal dialysis is technically more complicated for the patient, but the frequency of dialysis dementia associated with this method is lower. Dialysis dementia is associated with aluminum toxicity, so reducing the level of aluminum in the dialysate and treatment with the aluminum chelating agent deferoxamine may improve cognitive functioning. Despite the possibility of their precipitating encephalopathy in dialysis patients, the benzodiazepines clonazepam and diazepam may temporarily ameliorate speech and cognitive disturbances.

23–16. **Answer: A (1, 2, and 3).** Vitamin B_{12} (cobalamin), B_6 (niacin), and folic acid deficiency may all cause dementias that are at least partially reversible with supplementation. Ascorbic acid deficiency is not associated with dementia.

23–17. **Answer: B (1 and 3).** Dementia associated with systemic lupus erythematosus may respond dramatically to corticosteroids or electroconvulsive therapy. Normal-pressure hydrocephalus dementia occasionally responds to placement of an intraventricular shunt. Propranolol is slightly effective in the treatment of agitation associated with dementia.

23–18. **Answer: E (All).** Removal of the thyroid is occasionally indicated in severe hyperthyroidism or tumors. Surgical intervention is warranted for hyperparathyroidism secondary to tumors. Only 12% of patients with the classic triad of dementia, gait disturbance, and urinary incontinence will have normal-pressure hydrocephalus; the dementia associated with this condition may improve with placement of an intraventricular shunt. Subdural hematomas frequently require surgical drainage.

CHAPTER 24

Substance-Induced Persisting Dementia and Substance-Induced Persisting Amnestic Disorder

■ **DIRECTIONS: For questions 24–1 through 24–4, match each disease process to the correct statement(s). Each statement may be used once, more than once, or not at all.**

24–1. Marchiafava-Bignami disease

24–2. Korsakoff's syndrome

24–3. Wernicke's encephalopathy

24–4. Pellagra

a. Nicotinic acid deficiency is responsible for this process.

b. Symmetrical lesions in the mammillary bodies are present.

c. Dermatitis is a prominent symptom.

d. Demyelination of the corpus callosum occurs in this disorder.

e. Clinical symptoms of the disorder include aphasia.

f. Paresis of the sixth cranial nerve is the first sign that responds to treatment.

g. Confabulation may be a prominent feature.

h. Diarrhea is an associated feature.

i. Left-hand anomia may be seen as the disease progresses.

j. Initial treatment consists of parenteral thiamine 100 mg/day in divided doses.

■ **DIRECTIONS: For questions 24–5 through 24–11, select the single best answer.**

24–5. What percentage of individuals with chronic alcoholism have some level of intellectual deterioration?

1. 25%

2. 50%

3. 75%

4. 100%

24–6. What differentiates substance-induced persisting amnestic disorder (SIPA) from substance-induced persisting dementia (SIPD)?

  1. Judgment is impaired.
  2. Variable language impairment is present.
  3. Impairment in memory function is dominant.
  4. The ability to perform abstract thinking is markedly impaired.

24–7. Wernicke's encephalopathy is detected in what percentage of patients at autopsy?

  1. 0.05%
  2. 0.5%
  3. 1.0%
  4. 1.5%

24–8. Treatment of amnestic disorders for patients on chronic benzodiazepine medications consists of dose reduction and possibly discontinuation of the medication. What is the maximum daily dose reduction?

  1. 5% of the initial established dosage
  2. 10% of the initial established dosage
  3. 15% of the initial established dosage
  4. 20% of the initial established dosage

24–9. What percentage of elderly patients who receive tricyclic antidepressants will experience some degree of cognitive impairment?

  1. 10%
  2. 15%
  3. 25%
  4. 35%

24–10. Which of the following diagnostic studies are generally **not** useful in diagnosing SIPA or SIPD?

  1. Magnetic resonance imaging (MRI)
  2. Urine drug screen
  3. Electroencephalogram (EEG)
  4. Cerebrospinal fluid (CSF) examination

24–11. Depression is a frequent clinical complication of dementia. The psychomotor retardation and pseudodementia associated with depression worsen the cognitive deficits of individuals with dementia. Which of the following medications may be the most efficacious in the treatment of depression in patients with dementia?

  1. Sertraline
  2. Paroxetine
  3. Fluoxetine
  4. Amitriptyline

■ DIRECTIONS: **For questions 24–12 through 24–19, indicate**

    A if answers 1, 2, and 3 are correct.

    B if answers 1 and 3 are correct.

    C if answers 2 and 4 are correct.

    D if only answer 4 is correct.

    E if all are correct.

24–12. Evidence suggests that the registration, storage, and retrieval processes of memory involve which sites in the brain?

    1. Hypothalamus-diencephalon

    2. Periaqueductal

    3. Hippocampus

    4. Sylvian fissure

24–13. At what level does lithium carbonate produce a dementia syndrome?

    1. 1.5 mmol/L

    2. 0.7 mmol/L

    3. 2.5 mmol/L

    4. 0.2 mmol/L

24–14. Chronic solvent exposure may lead to irreparable damage to which of the following systems?

    1. Renal

    2. Respiratory

    3. Bone marrow

    4. Central nervous system

24–15. Treatment of lead poisoning includes which of the following?

    1. Ethylene diaminetetraacetic acid (EDTA)

    2. Aminoglycosides

    3. Dimercaprol (BAL)

    4. Levodopa

24–16. Neurological and neuropsychological symptoms of manganese toxicity include which of the following?

    1. Depressed mood

    2. Increased muscle tone

    3. Passivity

    4. Extrapyramidal signs

24–17. Which of the following toxins may be removed by chelation therapy?

    1. Arsenic

    2. Manganese

    3. Mercury

    4. Lead

24–18. Diagnosis of arsenic poisoning can be made by sampling which of the following?

    1. Hair

    2. Blood

    3. Nails

    4. Skin

24–19. Treatment of alcohol-related cognitive deficits includes replacement therapy with which of the following?

    1. Thiamine

    2. B_{12}

    3. Folic acid

    4. Magnesium

■ ANSWERS:

24–1. Marchiafava-Bignami disease: **d, e, i**

24–2. Korsakoff's syndrome: **b, g, j**

24–3. Wernicke's encephalopathy: **b, f, j**

24–4. Pellagra: **a, c, h**

24–5. **Answer: 2.** Approximately half of individuals with chronic alcoholism have some level of intellectual deterioration.

24–6. **Answer: 3.** In SIPA, impairments are confined to memory function, with other cognitive functions, such as judgment, language, executive functioning, and abstract thinking, being spared.

24–7. **Answer: 3.** In general hospital admissions, Wernicke's encephalopathy is diagnosed in 0.05% of patients. At autopsy, 1.0% of patients are diagnosed with Wernicke's syndrome.

24–8. **Answer: 2.** The maximum daily dose reduction should be less than 10% of initial established dosage. Too rapid withdrawal may increase cognitive deficits.

24–9. **Answer: 4.** As many as 10%–15% of all patients and 35% of elderly patients who receive tricyclic antidepressants will experience some degree of cognitive impairment.

24–10. **Answer: 3.** In the diagnosis of SIPA or SIPD, computed tomography scanning or MRI is useful to rule out space-occupying lesions. Urine drug screens will detect numerous illicit substances that impair cognitive functioning. CSF examination is important if there is suspicion of an infectious etiology or an inflammatory or demyelinating disorder. An EEG is not helpful, because only nonspecific slow-wave activity is generally seen.

24–11. **Answer: 1.** The selective serotonin reuptake inhibitors are associated with fewer side effects and are as efficacious as the traditional tricyclic antidepressants. Fluoxetine markedly impairs drug metabolism at the cytochrome P450 system. Paroxetine has muscarinic effects comparable to those of imipramine, producing the potential for a similar side-effect profile. Sertraline has little tendency to impair the P450 system and virtually no muscarinic effects. Amitriptyline is strongly anticholinergic and may create cognitive deficits.

24–12. **Answer: B (1 and 3).** The hypothalamic-diencephalic and hippocampal regions are the most important sites for registration, storage, and retrieval of memory.

24–13. **Answer: A (1, 2, and 3).** Lithium carbonate may produce a dementia syndrome even with levels in the therapeutic window of 0.5–1.5 mmol/L.

24–14. **Answer: E (All).** End organ damage in the renal, bone marrow, respiratory, and central nervous systems may occur with chronic solvent exposure.

24–15. **Answer: B (1 and 3).** EDTA and BAL are chelating agents that are used to treat lead poisoning. Aminoglycosides are a class of antimicrobial agents. Levodopa is used in the treatment of Parkinson's disease.

24–16. **Answer: C (2 and 4).** Neurological symptoms of manganese toxicity include extrapyramidal signs, ataxia, dysarthria, tremor, bradykinesia, and increased muscle tone. Neuropsychological symptoms include memory impairments, irritability, poor concentration, euphoria, hallucinations, and aggressiveness.

24–17. **Answer: E (All).** Mercury poisoning is treated by chelation with penicillamine. Manganese toxicity is treated with EDTA. Arsenic poisoning is treated with BAL. Lead poisoning is treated with EDTA or BAL.

24–18. **Answer: A (1, 2, and 3).** Diagnosis of arsenic poisoning is made by identifying levels above 0.01 mg/100 mL of blood or 0.1 mg/100 g in the hair or nails.

24–19. **Answer: E (All).** An essential feature of the treatment of alcohol-related cognitive deficits includes replacement of thiamine, B_{12}, folic acid, and, if there is concern about seizure risk, magnesium.

CHAPTER 25

Amnestic Disorder Due to a General Medical Condition and Amnestic Disorder Not Otherwise Specified

■ **DIRECTIONS:** For questions 25–1 and 25–2, match each type of memory to the most appropriate description(s). Each description may be used once, more than once, or not at all.

25–1. Declarative

25–2. Nondeclarative

a. A verbal narrative description of a sporting event

b. Tying one's shoelaces

c. Seeing a notebook and recalling several other uses for notebooks, exams, and other events associated with books

d. Recitation of facts

e. Pavlov well known for this type of memory

f. Necessary for high academic achievement

■ **DIRECTIONS:** For questions 25–3 through 25–5, match the central nervous system structure affected to the medical condition or event. Each condition or event may be used once, more than once, or not at all.

25–3. Medial temporal lobe

25–4. Hypothalamus-diencephalon

25–5. Entire brain

a. Closed head trauma

b. Malnutrition

c. Herpes simplex encephalitis

d. Hypoxia

e. Hypoglycemia

f. Transient global amnesia

g. Aneurysm of anterior communicating artery

    h. Wernicke-Korsakoff syndrome
    i. Neurosarcoidosis
    j. Posterior cerebral artery occlusion
    k. Pregnancy
    l. Severe vomiting
    m. Electroconvulsive therapy (ECT)
    n. Thalamoperforant artery occlusion
    o. Subarachnoid hemorrhage
    p. Temporal lobectomy
    q. Trauma other than simple closed head injury
    r. Hypoxia

■ **DIRECTIONS: For questions 25–6 through 25–8, indicate**

    A   if answers 1, 2, and 3 are correct.
    B   if answers 1 and 3 are correct.
    C   if answers 2 and 4 are correct.
    D   if only answer 4 is correct.
    E   if all are correct.

25–6. Practice and exercise drills have been analogically likened to training a "mental muscle." What are the drawbacks of this form of treatment for amnestic disorders?

    1. The training requires a computer.
    2. The presented material usually has no practical relevance.
    3. Simple repetition is poorly tolerated by patients.
    4. This process does not generalize to other tasks or situations.

25–7. Which of the following are components of the "ancient art of memory" as invented by Simonides in 477 B.C.?

    1. The basic mnemonic strategy involves creating a series of memory "pegs."
    2. The more concrete the image to be remembered, the better the recall ability.
    3. The more ridiculous the mental image associated with the item, the more easily the subject remembers.
    4. This technique is easily taught to individuals with amnestic disorders.

25–8. The creation and use of a memory book is a complex process that has had some success in individuals with amnestic disorders. Which of the following statements regarding memory books are **true**?

    1. The acquisition stage of the memory book process is dependent on some residual declarative memory skill.
    2. Prospective memory is essential for the memory book to have any practical application.
    3. Nondeclarative memory is important in the use of a memory book.
    4. The method of vanishing clues is essential to the creation of a memory book.

■ **ANSWERS:**

25–1. Declarative (explicit): **a** (events), **d** (facts), **f**

25–2. Nondeclarative (implicit): **b** (skills and habits), **c** (priming), **e** (classical conditioning), **f**

25–3. Medial temporal lobe: **c, d, e, i, p, q**

25–4. Hypothalamus-diencephalon: **b, h, k, l, n, q**

25–5. Entire brain: **a, f, g, m, o**

25–6. **Answer: C (2 and 4).** Computers are not essential in training involving practice and exercise drills. Although well tolerated by these patients, simple repetition does not circumvent the basic defect for encoding information and an inability to learn. The presented material generally has no practical relevance. The process of practice and exercise drills does not generalize to other tasks or situations.

25–7. **Answer: A (1, 2, and 3).** The first task in the process of Simonides is to create and recall a set of memory "pegs," which represents a formidable task for individuals with amnestic disorders. In general, the more concrete the item to be recalled and the more ridiculous the associated mental image, the more the subject remembers.

25–8. **Answer: A (1, 2, and 3).** The economics of the memory-book process are not well documented. This labor-intensive process relies on residual declarative memory, prospective memory (remembering to use the book), and nondeclarative memory. The method of vanishing clues is not part of the memory-book process. The vanishing clue method relies on priming to help the patient recall events.

SECTION 4

Substance-Related Disorders

CHAPTER 26

Overview of Treatment

■ **DIRECTIONS: For questions 26–1 through 26–8, indicate**

A if answers 1, 2, and 3 are correct.

B if answers 1 and 3 are correct.

C if answers 2 and 4 are correct.

D if only answer 4 is correct.

E if all are correct.

26–1. Which of the following are patient- and client-oriented goals in the treatment of substance abuse?

1. Abstinence

2. Major shifts in character structure

3. Adjustment to the "mundane" aspects of daily living

4. Pharmacological relief of symptoms

26–2. Which of the following populations have higher rates of substance abuse than have the general population?

1. Individuals with bipolar illness

2. Individuals with schizophrenia

3. Individuals with antisocial personality disorder

4. Individuals with major depression

26–3. Which of the following issues must be addressed in a substance-abuse/dependence program?

1. The need for placement after completing the program

2. Medical complications created or worsened by the substance

3. Assistance with financial management and vocational rehabilitation

4. Spirituality

26–4. Which of the following statements concerning the use of psychotropic medications in substance-dependent individuals are **true**?

1. Generalized anxiety observed during intoxication should be aggressively treated.

    2. Methadone may be an appropriate treatment for severely impaired opiate-dependent patients.

    3. Depression should be aggressively managed with antidepressants.

    4. Patients with bipolar disorder should be treated with a mood-stabilizing agent.

26–5. Which of the following patient characteristics lead physicians astray from the appropriate diagnosis of substance abuse or dependence?

    1. Being female

    2. Having health insurance

    3. Holding a job

    4. Being widowed

26–6. Which of the following laboratory measures should be included in the evaluation and treatment of substance abuse?

    1. Complete cell count

    2. Human immunodeficiency virus (HIV) and VDRL

    3. PPD (purified protein derivative)

    4. Liver enzymes

26–7. Which of the following drugs may cause persistent or permanent memory deficits and other cognitive impairments?

    1. Alcohol

    2. Benzodiazepines

    3. Cocaine

    4. Opioids

26–8. Which of the following are signs of **early** problematic alcohol or drug use?

    1. Medical problems

    2. Impaired relationships with family

    3. Disruptions of occupational functioning

    4. Guilty feelings about the behaviors engaged in while using alcohol or drugs

◼️ ANSWERS:

26–1. **Answer: B (1 and 3).** Abstinence is accepted as the **only** clinically relevant goal for treatment programs that focus on treatment for dependence on any substance. Small pilot programs are investigating the use of teaching controlled alcohol use to individuals who do *not* meet the criteria for dependence but who express concern over their occasional heavy intake of alcohol. In general, individuals with a history of substance abuse rapidly learn that "rules for intake" can be bent, leading to an escalation in intake of the substance. Helping the individual adjust to a substance-free lifestyle is critical. This assistance includes dealing with free time that is no longer spent in pursuit of the substance, finding and maintaining substance-free friends, adjusting to the more "mundane" aspects of daily living without the roller-coaster ride of crisis-oriented substance-use style, and reestablishing rewarding relationships with family members. Obtaining major shifts in character structure is outside the scope of most substance-abuse programs and their clientele. Pharmacological interventions are not part of the overall goals of treatment in substance-abuse/dependence programs, although such interventions may be part of a withdrawal or detoxification program.

26–2. **Answer: A (1, 2, and 3).** Patients with bipolar disorder and schizophrenia constitute a minority of substance-abusing and substance-dependent individuals, but there is a higher risk for substance abuse in these populations. Individuals with antisocial personality disorder are also at greater risk for substance abuse than is the general population. Individuals with major depression are not more likely to develop a substance-abuse disorder.

26–3. **Answer: A (1, 2, and 3).** Homelessness was previously a topic that applied only to inner-city, skid-row programs. In this time of limited financial resources, the type of available aftercare must be carefully investigated as well as the risk for relapse and the need for future treatment. By the time they reach treatment, many individuals with substance use problems have serious financial situations and have lost their previous occupations. Assistance with financial management and vocational rehabilitation is critical to rehabilitation programs. Medical conditions, such as cardiovascular disease and diabetes, may be worsened by substance abuse. Other conditions, such as HIV infection or cellulitis from dirty needles, cardiomyopathy, and pancreatitis, may be created by substance use and must be carefully investigated and treated. Many treatment programs have grown out of the Alcoholics Anonymous (AA) tradition, which recognizes the importance of a "supreme being." There is a debate about whether spirituality is an essential aspect of treatment.

26–4. **Answer: C (2 and 4).** The body does not reach its optimal level of functioning in a substance-free environment for 3 to 6 months following abstinence. Generalized anxiety, insomnia, and depression seen during this time are best managed with behavioral techniques, cognitive-behavior therapy, and counseling. Medications may be used to treat the acute withdrawal states and to treat those individuals with a documented history of schizophrenia or bipolar disorder. Methadone maintenance may be required in the long-term treatment of the severely opioid-dependent individual. Disulfiram may be used with alcohol-dependent individuals.

26–5. **Answer: A (1, 2, and 3).** Patients who are female, employed, insured, married, or white are most likely to be missed in diagnosing substance abuse or dependence. Covert and overt attitudes of physicians about drug and alcohol dependence may interfere with timely diagnosis and treatment of these disorders. Among these attitudes are a reluctance to recognize the harmful effects of a patient's substance abuse because of the physician's own pattern of use, a tendency to view addictive disorders as moral shortcomings, and concerns about labeling a patient.

26–6. **Answer: E (All).** Initial evaluation for substance abuse should include a urinalysis (renal damage), creatinine/blood urea nitrogen (renal damage and nutritional status), complete cell count (blood dyscrasias), electrolytes, serology (VDRL and hepatitis antibody and antigen), testing for tuberculosis (PPD), and, after appropriate counseling, testing for HIV.

26–7. **Answer: B (1 and 3).** Alcohol and cocaine may cause permanent cognitive and memory deficits.

26–8. **Answer: D (Only 4).** Late sequelae of problematic alcohol or drug use include medical and legal problems, impaired relationships with family and co-workers, loss of nonusing friends, and disruptions in occupational functioning. Early signs include blackouts, guilt feelings about the behaviors engaged in while under the influence of the substance, accidental overdose, and behavior changes.

CHAPTER 27

∎

Alcohol and Other Depressant Drugs

∎ **DIRECTIONS: For questions 27–1 through 27–10, indicate whether the statement is true or false.**

27–1. _____ The treatment of alcohol withdrawal symptoms is independent of motivating the patient to enter rehabilitation.

27–2. _____ Inadequately treated alcohol withdrawal episodes may predispose the patient to more severe alcohol withdrawal in the future.

27–3. _____ Clonidine, an alpha-adrenergic agonist, is successful in suppressing seizures associated with alcohol withdrawal.

27–4. _____ Patients with schizophrenia and comorbid alcoholism should never receive disulfiram.

27–5. _____ Individual psychotherapy or self-help recovery is usually not necessary in the treatment of benzodiazepine addiction.

27–6. _____ For patients who abuse high doses of barbiturates, treatment is best accomplished in an inpatient setting.

27–7. _____ Protracted withdrawal syndromes of benzodiazepines and alcohol are similar.

27–8. _____ High-dose benzodiazepine withdrawal occurs for patients who have taken more than the recommended therapeutic doses for more than 1 month.

27–9. _____ The maximum starting phenobarbital dose for sedative-hypnotic withdrawal is 500 mg/day.

27–10. _____ Sustained nystagmus is the least reliable sign of phenobarbital intoxication.

∎ **DIRECTIONS: For questions 27–11 through 27–21, indicate**

A if answers 1, 2, and 3 are correct.
B if answers 1 and 3 are correct.
C if answers 2 and 4 are correct.
D if only answer 4 is correct.
E if all are correct.

■ **For questions 27–11 through 27–18, use the following case material:**

Mr. K. is a 38-year-old with a long-standing history of alcohol abuse. He presents for alcohol detoxification and treatment. He has a past history of alcohol withdrawal seizures and multiple attempts at treatment. Admission laboratory reveals the following information: serum glutamic-oxaloacetic transaminase (SGOT) 350 IU/L (range 5–40 IU/L), serum glutamic-pyruvic transaminase (SGPT) 325 IU/L (range 7–53 IU/L), lactate dehydrogenase (LDH) 250 IU/L (range 90–250 IU/L), hematocrit 35% (range 40.7%–50.3%), hemoglobin 10.2 g/dL (range 13.8–17.2 g/dL), mean corpuscular volume 120 mm^3 (range 80.0–97.6 mm^3), mean corpuscular volume 37.1 pg/cell (range 26.7–33.7 pg/cell), platelet count 124 mm^3 (range 190–405 mm^3), sodium 134 mmol/L (range 135–145 mmol/L), potassium 3.0 mmol/L (range 3.3–4.9 mmol/L), magnesium 0.9 mEq/L (range 1.3–2.1 mEq/L), chloride 99 mmol/L (range 97–110 mmol/L), and glucose 45 mg/dL (range 65–11 mg/dL).

27–11. What other history would you want to obtain from Mr. K.?

    1. Age at onset of his alcohol consumption

    2. Time of his last ingestion of alcohol

    3. Family history of alcohol use

    4. Amount of alcohol consumed per day

27–12. Which of the following benzodiazepines would be the most appropriate for alcohol detoxification for Mr. K.?

    1. Oxazepam

    2. Diazepam

    3. Lorazepam

    4. Chlordiazepoxide

27–13. Mr. K. has severe emesis and is unable to tolerate oral medication. Which of the following medications may be used intramuscularly for alcohol detoxification?

    1. Diazepam

    2. Clonidine hydrochloride

    3. Chlordiazepoxide

    4. Lorazepam

27–14. You have learned that Mr. K. is also abusing benzodiazepines. Which of the following medications are indicated for management of his withdrawal symptoms?

    1. Phenytoin

    2. Diazepam

    3. Phenobarbital

    4. Carbamazepine

27–15. Mr. K. would like to be placed on disulfiram. Which of the following statements concerning disulfiram are **true**?

1. Disulfiram will worsen Mr. K.'s hepatic damage.
2. Peripheral nerve damage is quite rare and usually associated with dosages of more than 250 mg/day.
3. There are no studies documenting the efficacy of disulfiram.
4. Liver function tests should be routinely checked for patients receiving disulfiram.

27–16. Mr. K. complains of early and late insomnia, extreme dysphoria, and a loss of interest in all activities. He has a childhood history of separation anxiety disorder. He has been in an inpatient alcohol treatment program for 45 days. Which medications, if any, may be effective for treating his insomnia and affective symptoms?

1. Doxepin
2. Fluoxetine
3. Trazodone
4. Sertraline

27–17. What dietary supplements are indicated for Mr. K.?

1. Folic acid
2. Thiamine
3. Magnesium
4. No dietary supplements

27–18. On endoscopy, Mr. K. is found to have several large esophageal varices. Which medications are recommended?

1. Clonidine hydrochloride
2. Propylthiouracil
3. Naltrexone
4. Propranolol

27–19. Which of the following are **not** signs and symptoms of sedative-hypnotic withdrawal?

1. Carbohydrate craving
2. Anxiety
3. Gooseflesh
4. Seizures

27–20. Which of the following are treatment strategies for high-dose benzodiazepine withdrawal?

1. Phenobarbital is substituted and tapered.
2. Decreasing doses of the agent of dependence are used.
3. Chlordiazepoxide is substituted and tapered.
4. The agent of addiction is abruptly discontinued.

27–21. If sustained nystagmus, slurred speech, and ataxia are present in a patient who is receiving phenobarbital for treatment of sedative-hypnotic withdrawal, what should be done?

    1. The next two doses of phenobarbital should be withheld.

    2. The next dose of phenobarbital should be withheld.

    3. The daily dosage of phenobarbital should be halved after the medication is reinitiated.

    4. The daily dosage of phenobarbital should remain the same after the medication is reinitiated.

■ ANSWERS:

27–1. **False** A positive correlation exists between treatment of withdrawal symptoms and motivation to enter rehabilitation.

27–2. **True** There is an increased risk for more severe alcohol withdrawal symptoms if previous episodes were inadequately treated.

27–3. **False** Clonidine does *not* suppress seizures.

27–4. **False** Some patients with both schizophrenia and alcoholism may be treated with disulfiram; however, careful monitoring is required for those patients on neuroleptics.

27–5. **False** Individuals addicted to benzodiazepines will benefit from both individual treatment and self-help groups.

27–6. **True** The morbidity and mortality, as well as the technical difficulty, associated with high-dose barbiturate withdrawal require an inpatient setting.

27–7. **False** Protracted withdrawal symptoms for benzodiazepines are more severe compared with those for alcohol.

27–8. **True** More than 1 month of benzodiazepine use above the recommended dose level may precipitate high-dose withdrawal.

27–9. **True** The maximum starting dose of phenobarbital is 500 mg/day.

27–10. **False** Sustained nystagmus is among the most reliable signs of phenobarbital intoxication.

27–11. **Answer: E (All).** To successfully detoxify a patient and to recommend appropriate treatment, one must obtain a careful history of drinking patterns, including time of last alcohol ingestion, age at which the patient started drinking, the style of the patient's drinking (Do they drink alone? after work with friends? only on the weekends? etc.), and the amount of alcohol consumed in a given amount of time. Alcoholism has a strong familial component, and determining the family history of drinking patterns is critical to make an appropriate choice in treatment.

27–12. **Answer: B (1 and 3).** Oxazepam and lorazepam do not undergo hepatic oxidation and therefore are less affected by hepatic dysfunction. Mr. K. has moderately elevated liver function tests; thus, oxazepam or lorazepam would be the most appropriate benzodiazepine for alcohol detoxification.

27–13. **Answer: D (Only 4).** Diazepam and chlordiazepoxide are poorly and erratically absorbed when they are administered intramuscularly. Lorazepam is evenly absorbed via an intramuscular route. Clonidine hydrochloride is not available in an intramuscular form.

27–14. **Answer: D (Only 4).** The use of phenytoin has not been well established for the management of alcohol withdrawal seizures. Diazepam is not the best choice in this patient because of the significant hepatic insufficiency. Phenobarbital is not indicated. Carbamazepine is effective for the management of combined alcohol-benzodiazepine withdrawal.

27–15. **Answer: C (2 and 4).** There are numerous studies documenting the efficacy of disulfiram therapy, especially if this approach is combined with supportive therapies and supervision of the medication. There are documented reports of disulfiram hepatitis—25 in the world literature. Patients who receive disulfiram should have regular monitoring of liver functions. Disulfiram in doses of 250 mg/day or less is not associated with increased liver damage. Peripheral nerve damage is quite rare and is usually observed when doses of more than 250 mg/day are used.

27–16. **Answer: B (1 and 3).** Affective disorders and alcoholism may start at the same age, and it is often difficult to discern if the excessive use of alcohol created the depression or if the patient is self-medicating a depression. If the affective symptoms continue beyond 1 to 2 months despite psychotherapeutic interventions, then pharmacotherapeutic intervention for depression may be indicated. If the patient has a history of major depression preceding the onset of alcoholism, or if the affective disorder occurs during periods of sustained abstinence, then specific treatment for depression is indicated. Other indications for a diagnosis of major depression or bipolar disorder are 1) history of separation anxiety disorder, 2) hypomanic or manic reaction to antidepressant medication, 3) family history of bipolar disorder, 4) multigenerational family history of major depression, or 5) a positive dexamethasone suppression test. The selective serotonin reuptake inhibitors, such as fluoxetine and sertraline, are effective in the treatment of depression. They tend to be activating and, as such, may not be the medications of choice for the treatment of insomnia and depressive symptoms. Doxepin and trazodone are relatively more serotonergic compared with other traditional antidepressants and are highly sedating.

27–17. **Answer: A (1, 2, and 3).** Mr. K. has mild megaloblastic anemia. This type of anemia is associated with vitamin B_{12} and/or folic acid deficiency, and both of these deficiencies are associated with alcoholism. Thiamine deficiency is frequently associated with alcoholism and, clinically, manifests as amblyopia and peripheral neuropathy. Depletion in magnesium is seen in alcoholic individuals. Mr. K. has a mildly decreased magnesium level. Low magnesium and sodium levels are both associated with seizures.

27–18. **Answer: C (2 and 4).** Both clonidine hydrochloride and naltrexone are efficacious in the treatment of alcohol withdrawal symptoms, except for seizures. Neither medication is indicated for the treatment of esophageal varices. Propranolol has been shown to reduce variceal bleeding deaths and overall fatality. Similarly, propylthiouracil has been shown to decrease the mortality associated with variceal bleeding in those patients who remained abstinent.

27–19. **Answer: B (1 and 3).** Signs and symptoms of sedative-hypnotic withdrawal include anxiety, tremors, seizures, delirium, nausea, anorexia, emesis, postural hypotension, hyperpyrexia, insomnia, and nightmares. Carbohydrate craving is seen with cannabis intoxication. Gooseflesh is commonly seen with heroin withdrawal.

27–20. **Answer: A (1, 2, and 3).** There are three methods for the treatment of high-dose benzodiazepine withdrawal. Phenobarbital is a long-acting and relatively safe medication that is cross-tolerant with benzodiazepines. This medication may be substituted and then gradually tapered. Chlordiazepoxide is a long-acting benzodiazepine that may be substituted for shorter-acting ones and then gradually tapered. Finally, a slow taper of the agent of abuse may be employed. The one strategy that may be lethal is the abrupt discontinuation of the benzodiazepine.

27–21. **Answer: B (1 and 3).** Before receiving each dose of phenobarbital, the patient should be checked for signs of phenobarbital intoxication: sustained nystagmus, slurred speech, and ataxia. If all three signs are present, the next two doses should be withheld and withdrawal should be reinitiated at half the dose of phenobarbital. If only nystagmus is present, the next dose should be withheld and withdrawal should then be restarted at the same dose of phenobarbital.

CHAPTER 28

The Hallucinogens and Cannabis

■ **DIRECTIONS: For questions 28–1 through 28–5, select the single best response.**

28–1. Which of the following drugs have no abstinence syndrome after repeated use?

1. Alcohol
2. Benzodiazepines
3. Opioids
4. Psilocybin

28–2. The emotional responses to the hallucinogens can vary. What is the most frequent initial response?

1. Euphoria
2. Depression
3. Intense anxiety
4. Rage

28–3. Lysergic acid diethylamide (LSD) is absorbed rapidly in the gastrointestinal tract and diffuses rapidly to all tissues **except**

1. Brain.
2. Placenta.
3. Liver.
4. None of the above.

28–4. What may be lasting effects after the use of LSD?

1. Memory deficits
2. Cognitive impairments
3. Personality changes
4. Anxiety disorders

28–5. What is the treatment of choice for chronic hallucinogen abuse not associated with a schizophreniform reaction?

1. Neuroleptics to guard against the possibility of psychosis
2. Group-home setting

3. Anxiolytics to ameliorate the effects of flashbacks
4. Long-term psychotherapy

◼ **DIRECTIONS: For questions 28–6 through 28–10, indicate**

A if answers 1, 2, and 3 are correct.
B if answers 1 and 3 are correct.
C if answers 2 and 4 are correct.
D if only answer 4 is correct.
E if all are correct.

28–6. Which of the following are physical signs of chronic cannabis use?

1. A normal physical examination
2. Conjunctival vascular injection
3. Swollen uvula
4. Chronic bronchitis

28–7. Phencyclidine (PCP) psychosis may be differentiated from other psychoto-mimetic reactions and other psychotic states by which of the following?

1. Auditory hallucinations
2. Vertical nystagmus
3. Synesthesia
4. Ataxia

28–8. Which of the following are **true** statements regarding the early recovery period in the treatment of cannabis dependence?

1. The recovery period may last 2 to 12 months.
2. The patient must avoid situations that are associated with drug use.
3. The patient must learn to identify internal feeling states.
4. Anxiolytics may be used.

28–9. What are the criteria for inpatient treatment of cannabis abuse?

1. Failure to respond to outpatient treatment
2. Presence of psychosis
3. Absence of adequate psychosocial supports
4. The need to make a point to the adolescent patient

28–10. Which of the following statements regarding flashbacks are **false**?

1. If no flashbacks have occurred after 1 to 2 years of abstinence, then it is unlikely that the person will have flashbacks.
2. A "good trip" or experience confers immunity from a "bad" flashback.
3. Flashbacks may be precipitated by stress or by ingestion of another psyche-delic drug.
4. Cannabis abuse is not associated with flashbacks.

◼ **DIRECTIONS: For questions 28–11 through 28–15, match the drug to the appropriate descriptive phrase(s). Each descriptive phrase may be used once, more than once, or not at all.**

28–11.	Psilocybin	a.	Dilated pupils
28–12.	Methylenedioxy-methamphetamine (MDMA)	b.	Hemiplegia
28–13.	Lysergic acid diethylamide (LSD)	c.	Sore jaw muscles
28–14.	Cannabis	d.	No abstinence syndrome
28–15.	Dimethyltrypta-mine (DMT)	e.	Magic mushrooms
		f.	Businessman's LSD
		g.	Panic attacks
		h.	Depersonalization
		i.	Amotivational syndrome
		j.	Delirium

◼ **ANSWERS:**

28–1. **Answer: 4.** The hallucinogens, such as psilocybin, have no abstinence syndrome; therefore, no detoxification is required for the chronic effects of the hallucinogens.

28–2. **Answer: 1.** Elation or euphoria is the most frequent initial response to a hallucinogen. The affective state is quite labile, and an inappropriate emotional response may be elicited either by an internal or by an external cue. Initial mild anxiety may also occur.

28–3. **Answer: 4.** LSD diffuses to *all* tissues.

28–4. **Answer: 3.** Personality changes may occur after a single use of LSD or, perhaps, PCP. Repeated use of other hallucinogens may lead to personality changes. Schizophreniform reactions lasting from weeks to years have followed the use of hallucinogens. The management of these psychotic reactions does not differ from that of schizophrenia. Memory deficits and other cognitive impairments are not associated with hallucinogen use. Anxiety disorders also are not associated with hallucinogen use.

28–5. **Answer: 4.** The treatment of chronic hallucinogen abuse usually involves long-term psychotherapy to determine what needs are being fulfilled by the long-term use of the drug. Neuroleptics are not indicated when psychosis is absent. Anxiolytics are not indicated for flashbacks. Indeed, anxiolytics may only worsen the effects of a flashback and fuel secondary drug dependence. Treatment of flashbacks is reassurance that the condition will pass and that the brain is not damaged. Group-home settings are not necessarily indicated.

28-6. **Answer: E (All).** The physical examination in chronic cannabis use may be completely unremarkable. Conjunctival vascular injection, a swollen uvula, or chronic bronchitis may be present.

28-7. **Answer: B (2 and 4).** Auditory hallucinations are relatively rare in psychotomimetic-induced reactions. Hyperacusis is common. Synesthesia involves the overflow from one sensory system to another (e.g., colors are heard and sounds are seen). Synesthesia has been described in PCP and LSD perceptual alterations. Vertical nystagmus, ataxia, and autonomic dysregulation are the differentiating features of PCP psychosis.

28-8. **Answer: A (1, 2, and 3).** The recovery period of treatment may last 2 to 12 months. During the early recovery phase, avoidance of environmental cues (i.e., people, places, and things) associated with drug use is important. Insulating "slips" so that they do not become full-blown relapses, learning new methods to cope, and identifying internal feeling states are critical features of treatment. The use of psychotropic medications is not usually a part of the early phase of treatment unless there is a preexisting psychiatric condition.

28-9. **Answer: A (1, 2, and 3).** The criteria for inpatient treatment of cannabis abuse include 1) failure to respond to outpatient treatment, 2) severe depression or psychosis, 3) the absence of adequate psychosocial supports that may be mobilized to facilitate the cessation of drug use, 4) the necessity to interrupt a living situation that reinforces drug use, and 5) the need to enhance motivation. Intermittent or experimental marijuana use is normative for an adolescent peer group, and if there is no impact on the adolescent's psychosocial adjustment, then coercing him or her into treatment may serve only to disrupt his or her development.

28-10. **Answer: B (2 and 4).** Flashbacks are apparently spontaneous recrudescences of the same drug effects that were experienced during the psychotomimetic state. Flashbacks are usually brief visual, temporal, or emotional recurrences. They usually are treated with reassurance. LSD, PCP, cannabis, and other hallucinogens are all associated with flashbacks. There is no immunity conferred by having "good trips." Generally, flashbacks decrease in intensity and frequency over time. Emotional stress and the ingestion of hallucinogens may precipitate the occurrence of flashbacks.

28-11. Psilocybin: **a, d, e** (street name), **h, j**

28-12. MDMA: **a, d, h, j**

28-13. LSD: **a, b** (due to vasospasm), **d, h, j**

28-14. Cannabis: **i, j**

28-15. DMT: **d, f** (because of its rapid onset and its 1- to 2-hour duration of action, it must be injected, sniffed, or smoked), **h, j**

CHAPTER 29

Stimulants and Related Drugs

■ DIRECTIONS: **For questions 29–1 through 29–5, match each drug to the appropriate statement(s). Each statement may be used once, more than once, or not at all.**

29–1. Methamphet-
amine

29–2. Cocaine

29–3. Crack

29–4. Phencyclidine
(PCP)

29–5. Tobacco

a. This drug has centrally mediated effects on mood.

b. Ataxia may occur.

c. There is a clear sensorium during the period of intoxication.

d. There has been very little street activity for 20 years.

e. There is no intoxication syndrome.

f. Interpersonal communication is facilitated by this drug.

g. Black males constitute the largest number of those addicted.

h. There are 2.5 million addicted individuals.

i. A higher dosage of neuroleptics is required to ameliorate psychotic symptoms.

j. There are serotonergic effects.

k. Dissociative psychotic reactions may occur in response to ingestion of this drug.

l. A "patch" is available to treat withdrawal symptoms.

m. Hypertension is a documented side effect.

n. This drug is a cataleptoid anesthetic.

o. This drug activates mesolimbic and mesocortical pathways.

p. This drug has anxiolytic effects.

q. Nystagmus results from ingestion.

r. "Talk down" techniques are a form of treatment.

s. Acute renal failure is a potential side effect.

t. "Crank" is the street name.

u. Average weight gain during withdrawal is 2–3 kg.

v. Psychosis with a clouded sensorium is not unusual after ingestion.

w. This is a glamour drug that fulfills narcissistic needs.

x. Treatment may include hypothermic blankets.

y. Antidepressants may be helpful in treating symptoms of withdrawal from this agent, although antidepressants have not been approved by the Food and Drug Administration for such use.

z. Barbiturates are used for intoxication symptoms.

■ **DIRECTIONS: For questions 29–6 through 29–11, select the single best answer.**

29–6. Which of the following statements is **true** regarding inpatient versus outpatient treatment for stimulant abuse?

1. Inpatient treatment is never indicated.

2. Inpatient treatment is more successful than outpatient treatment.

3. Inpatient treatment allows patients to "practice" controlling their drug craving.

4. Inpatient treatment is indicated for neurovegetative depression.

29–7. When do the signs and symptoms of nicotine withdrawal begin?

1. 12 hours after the last intake

2. 24 hours after the last intake

3. Onset depends on the amount of nicotine in each cigarette

4. 72 hours after the last intake

29–8. What method of drug ingestion is **not** usually used to administer PCP?

1. Intramuscular

2. Intravenous

3. Oral

4. Insufflation

29–9. When smoking is being addressed in a patient with severe alcoholism, when should a smoking cessation program begin?

1. Never. Once an individual manages to become abstinent from alcohol, the smoking issue is irrelevant.

2. Immediately. Smoking represents such a health threat that it must be addressed along with the alcoholism.

3. After 6 to 12 months of abstinence.

4. After more than 12 months of abstinence.

29–10. Which of the following statements is **true** regarding stimulant intoxication?

    1. Medical emergencies are common.

    2. Hallucinations are common.

    3. No treatment may be required.

    4. Bipolar mania can be consistently distinguished from intoxication.

29–11. Which of the following statements is **true** regarding treatment of patients who smoke and also have psychiatric disorders?

    1. Smoking may decrease the dosage required of neuroleptics.

    2. Smoking does not affect drug-related movement disorders.

    3. Patients who are depressed are less likely to smoke.

    4. None of the above.

■ **DIRECTIONS: For questions 29–12 through 29–16, indicate**

    A if answers 1, 2, and 3 are correct.

    B if answers 1 and 3 are correct.

    C if answers 2 and 4 are correct.

    D if only answer 4 is correct.

    E if all of the above are correct.

29–12. Which of the following types of therapy are generally used to treat individuals with cocaine addiction?

    1. Supportive therapy

    2. Pharmacotherapy

    3. Behavior therapy

    4. Psychodynamic therapy

29–13. Nicotine replacement therapy includes nicotine-containing gum and the transdermal patch. Both have proven efficacy in aiding cessation of smoking. Which of the following statements apply to nicotine replacement therapy?

    1. The gum may be chewed too vigorously.

    2. Both the gum and the patch must be continued for 3 to 6 months.

    3. The recommended number of pieces of gum is half that of the number of cigarettes.

    4. Nicotine replacement therapy offers a complete cure for smoking.

29–14. Behavior therapy helps the individual who abuses stimulants understand the deleterious effects of these drugs. Contingency contracting has two basic elements: 1) agreement to participate in urine drug screen monitoring and 2) agreement to accept an aversive consequence for failure to give a urine sample or for showing a positive sample. Which of the following statements are **true** regarding this technique?

    1. 80% of individuals who abuse cocaine are cocaine abstinent during the contract.

    2. This program has excellent follow-through when the program is discontinued.

   3. Contingencies are derived from the patient's beliefs and expectations.

   4. 75% of individuals who abuse cocaine agree to this type of intervention.

29–15. PCP delirium is one of the most common causes of emergency room admissions for drug-induced psychosis. Treatment approaches include which of the following?

   1. Admission to a closed psychiatric unit

   2. Administration of furosemide

   3. Use of neuroleptics

   4. Avoidance of benzodiazepines

29–16. Which of the following statements are **true** regarding acidification of the urine for PCP-toxigenic–induced coma or delirium?

   1. Ascorbic acid should be given, 2 g in 500 cc every 6 hours intravenously or 1 g orally four times a day.

   2. Acidification is contraindicated if hepatic or renal insufficiency is present.

   3. Ammonium chloride 2.75 mEq/kg should be given in 60 cc normal saline every 6 hours intravenously or 500 mg/5 cc given in 10-cc increments orally four times a day.

   4. Urine pH and serum electrolytes should be monitored daily.

■ ANSWERS:

29–1. Methamphetamine: **a, c, f, j, m, o, r, z**

29–2. Cocaine: **c, m, w, y**

29–3. Crack: **h, m, t, y**

29–4. Phencyclidine: **b, d, g, k, m, n, q, s, v, x**

29–5. Tobacco: **e, i, l, m, p, u**

29–6. **Answer: 4.** Inpatient treatment is indicated for severe neurovegetative depression or psychotic symptoms lasting beyond the 1 to 3 days of the postcocaine crash or in cases of outpatient treatment failure. Outpatient treatment alone, compared with inpatient treatment alone, is more successful. Hospital environments are devoid of social and environmental cues that may initiate craving and, thus, do not fully allow patients to control their drug craving.

29–7. **Answer: 2.** Signs and symptoms of nicotine withdrawal begin within 24 hours of cessation or significant reduction in the amount of nicotine used. The syndrome increases over 3 to 4 days, with a gradual decrease over 1 to 3 weeks.

29–8. **Answer: 1.** PCP may be injected intravenously, taken orally, taken by insufflation (i.e., snorting), or smoked. Intramuscular injection of any street drug is relatively rare.

29–9. **Answer: 3.** The incidence of smoking is 85% to 90% in studies of alcoholic patients. The majority of these patients smoke to such an extent that the smoking poses a serious threat to their health. Data indicate that fears of jeopardizing abstinence are groundless, and some studies indicate that smoking cessation is associated with a decreased relapse rate. Empirical data are relatively sparse as to when to initiate smoking cessation programs. Such programs are commonly begun after 6 to 12 months of abstinence.

29–10. **Answer: 3.** Stimulant intoxication is characterized by heightened interest in the environment, feelings of increased competence and self-esteem, and a clear sensorium without hallucinations. Medical emergencies are relatively rare. Stimulant intoxication may be indistinguishable from hypomania or frank mania. If stimulant activation persists longer than 24 hours in a stimulant-free environment, then mania is possibly present. Uncomplicated stimulant intoxication requires no treatment.

29–11. **Answer: 4.** There is a much higher prevalence of smoking in psychiatric populations. Patients who are depressed are more likely to smoke and less likely to quit. Minor tranquilizer and imipramine metabolism, as well as neuroleptic bioavailability, may be affected by nicotine. The effect may be so pronounced with neuroleptics that an increase in the dosage may be required. This is especially important to realize as many inpatient units where the medication may be initiated and/or titrated frequently ban smoking. After discharge, the patient may then resume smoking, and a dosage adjustment may be necessary. Smoking may also affect drug-related movement disorders.

29–12. **Answer: E (All).** The immediate treatment goal for stimulant addiction is breaking the cycle of recurrent stimulant binges. Supportive, behavior, and psychodynamic therapies are efficacious in the treatment of individuals with cocaine addiction. These approaches may be used sequentially or in combination with each other. Behavior therapy with contingency contracting is successful in 80% of patients while they are actively engaged in the contractual arrangement. Supportive therapy that assists in eliminating paraphernalia and drug caches, developing relationships that are drug free, and reintegrating with appropriate family members and counseling and educating family members are all useful elements in treatment. Obtaining regular random urine drug screens is also a supportive/behavioral technique that helps maintain sobriety. Psychodynamic therapy best addresses the underlying intrapsychic issues involved in substance abuse, including narcissistic gratification associated with cocaine as a glamour drug and stimulant compensation for interpersonal or professional failures. Although no long-term pharmacotherapy confers enduring immunity to stimulant abuse, administration of antidepressants for 6 to 8 weeks on an outpatient basis has been found to facilitate initiation and/or engagement of abstinence in cocaine-abusing individuals.

29–13. **Answer: A (1, 2, and 3).** There are several problems associated with the gum system of nicotine replacement therapy: chewing the gum too vigorously rather than "parking" it between the cheek and gum, which results in poor nicotine absorption and mucosal irritation, and chewing too few pieces (number of pieces equals one-half the number of cigarettes smoked). The transdermal system offers the advantages of no oral or gastrointestinal symptoms. Both systems should be continued for 3 to 6 months, and neither system offers a cure for smoking. The nicotine replacement systems allow smokers to decrease nicotine withdrawal symptoms while they learn to be nonsmokers.

29–14. **Answer: B (1 and 3).** Approximately half of an outpatient sample are willing to participate in a behavioral treatment program. This type of program is dependent upon creating aversive consequences that are based upon the patient's own statements concerning what he or she expects to result from continued substance use. During the duration of the contract, 80% of the participants are abstinent. This type of therapy is effective only as long as the contract is in effect.

29–15. **Answer: A (1, 2, and 3).** Treatment of PCP-induced delirium includes prevention of injury, facilitation of the excretion of PCP from urine, and amelioration of the psychosis. Patients should be admitted to a closed psychiatric unit. Physical restraints should be avoided because the patient will continuously struggle against the restraints, causing rhabdomyolysis and creating a risk of renal failure. The patient should be hydrated and the urine acidified to pH 5.5 or less. Patients with a delirium may take oral furosemide to enhance diuresis of the PCP once the urine is acidified. The use of benzodiazepines to treat the severe agitation and the use of neuroleptics to treat the psychotic symptoms are both warranted.

29–16. **Answer: A (1, 2, and 3).** To promote excretion of PCP, the urine must be acidified, the patient well hydrated, and diuresis enhanced by the use of intravenous or oral furosemide. Acidification of the urine is contraindicated in the presence of hepatic or renal insufficiency. The urine pH should be monitored two to four times a day. Electrolytes should be examined daily. The use of loop diuretics, such as furosemide, may necessitate adding oral potassium supplement to the treatment regimen. The urine may be acidified using cranberry juice 8 to 16 oz four times a day, or ascorbic acid 2 g in 500 cc every 6 hours intravenously or 1 g orally four times a day or ammonium chloride 2.75 mEq/kg in 60 cc normal saline every 6 hours intravenously or 500 mg/5 cc given in 10-cc increments orally 4 times a day. As a general rule, if the patient is able to take oral fluids and acidification agents, then oral administration is preferred over intravenous administration.

CHAPTER 30

Pharmacological Treatments for Narcotic and Opioid Addictions

DIRECTIONS: For questions 30–1 through 30–16, indicate

    A if answers 1, 2, and 3 are correct.

    B if answers 1 and 3 are correct.

    C if answers 2 and 4 are correct.

    D if only answer 4 is correct.

    E if all are correct.

30–1. Which of the following populations are particularly amenable to naltrexone therapy for treatment of opioid addiction?

    1. Individuals with a history of recent employment and a good educational background

    2. Parolees in an early work-release program

    3. Physicians

    4. Individuals addicted to street heroin

30–2. Which of the following statements are **true** regarding methadone?

    1. Methadone reduces use of nonprescribed opioids in heroin-abusing individuals.

    2. Methadone improves self-esteem in heroin-abusing individuals.

    3. Methadone suppresses narcotic withdrawal and craving for 24 to 36 hours.

    4. Methadone, even in doses prescribed by maintenance programs, produces an intoxication.

30–3. Federal and state eligibility for prescribing methadone include which of the following criteria?

    1. Methadone may be prescribed only by a licensed physician who holds a current Drug Enforcement Agency registration.

    2. Special requirements are necessary to prescribe methadone as an analgesic.

    3. Methadone used for the treatment of opioid dependence may be prescribed only by a physician working in a treatment facility licensed by the state.

    4. Special requirements must be met if methadone is used for a methadone maintenance program.

30–4. Which of the following statements are **false** regarding detoxification from opioids in preparation for treatment with an opioid antagonist?

   1. Detoxification should take place on an outpatient basis.

   2. Detoxification with clonidine may have the patient ready for opioid antagonist therapy in less than 48 hours.

   3. Detoxification using methadone should be done gradually over 2 to 3 weeks.

   4. A test dose of naloxone 0.4 mg to 1.4 mg subcutaneously or intramuscularly should be given before initiating therapy.

30–5. Which of the following patients would meet the criteria for entrance into a methadone maintenance program?

   1. A 16-year-old adolescent who has had one attempt at drug detoxification but whose parents do not wish to sign consent documents stating that "if he is old enough to use the stuff, then he can decide on his treatment"

   2. A 26-year-old pregnant woman who has been physiologically dependent for 3 months

   3. A 34-year-old man who had been successfully detoxified in a methadone program and was maintained for 2 years and who returns 3 years after leaving treatment and does not meet the criteria for physiological dependence

   4. A 19-year-old man who has track marks, a 1-year history of opioid dependence, and no current physiological dependence and is incarcerated

30–6. Which of the following medications speed the biotransformation of methadone?

   1. Rifampin

   2. Phenobarbital

   3. Imipramine

   4. Pentazocine

30–7. Under which of the following conditions would the initial dose of methadone be 10 mg–20 mg?

   1. The patient has dilated pupils (miosis), rhinorrhea, and tearing.

   2. The patient has pupillary constriction and dry mouth.

   3. The patient has used heroin more than once a day for the past 3 weeks.

   4. The patient has used heroin once a day for the past 3 weeks.

30–8. Which of the following statements characterize naloxone?

   1. It is well absorbed from the gastrointestinal tract.

   2. An active metabolite, 6-β-naltrexol, has a plasma half-life of 12 hours.

   3. Pharmacological duration is longer than that predicted by plasma kinetics.

   4. It is useful to treat opioid overdose.

30–9. Which of the following statements are **true** regarding methadone use and opioid-dependent populations with psychiatric disorders?

   1. Methadone may worsen a comorbid major depressive disorder.

   2. Generalized anxiety disorder may be found more frequently in opioid-addicted individuals than in the general population.

3. Methadone may worsen psychotic symptoms.

4. Antisocial personality disorder is found more frequently in opioid-addicted individuals than in the general population.

30–10. Which of the following characterize relapse prevention programs involving naltrexone?

1. Psychotherapy programs should be initiated early in treatment.

2. Doses of 100 mg, 100 mg, and 150 mg are given on Monday, Wednesday, and Friday, respectively.

3. Random urine drug screens are an important part of treatment.

4. Some individuals may deactivate their naltrexone by placing the tablets in a microwave oven.

30–11. Which of the following statements are **true** regarding the effects of naltrexone on blood chemistry and the monitoring required?

1. There is a surge in luteinizing hormone (LH).

2. Liver function tests should be measured at baseline and monthly for the first 3 months.

3. Transaminase levels should be less than two times normal before initiating therapy.

4. Elevation in transaminase levels is routinely observed.

30–12. Which of the following are considered priorities in methadone maintenance programs?

1. Maintaining as low a daily dose as possible

2. Having patients understand that they must withdraw from the program in 2 years

3. Satisfying drug hunger or craving

4. Stopping illegal activity

▪ **DIRECTIONS: For questions 30–13 through 30–16, use the following case vignette:**

J.K. is an 18-year-old male who dropped out of school in the sixth grade and has a long history of petty theft and assault and battery. He has a history of substance abuse, but he refuses to discuss which drugs. Twelve hours after being arrested by the police, he is brought to the emergency room with nausea, vomiting, and abdominal cramps.

30–13. Physical examination of an opioid-addicted patient experiencing withdrawal would reveal which of the following?

1. Tachycardia

2. Needle tracks

3. Hypertension

4. Dry mouth

30–14. Which of the following could be positive laboratory findings for this patient?

   1. Tuberculin skin test

   2. HIV

   3. Hepatitis screen

   4. Abnormal white cell count

30–15. J.K. has a seizure 28 hours after he is taken into custody. Which of the following are possible?

   1. The seizure may be caused by alcohol withdrawal.

   2. The patient may have epilepsy.

   3. The patient may have a head injury.

   4. The seizure may be related to opioid withdrawal.

30–16. The decision was made to use clonidine for this patient's withdrawal. Which of the following statements are valid regarding the use of clonidine for opioid withdrawal?

   1. Clonidine should be given every 4 hours for the first 4 days.

   2. Clonidine is not approved by the Food and Drug Administration (FDA) for opioid withdrawal.

   3. An electrocardiogram should be obtained before treatment is initiated.

   4. Clonidine reduces the autonomic components of opioid withdrawal.

■ ANSWERS:

30–1.   **Answer: A (1, 2, and 3).** Only 10%–15% of all opioid-addicted individuals are interested in any medication that can "keep them from getting high." This type of treatment is most appealing to opioid-dependent health care professionals, opioid-dependent middle-class individuals, and formerly addicted individuals given an early parole from prison. Methadone requires much less motivation because treatment involves only a relatively small gradual shift from daily use of heroin to daily use of another opioid agonist, methadone.

30–2.   **Answer: B (1 and 3).** Methadone does not improve self-esteem, affect psychopathology, or affect any of the multitude of social problems that frequently accompany opioid dependence. If methadone is used in prescribed doses, it is not intoxicating or sedating. Methadone suppresses narcotic withdrawal and craving for 24 to 36 hours and reduces the use of nonprescribed opioids in heroin-abusing individuals.

30–3.   **Answer: B (1 and 3).** Methadone may be prescribed as an analgesic by any licensed physician who holds a current Drug Enforcement Agency registration. By federal mandate, each state must designate a single agency that licenses and coordinates drug treatment and prevention programs, including methadone maintenance. The use of methadone for the treatment of narcotic dependence for 90 days falls under the direction of methadone maintenance. To prescribe methadone for maintenance treatment, the physician must be employed by the state-directed treatment facility.

30–4.　**Answer: B (1 and 3).** Detoxification from opioids in preparation for treatment with an opioid antagonist should be carried out in an inpatient setting where access to opioids is better controlled and where complete psychological assessment of the individual and evaluation of the patient's environment can be conducted. A highly motivated patient who has been using short-acting opioids can be detoxified with clonidine and ready for antagonist therapy in 48 hours. Detoxification from methadone takes 5 to 10 days. A test dose of naloxone 0.4 mg to 1.4 mg subcutaneously or intramuscularly is given to determine the extent of continued physical dependence on opioids. An oral dose of naloxone (12.5 mg to 25 mg) may be given; however, the drawback of this approach is that even mild withdrawal symptoms will persist for several hours.

30–5.　**Answer: C (2 and 4).** In general, criteria include a 1-year history of physiological dependence on opioids and current physiological dependence as demonstrated by positive urine drug screens for opioids, needle tracks, and signs and symptoms of opioid withdrawal. Individuals in the penal system who previously met the criteria for methadone maintenance programs may be admitted without current physiological dependence. Pregnant patients can be placed on methadone maintenance if they are currently physiologically dependent on opioids or if they were dependent in the past and there is a threat of returning to opioid dependence. There is no stipulation that the dependence must have existed for any particular duration. During the 2 years following treatment on methadone maintenance, a patient may be readmitted without evidence of current physiological dependence if there is evidence that return to opioid dependence is imminent. If patients are younger than 18 years of age, they must have two documented attempts at drug detoxification, they must show evidence of current physiological dependence, and their legal guardian must complete and sign an official FDA consent form. These are minimum standards, and individual states may elect to make their criteria more stringent.

30–6.　**Answer: A (1, 2, and 3).** Rifampin, barbiturates (e.g., phenobarbital), and tricyclic antidepressants (e.g., imipramine) may induce live enzymes that increase the biotransformation of methadone. Pentazocine is a mixed agonist-antagonist opioid receptor anesthetic that may have antagonist actions and cause or worsen withdrawal.

30–7.　**Answer: B (1 and 3).** If an addicted patient is not going to be observed for the first several hours after the initial administration of methadone, then one should start on the low side of the recommended range for initial dose, because giving a higher dose may subject the patient to excessive sedation. Indications for a 10 mg to 20 mg initial dose include 1) there are signs of withdrawal, dilated pupils, rhinorrhea, lacrimation (as opposed to intoxication, pupillary constriction, and dry mouth), 2) the heroin used was of medium potency, and 3) the heroin has been used more than once per day for the past 3 weeks.

30–8.　**Answer: D (Only 4).** Naloxone is poorly absorbed from the gastrointestinal tract. It is available parenterally by the following routes: subcutaneously, intravenously, and intramuscularly. Its onset of action is minutes, and its duration of action is 20–30 minutes. In contrast, naltrexone is well absorbed from the gastrointestinal tract and its pharmacological duration is longer than that predicted by plasma kinetics. 6-β-Naltrexol is an important active metabolite of naltrexone, not naloxone, and has a half-life of 12 hours.

30–9. **Answer: C (2 and 4).** The prevalence of antisocial personality disorder and of all types of anxiety disorders is higher in the opioid-dependent population than in the general population. Methadone is not an effective treatment for antisocial personality disorder or anxiety disorders, but with its use the frequency of antisocial activities used to obtain opioids may decrease. Methadone will not worsen or, in general, improve depression or psychosis.

30–10. **Answer: E (All).** Progress in treatment for opioid dependence is determined by engagement in psychotherapy, performance on the job, and absence of drug abuse as determined by random urine drug tests. Monitoring of the patient's medication may be done by a colleague or family member. Patients may take 100 mg, 100 mg, and 150 mg (50-mg tablets) on Monday, Wednesday, and Friday, respectively. Physicians and pharmacists have been well known to deactivate their naltrexone by using the microwave oven. Consequently, physicians who treat these professionals should keep a supply of naltrexone in their offices as "test doses."

30–11. **Answer: A (1, 2, and 3).** Studies involving high-dose naltrexone (300 mg/day) revealed dose-related, reversible elevations in transaminase levels (SGOT, SGPT). Elevations have *not* been routinely observed secondary to naltrexone use. The most common reason for elevated transaminase levels in heroin-addicted individuals on naltrexone is concomitant use of alcohol. The guidelines for naltrexone management include assessment of liver function at baseline, every month for the first 3 months, then every 3 to 6 months during drug treatment. Before initiation of naltrexone, transaminase levels should be less than twice normal, and if they rise to three times normal, then naltrexone should be stopped.

30–12. **Answer: D (Only 4).** The first priority in methadone maintenance programs is to stop illegal activity and needle sharing. The drug hunger or craving may or may not be related to actual signs of opioid withdrawal. Increasing the dose should be at least based somewhat on the signs of opioid withdrawal; however, when urine drug screens are positive and the patient is reporting drug craving, consideration should be given to increasing the daily dose to attempt to lessen the risk of illegal activity and needle sharing.

30–13. **Answer: A (1, 2, and 3).** Opioid intoxication is notable for pulse and blood pressure decrease, constipation, dry eyes and mouth, and subjectively feeling no anxiety. Opioid withdrawal is associated with tachycardia, hypertension, nausea, diarrhea, vomiting, abdominal cramps, muscle spasm, lacrimation, rhinorrhea, yawning, anxiety, dysphoria, and craving.

30–14. **Answer: E (All).** Sharing needles is a common occurrence among street addicts and leads to transmission of hepatitis, HIV, and bacterial infections. Leukocytosis with counts greater than $14,000/mm^3$ is not unusual. Tuberculosis is more common among heroin-addicted individuals than in the general population.

30–15. **Answer: A (1, 2, and 3).** Seizures are not usually part of opioid withdrawal in adults. Seizures may be part of alcohol, barbiturate, or benzodiazepine withdrawal. The seizure may be factitious or due to trauma or epilepsy.

30–16. **Answer: E (All).** Clonidine hydrochloride is not approved by the FDA for opioid withdrawal. Clinically, it has been noted to be efficacious in the treatment of opioid withdrawal for both street addicts and those individuals who are discontinuing a methadone maintenance program. For the first 4 days, it is given every 4 hours. Sedation and hypotension are not uncommon side effects. Because clonidine acts by binding to central and peripheral α_2 receptors, cardiac arrhythmias are a contraindication for its use.

CHAPTER 31

■

Individual Treatment

■ **DIRECTIONS: For questions 31–1 through 31–19, indicate**

A if answers 1, 2, and 3 are correct.

B if answers 1 and 3 are correct.

C if answers 2 and 4 are correct.

D if only answer 4 is correct.

E if all are correct.

31–1. Which of the following statements are **true** regarding network therapy?

1. The therapist's relationship with the network is one of task-oriented team leader.

2. Network members can expect symptom relief for themselves.

3. It is important to avoid asking why someone has volunteered to serve as a network member.

4. Exploration of the family history is imperative.

31–2. Which of the following statements are **true** regarding psychotherapy of addicted individuals?

1. The focus may be on intrapsychic conflicts.

2. Services for legal aid, job counseling, and medical attention are provided.

3. Symptoms such as shame, guilt, and isolation may be treated by psychotherapy.

4. Psychotherapy is not efficacious for the treatment of depression.

31–3. Which of the following patients will especially benefit from psychotherapy?

1. A 52-year-old alcoholic business executive who expresses dismay over not achieving what he had hoped professionally and personally and who is on the brink of losing his current employment. He has a past history of major depression and currently has what he calls "the same feelings" as he had during his previous major depression.

2. An 18-year-old heroin-addicted individual who has no social support system and who dropped out of school in the fifth grade.

167

    3. A 30-year-old, never-married emergency room nurse who craves not only the meperidine she steals from the narcotics supply but also the excitement that an emergency provides. Her nursing license is at risk, and she is isolated from her family.

    4. A 29-year-old mother of four children (all younger than 6 years of age) who completed high school and 2 years of college, was abandoned by her abusive husband, and now finds herself addicted to benzodiazepines, homeless, and without career skills.

31–4. *Relapse* is defined by a return to substance use and secondary behaviors associated with substance use. Which of the following are high-risk situations for relapse?

    1. Being frustrated
    2. Experiencing the breakup of a significant relationship
    3. Undergoing withdrawal and craving the substance
    4. Being around the "same old crowd," all of whom abuse substances

31–5. What are the priorities of network therapy?

    1. Maintaining abstinence
    2. Supporting the network's integrity
    3 Maintaining appropriate behavior in the addicted individual
    4. Exploring psychological issues of substance abuse

31–6. Abstinence violation effect (AVE) accounts for the reaction to the transgression of an absolute rule, such as abstinence. Before the first lapse, the individual is committed to a period of abstinence. What are the operational elements that determine the intensity of the AVE?

    1. The duration of abstinence
    2. The importance of the prohibited behavior to the individual
    3. The presence of guilt
    4. The cause of the relapse being blamed on others

31–7. Which of the following are strategies for relapse prevention?

    1. Restructuring AVEs
    2. Mindfulness
    3. Behavioral responses to cope with high-risk situations
    4. Meditation

31–8. Which of the following are **not** principles of network therapy?

    1. Arrangements for assembling a network should begin the first time the patient is seen.
    2. The tone should be explorative and collegial.
    3. The spouse should be involved immediately.
    4. Fellow substance abusers make good allies for the network team.

31–9. Which of the following statements are **true** regarding the efficacy of psychotherapy for substance abuse?

    1. Psychotherapy is most effective when combined with other treatment services.

2. Psychotherapy should be delivered at a high level of intensity.

3. Patients who have high levels of psychiatric symptoms do better with psychotherapy than with drug counseling.

4. The match of therapist and patient has no effect on outcome.

31–10. Which types of psychotherapy are more helpful than others in the treatment of addiction?

1. Interpersonal psychotherapy

2. Cognitive-behavior therapy

3. Supportive/dynamic therapy

4. No one approach has proven efficacy over another.

31–11. What special emphases are particularly important in treatment for substance abuse?

1. Keeping abreast of the patient's compliance with abstinence

2. Determining the time of day for conducting therapy with regard to methadone dosing

3. Formulating clear treatment goals early and keeping them in sight

4. Engaging the patient in treatment requires no special efforts.

31–12. Which of the following statements characterize individual psychotherapy for alcoholism?

1. Deep interpretations of unconscious thoughts and feelings

2. Guidance and direction

3. An attitude of exploration

4. Suggestions regarding the need to maintain sobriety

31–13. Which defense mechanisms are especially used by alcoholic individuals?

1. Denial

2. Sublimation

3. Repression

4. Reaction formation

31–14. For alcoholism to develop, what other factors in addition to psychological conflict must be present?

1. Familial prohibition against relaxation

2. Genetic predisposition

3. Legally available alcohol

4. Sanctioned use of alcohol by the society

31–15. Group therapy is the most frequently recommended form of therapy for individuals with alcoholism. What are the advantages of individual therapy for alcoholic individuals?

1. Sensitive life events may be more easily disclosed.

2. Cognitive relapse-prevention strategies specific for an individual may be created.

3. Because 57% of all alcoholic patients have a comorbid diagnosis, individual therapy will allow the patient to receive a careful and lengthy evaluation.

4. Individual therapy will allow the alcoholic patient to identify with recovering alcoholic individuals.

31–16. Which of the following are characteristics required of the patient for a good outcome in individual psychotherapy for substance abuse?

1. An awareness of self-destructive patterns in the substance use

2. A wish to understand or find meaning in the behavior

3. A wish to change aspects of the self that are not acceptable

4. The active use of substances

31–17. What are the typical countertransference issues involved in working with an alcoholic patient engaged in individual therapy?

1. The therapist's feelings of inadequacy regarding his or her knowledge of addiction

2. The therapist's attitudes (conscious and unconscious) about substances of abuse

3. The therapist's identification with critical attitudes projected by the patient

4. The therapist's reactions to conflicts that many alcoholic patients have regarding authority figures

31–18. Scaffolding therapy consists of structural components that must be accepted by the patient for the primary goal of abstinence to be achieved. What are the essential components of scaffolding therapy?

1. Family and spouse

2. Alcoholics Anonymous

3. Therapist

4. Disulfiram

31–19. Which of the following statements characterize the second stage of psychotherapy with alcoholic patients?

1. The patient has established an internalized sense of sobriety.

2. Dreams about drinking are common.

3. The patient attains a mature recognition of his or her own limitations.

4. The goal is for the patient to arrive at the conclusion "I don't have to drink."

■ ANSWERS:

31–1. **Answer: B (1 and 3).** Network members have volunteered their time and services, so their motives must not be scrutinized. Network volunteers should not expect symptom relief or other gains for themselves. Family history and dynamics are not the focus of network therapy.

31–2. **Answer: B (1 and 3).** Psychotherapy addresses issues related to conflicts in patients' lives, past and present, under the assumption that these conflicts may be contributing to their current situation. Symptoms such as shame, guilt, lone-liness, isolation, anxiety, dysphoria, and depression may be effectively treated by psychotherapy. Unlike counseling, psychotherapy does not generally include management of the patient's behavior or provide specific concrete services.

31–3. **Answer: B (1 and 3).** The 52-year-old alcoholic business executive may have a major depressive disorder or dysthymia, both of which are amenable to treat-ment with psychotherapy. This patient has the ego integrity to maintain a psy-chotherapeutic alliance. The 30-year-old, never-married, and socially isolated emergency room nurse may have a dysthymia, depression, or characterological structure that creates the opportunity for her to self-medicate with meperidine while also using the emergency room as a source of stimulation. The 18-year-old heroin-addicted individual would most likely benefit from a highly struc-tured living arrangement and a more concrete counseling approach. The 29-year-old mother of four may indeed benefit from psychotherapy after basic needs of shelter and provisions are addressed.

31–4. **Answer: E (All).** Negative emotional states (e.g., frustration, anger, anxiety, depression, boredom) before or simultaneously with the first lapse are associ-ated with the highest risk of relapse. Interpersonal conflict is also associated with relapse, as is overt or covert social pressure. Negative physical states (i.e., withdrawal), testing of personal control, and cravings are all associated with relapse.

31–5. **Answer: A (1, 2, and 3).** Maintaining abstinence is critical in network therapy. The patient and network members should report at the start of each session any events related to the addicted patient's exposure to alcohol and drugs. The patient is expected to make sure that each of the network members keeps meet-ing appointments and stays involved. The therapist supports the integrity of the network by setting meeting times and summons the network for any emer-gency. The therapist should combine any and all modalities necessary to ensure the patient's stability. Exploration of intrapsychic and interpersonal conflicts is not a major focus of network therapy.

31–6. **Answer: A (1, 2, and 3).** Individuals who experience intense AVE following a lapse often experience a motivation crisis that undermines their commitment to abstinence goals. The intensity of AVE varies with the duration of abstinence (with greater intensity associated with longer abstinence), the degree of impor-tance placed on the prohibited behavior, cognitive dissonance (conflict and guilt), and personal attribution effect (i.e., blaming oneself as the cause of the transgression).

31–7. **Answer: E (All).** The three main components of relapse prevention are 1) skill-training strategies, including behavioral and cognitive responses for coping with high-risk situations; 2) cognitive reframing procedures to provide the in-dividual with a different view of the situation, that is, as a learning process and reframing reaction to the initial lapse (restructuring the AVE); and 3) lifestyle-balancing strategies such as meditation, mindfulness, and exercise.

31–8. **Answer: C (2 and 4).** In network therapy, the tone of the first meeting and of subsequent ones should be directive. Explicit instructions to support and en-sure abstinence should be given. Fellow abusers, no matter how close the rela-tionship, do not make good network members because they cannot be relied upon to give unbiased support.

31–9. **Answer: A (1, 2, and 3).** Psychotherapy is most effective when it is combined with other treatment services such as pharmacotherapy, support groups (e.g., Alcoholics Anonymous, Narcotics Anonymous), group living arrangements, and so forth. Psychotherapy conducted twice a week following intensive 12-step–oriented programs is associated with higher rates of abstinence than is once-per-week outpatient therapy following intensive 12-step programs. Patients who have high levels of psychiatric symptoms are helped by psychotherapy with life adjustment issues as well as abstinence. The patient-therapist match, therapist skill, and desire to be helpful all determine the outcome of therapy.

31–10. **Answer: D (Only 4).** Supportive-expressive and interpersonal psychotherapies derived from psychoanalysis, cognitive-behavior therapy, and supportive/dynamic therapy *all* have proven efficacy, and to date, no one approach appears superior to another.

31–11. **Answer: A (1, 2, and 3).** For substance-abusing patients, treatment goals must be formulated clearly and early in treatment. Keeping abreast of the patient's compliance with his or her abstinence and of other aspects of the treatment (e.g., attending school, seeking employment) is particularly important. Methadone is a central part of the opioid-addicted patient's life, so therapy appointments may need to be scheduled around the time the patient feels the most comfortable and cognitively alert. Substance-abusing patients generally require more supportive interactions (e.g., calling if an appointment is missed) and education about the therapy process. These measures require the therapist to devote more than the usual amount of time to engaging the patient in treatment.

31–12. **Answer: C (2 and 4).** Deep, probing interpretations of unconscious conflicts are not usually addressed early in the treatment of alcoholic patients. An attitude of exploration should be tempered with guidance, direction, and suggestions regarding the need to maintain sobriety.

31–13. **Answer: B (1 and 3).** The low self-esteem and feelings of worthlessness and inadequacy are denied and repressed, leading to unconscious needs to be cared for and accepted. Other primitive defenses such as projection, projective identification, rationalization, and splitting are used. With treatment, higher defenses such as sublimation, reaction formation, and intellectualization are used.

31–14. **Answer: C (2 and 4).** Psychological conflict, a genetic predisposition, and sanction of alcohol use by the society create a constellation in which an individual may develop alcoholism.

31–15. **Answer: A (1, 2, and 3).** Individual therapy can be more effective for people who fear groups and/or are unable to disclose sensitive life events in a group setting. Individualized cognitive relapse-prevention strategies may be developed. Approximately 57% of all alcoholic patients have a comorbid psychiatric disorder, many of which will not be apparent in a group setting or during brief medication evaluations. Individual therapy allows careful observation and scrutiny of the patient over time. Individual therapy does *not* provide peer group support or identification with recovering alcoholic individuals, both of which a group therapy or support group may provide.

31–16. **Answer: A (1, 2, and 3).** Positive characteristics for insight-oriented psychotherapy for substance abuse include a high level of intellect, a wish to understand or find meaning in the behavior, a wish to change aspects of the self that are not acceptable, a capacity for intimacy, the time available for the process, an awareness of conflicts and patterns of self-destructive behavior, socioeconomic security, marital stability, and a low level of sociopathy. Individuals are encouraged to arrive at their sessions sober. The active use of substances is not a good prognostic indicator.

31–17. **Answer: E (All).** The therapist's lack of knowledge about addiction and its treatment may enhance his or her negative reaction toward the patient. The therapist's attitudes and beliefs about the substance in question may affect how he or she views the patient. Many alcoholic patients grew up in households with punitive, overly harsh authority figures, and the patient may project these attitudes onto the therapist, resulting in the therapist's feeling rage, despair, and fear. Alcoholic patients may trust sibling relationships, such as those with fellow alcoholics, more than the authority figure of the therapist, and this will affect the transference and countertransference.

31–18. **Answer: E (All).** Changes produced in psychotherapy with an alcoholic patient occur from the outside in, rather than from the inside out as in traditional psychodynamic/psychoanalytic therapy. Scaffolding therapy consists of creating the "outside in" component of therapy, which includes family/spouse involvement (as sources of information as to the patient's sobriety and as support to maintain sobriety), Alcoholics Anonymous, the therapist, and disulfiram.

31–19. **Answer: A (1, 2, and 3).** During the middle phase of therapy with alcoholic patients, a firmly established sense of internalized sobriety should be established. Dreams and fantasies about drinking are common. Interpretation should include dealing with the issues of controlling the impulse to drink. Egocentrism is decreased, and a mature recognition by the individual of his or her own limitations is attained. The goal of the third, and final, stage of therapy is for the patient to arrive at the conclusion "I don't have to drink."

CHAPTER 32

Group and Family Treatments

■ **DIRECTIONS: For questions 32–1 through 32–5, match the treatment to the appropriate statement(s). Each statement may be used once, more than once, or not at all.**

32–1. Alcoholics Anonymous

32–2. Psychodynamic group therapy

32–3. Recovery training/ self-help

32–4. Psychoeducational group

32–5. Family therapy

a. This is a form of cognitive-behavior therapy.

b. Substance abuse may be controlled or stopped by engaging parents in the process.

c. Addiction is related to ego deficits involving affects, self-esteem, self-care, and relationships.

d. Take one day at a time.

e. Give oneself over to a higher power.

f. A didactic group is used.

g. Parenting skills are routinely addressed.

h. Reframing techniques are important.

i. This therapy is based on psychoanalytic principles.

j. Contracts are initiated in the first few sessions.

k. Multigenerational issues are addressed.

l. It is assumed that the addictive behavior is conditioned.

■ **DIRECTIONS: For questions 32–6 through 32–11, select the single best answer.**

32–6. When would a paradoxical technique be indicated?

1. A non–substance-abusing child in the family is threatening suicide.

2. There is an allegation of child abuse, and the children may be removed from the home.

    3. Charges of battery are filed the afternoon of the first therapy session.

    4. Both partners in the marriage are alcoholic and have been ordered by the court into their eighth treatment process.

32–7. What type of attitude must the group therapist in an addictions group exhibit?

    1. Passive

    2. Blank screen

    3. Facilitative

    4. Active

32–8. Which of the following is true regarding the efficacy of group therapy for addictions?

    1. There are numerous well-controlled studies.

    2. Common sense allows us to appreciate the usefulness of group therapy.

    3. There are few controlled studies.

    4. Group therapy is not efficacious.

32–9. Alcoholics Anonymous is successful because it offers what type of approach?

    1. Corrective spiritual approach

    2. Insight into intrapsychic conflicts

    3. An understanding of the intergenerational family conflicts

    4. Social skills training

32–10. Dyads are the most difficult unit to treat in family therapy for substance abuse. Which of the following dyads is the most difficult?

    1. Mother–addicted daughter

    2. Father–addicted son

    3. Mother–addicted son

    4. Father–addicted daughter

32–11. Which of the following statements is **false** regarding families of alcoholic individuals?

    1. Alcoholism is a familial condition.

    2. There are two distinct interactional styles in the family based on whether the family member is sober or intoxicated.

    3. Family patterns of behavior have been organized around the alcoholic family member's behavior.

    4. Clinicians usually see the alcoholic individual early in the course of the illness.

■ **DIRECTIONS: For questions 32–12 through 32–15, indicate**

    A if answers 1, 2, and 3 are correct.

    B if answers 1 and 3 are correct.

    C if answers 2 and 4 are correct.

    D if only answer 4 is correct.

    E if all are correct.

32–12. According to the strategic-structural model of family therapy, symptoms develop into a homeostatic life of their own and regulate family transactions. Which of the following are techniques used in this process?

　　1. Emphasis is placed on change outside the sessions.

　　2. Aspects of the therapist will be internalized by every family member.

　　3. Metaphorical directives are used.

　　4. Emphasis is placed on the exploration of what creates triangulation.

32–13. Which of the following represent therapeutic communities in which an individual commits to a "total" group approach?

　　1. Synanon

　　2. Daytop

　　3. Phoenix House

　　4. River Ridge

32–14. What are the main areas of psychological vulnerability in the addicted individual that may be conceptualized as deficits in ego functioning?

　　1. Regulation of affects

　　2. Self-care

　　3. Interpersonal relationships

　　4. Self-esteem

32–15. Which of the following statements are **false** regarding family therapy?

　　1. Usually, families will easily and readily accept early recommendations for hospitalization.

　　2. The therapist should never terminate therapy with a family, because this would convey a sense of hopelessness.

　　3. The employer should never be involved in the treatment of an employee with ongoing substance abuse.

　　4. The spouse should never leave the substance-abusing individual.

■　**ANSWERS:**

32–1.　Alcoholics Anonymous: **d, e**

32–2.　Psychodynamic group therapy: **c, i**

32–3.　Recovery training/self-help: **d, f**

32–4.　Psychoeducational group: **a, f, l**

32–5.　Family therapy: **b, g, h, j, k**

32–6.　**Answer: 4.** Paradoxical techniques are reserved for highly resistant family systems with several prior treatment failures. These techniques are not used during times of crisis.

32–7.　**Answer 4.** An active mode of leadership is important because individuals with addictions need therapists who can help group members engage with each other, especially around their vulnerabilities and denial concerning substance abuse.

32–8.   **Answer: 3.** There are few well-controlled studies documenting the efficacy of group therapy for patients who are addicted to drugs or alcohol, despite the fact that group therapy is the most frequently prescribed treatment for addiction.

32–9.   **Answer: 1.** Alcoholics Anonymous is successful because it offers a corrective psychological, spiritual, and moral approach to the problem of addiction.

32–10.   **Answer: 3.** In family therapy for substance abuse, the mother-son dyad is the most difficult to treat.

32–11.   **Answer: 4.** Clinicians usually encounter the alcoholic patient after years of drinking and associated morbidity.

32–12.   **Answer: B (1 and 3).** Techniques used in strategic-structural therapy include the following: 1) using tasks to solve problems, 2) putting a problem into a solvable form, 3) placing emphasis on change outside the sessions, 4) learning to take the path of least resistance so that the family's existing behaviors are used positively, 5) using paradoxical techniques, 6) having changes occur in stages, and 7) using metaphorical directives in such a manner that the family will not realize that they have received a directive. In psychodynamic therapy, each of the family members will internalize aspects of the therapist. Bowen's systems family therapy emphasizes triangulation (i.e., that whenever there is emotional distance or conflict between two persons, tensions will be displaced onto a third party, issue, or substance) and what creates triangulation.

32–13.   **Answer: A (1, 2, and 3).** Synanon was established in the 1960s for heroin-addicted individuals. The group approach was used to change attitudes through confinement, structure, daily work assignments, and interpersonal confrontations. Daytop and Phoenix House are other therapeutic communities.

32–14.   **Answer E (All).** The areas of ego deficits that may potentiate characterological problems are 1) regulation of affects, 2) self-care, 3) interpersonal relationships, and 4) self-esteem.

32–15.   **Answer: E (All).** Families are usually most reticent to hospitalize the substance-abusing family member and will usually do so only after multiple treatment failures. Maintaining long-term ties with families in which there is ongoing substance abuse is imperative for treatment; on the other hand, terminating therapy may be indicated if family members continue abusing substances. In working with families with continued substance abuse, involving the employer of the substance-abusing family member will be important. The third step in working with families with ongoing substance abuse involves giving the spouse three choices: 1) maintain the current system, 2) detach emotionally from the substance abuser, or 3) get physically distant from the substance abuser.

CHAPTER 33

■

Special Programs

■ DIRECTIONS: For questions 33–1 through 33–18,
indicate whether the statement is true or false.

33–1. _____ Therapeutic communities (TCs) view substance abuse as a disease process.

33–2. _____ One goal of treatment in a TC is detoxification.

33–3. _____ Persons entering TCs usually have been successfully employed members of society who need rehabilitation from their substance abuse/dependence.

33–4. _____ Individuals who receive professional treatment before attending Alcoholics Anonymous (AA) generally have better treatment outcomes than those who do not receive professional treatment.

33–5. _____ In a TC, work and daily living tasks are considered educational and an integral part of therapy.

33–6. _____ The best way to prescribe AA is to dictate how often the individual will attend.

33–7. _____ The philosophy of a TC is that treatment is made available in the environment and that it is the individual's responsibility to make use of treatment.

33–8. _____ Some individuals will discontinue drinking on their own accord.

33–9. _____ The availability of alcohol is related to alcohol abuse.

33–10. _____ Workplace testing for drugs and alcohol may be used to intimidate employees.

33–11. _____ For alcohol abuse, day treatment is less effective than traditional inpatient treatment.

33–12. _____ The lifestyle of a traditional TC may be too intense for some individuals with substance-abuse issues and severe chronic mental illness.

33–13. _____ Age, gender, education, intelligence, marital status, and employment status determine who will benefit from AA.

33–14. _____ Social support from family/friends is crucial in recovery from alcoholism.

33–15. _____ The dropout rate in a TC is highest after the first 30 days.

33–16. _____ AA is absolutely essential to the treatment of every alcoholic patient.

33–17. _____ More adults than adolescents are legally referred for treatment in a TC.

33–18. _____ Inpatient treatment programs for alcoholism that have an intensive medical approach have the best treatment outcomes.

■ **DIRECTIONS: For questions 33–19 through 33–23, indicate**

> A if answers 1, 2, and 3 are correct.
> B if answers 1 and 3 are correct.
> C if answers 2 and 4 are correct.
> D if only answer 4 is correct.
> E if all are correct.

33–19. Which of the following are more likely to affiliate with an AA group?

1. Those who experience loss of control while drinking
2. Those who are obsessive-compulsive about their drinking
3. Those who use external sources of support
4. Those who engage in religious/spiritual activity

33–20. Which areas should be assessed when inpatient treatment is being considered for alcoholism?

1. Acute withdrawal potential
2. Relapse potential
3. Recovery environment
4. Physical illness

33–21. Which of the following characterize an individual who will have a good response to inpatient treatment for alcoholism?

1. The patient is married.
2. Alcohol is the sole drug of abuse.
3. Families agree to participate in treatment.
4. The patient is relatively youthful.

33–22. Which of the following are **not** a characteristic of individuals who enter a TC?

1. Male
2. History of criminal activity
3. Low self-esteem
4. High normal intelligence

33–23. Which of the following may be requested from a person at the time of admission to a TC?

1. Tuberculin test
2. HIV status
3. Hepatitis profile
4. Urine drug screen

■ **ANSWERS:**

33–1. **False** TCs view substance abuse as a lifestyle problem, not a disease process.

33–2. **False** Detoxification is not a goal for TCs.

33–3. **False** The typical TC client has a spotty record of employment.

33–4. **True** Individuals who have had no professional treatment before entering AA have higher dropout rates and more frequent relapses.

33–5. **True** In a TC, the daily tasks of living are essential to treatment.

33–6. **False** Frequency of attendance at AA meetings should be individualized.

33–7. **True** Treatment at a TC is the milieu provided by the environment.

33–8. **True** Some individuals will discontinue alcoholic consumption without formal treatment.

33–9. **True** The more available alcohol is, the more likely it will be consumed.

33–10. **True** Forced workplace drug screens may be used to intimidate employees.

33–11. **False** For alcohol abuse, day treatment is as effective as traditional inpatient treatment.

33–12. **True** Individuals with chronic mental illness, such as schizophrenia, may not tolerate the intense interpersonal relationships in a TC.

33–13. **False** None of these factors has a bearing on who will benefit from AA.

33–14. **True** A strong, sober support system is crucial for recovery from alcoholism.

33–15. **False** The TC dropout rate is highest in the first 30 days.

33–16. **False** Many alcoholic patients benefit from treatment modalities other than AA.

33–17. **False** Adolescents are frequently referred to TCs as part of a legal encounter.

33–18. **True** Medical-based inpatient treatment programs for alcoholism are the most successful.

33–19. **Answer: E (All).** Individuals who lose control when under the influence of alcohol, consume large quantities of alcohol on days when they drink, are anxious about their drinking behaviors, and are obsessive-compulsive about their drinking do well in AA. Those who engage in religious/spiritual activities are more likely to affiliate with an AA group.

33–20. **Answer: E (All).** The areas recommended for assessment when considering inpatient treatment for alcoholism are 1) acute intoxication and/or withdrawal potential, 2) biomedical conditions and complications, 3) emotional and behavioral conditions, 4) treatment acceptance or resistance, 5) relapse potential, and 6) recovery environment.

33–21. **Answer: A (1, 2, and 3).** Patients who do well in inpatient treatment for alcoholism are older, are married, abuse only alcohol, and have families that are willing participants in treatment.

33–22. **Answer: D (Only 4).** Individuals who arrive for treatment in a TC are typically male and more than 21 years of age. Fewer than one-third have been employed in the year prior to arrival, and two-thirds have engaged in criminal activity. They tend to have low self-esteem, have dull normal intelligence, and have been in previous drug treatments.

33–23. **Answer: E (All).** Urine drug screens and physical examinations are routinely required by TCs. Because of concern about communicable diseases in a residential setting, some TCs require tuberculin testing, hepatitis profile, and HIV status.

SECTION 5

Schizophrenia and Other Psychotic Disorders

CHAPTER 34

Basic Neuropharmacology of Antipsychotic Drugs

■ DIRECTIONS: For questions 34–1 through 34–7, select the single best answer.

34–1. What percentage of patients with schizophrenia respond to treatment with traditional antipsychotic medications?

    1. 30%

    2. 50%

    3. 70%

    4. 90%

34–2. What percentage of previously chronically hospitalized patients have returned to the community since the introduction of antipsychotic medications?

    1. 25%

    2. 50%

    3. 75%

    4. 90%

34–3. After its synthesis, dopamine is stored and bound in vesicles. What chemical is essential for the release of dopamine from the vesicles?

    1. Calcium

    2. Potassium

    3. Chloride

    4. Sodium

34–4. Although dopamine is normally released from intracellular vesicles, it may be released from extravesicular pools. Which of the following drugs can prompt such a release?

    1. Haloperidol

    2. Reserpine

    3. Methamphetamine

    4. Methadone

34–5. Antipsychotic drugs share all of the following properties **except**

     1. Being highly lipid soluble.

     2. Being 50% protein bound.

     3. Having first-pass metabolism.

     4. Being readily absorbed.

34–6. What is the defining characteristic of an atypical antipsychotic drug?

     1. Efficacy in the treatment of negative symptoms and disorganization

     2. Efficacy greater than that of traditional antipsychotic medications

     3. Efficacy equal to or greater than that of traditional antipsychotic medications and fewer extrapyramidal side effects

     4. Efficacy equal to or greater than that of traditional antipsychotic medications and no risk of tardive dyskinesia

34–7. Chlorpromazine was developed for what purpose?

     1. As an antipsychotic agent

     2. As a presurgical anesthetic agent

     3. For suppression of vagal stimulation after abdominal surgical procedures

     4. As an antihypertensive agent

■   **DIRECTIONS: For questions 34–8 through 34–11, match the type of receptor with its effect(s). Each effect may be used once, more than once, or not at all.**

34–8.	Muscarinic	a.	Weight gain
34–9.	Cholinergic	b.	Sedation
34–10.	Adrenergic	c.	Tachycardia
34–11.	Endocrine	d.	Tachypnea
		e.	Psychosis
		f.	Orthostatic hypotension
		g.	Lactation
		h.	Blurred vision
		i.	Retinitis pigmentosa
		j.	Menstrual irregularities
		k.	Parotitis
		l.	Blurred vision
		m.	Constipation
		n.	Diarrhea

■ DIRECTIONS: For questions 34–12 through 34–19, indicate

    A if answers 1, 2, and 3 are correct.
    B if answers 1 and 3 are correct.
    C if answers 2 and 4 are correct.
    D if only answer 4 is correct.
    E if all are correct.

34–12. Which of the following statements do **not** support the dopamine hypothesis of schizophrenia?

1. The clinical response to antipsychotics takes place in conjunction with dopamine blockade.
2. There is a subgroup of patients who meet the criteria for schizophrenia but do not respond to treatment with traditional antipsychotic medications.
3. Amphetamine and cocaine may cause psychosis.
4. Dopaminergic systems do not function independently of other neurotransmitter systems.

34–13. Which of the following statements are related to the long-length dopaminergic systems whose soma are located in the ventral mesencephalon?

1. A dysfunction results in Parkinson's disease.
2. Beta-endorphin, melanocyte-stimulating hormone, vasopressin, and oxytocin are released.
3. Performance of cognitive tasks is dependent on an intact system.
4. There is a relationship with the amacrine cells of the retina and the periglomerular neurons in the olfactory bulb.

34–14. Tryptophan is the precursor for which neurotransmitters?

1. Dopamine
2. Epinephrine
3. Norepinephrine
4. Serotonin

34–15. Which of the following compounds may modulate dopamine synthesis and release?

1. Tyrosine hydroxylase
2. Gamma-aminobutyric acid
3. Dihydroxyphenylalanine decarboxylase
4. Glutamate

34–16. What is (are) the major metabolite(s) of dopamine in humans?

1. Catechol-O-methyltransferase
2. Dihydroxyphenylacetic acid
3. Monoamine oxidase
4. Homovanillic acid

34–17. Research and clinical interest in the serotonin neurotransmitter system and its relationship to schizophrenia has grown recently. Which of the following statements are **true** regarding the serotonergic system?

    1. Clozapine may exert at least some of its action on the serotonergic system.

    2. Perception may be related to the 5-HT_{2A} receptor.

    3. Motor control may be, at least in part, regulated by the serotonergic system.

    4. Dopamine is regulated independently of serotonin.

34–18. Cyclic adenosine 3′,5′-monophosphate (cAMP) triggers a cascade of intracellular events. What are the interactions between the dopamine receptors and cAMP?

    1. D_4 increases cAMP.

    2. D_3 increases cAMP.

    3. D_2 increases cAMP.

    4. D_1 increases cAMP.

34–19. Autoreceptor regulation of dopamine is a target of investigation for novel antipsychotic medications. What are the relationships among autoreceptors, neuroanatomy, antipsychotics, and dopamine receptor subtypes?

    1. The D_4 receptor is particularly vulnerable to clozapine and is found chiefly in the limbic areas of the brain and in the mesolimbic area, where there are no autoreceptors.

    2. The D_2 receptor is vulnerable to traditional antipsychotics and is found in the nigrostriatal area of the brain, where there are no autoreceptors.

    3. The D_2 receptor is vulnerable to traditional antipsychotics and is found in the mesocingulate area of the brain, where autoreceptors are found.

    4. The D_3 receptor is particularly vulnerable to clozapine and is found chiefly in the limbic areas of the brain and in the mesolimbic area, where there are no autoreceptors.

■ **ANSWERS:**

34–1. **Answer: 3.** Approximately 70% of patients with schizophrenia who are treated with traditional antipsychotic medications will experience a relief of the positive symptoms of schizophrenia (i.e., hallucinations, delusions, thought disorders).

34–2. **Answer: 4.** Since the introduction of antipsychotic medications, approximately 90% of previously hospitalized patients have returned to the community.

34–3. **Answer: 1.** An influx of calcium is required to promote fusion of the dopamine-containing vesicle to the presynaptic membrane that allows the dopamine to be released into the extracellular space.

34–4. **Answer: 3.** Amphetamines can release dopamine from extravesicular pools in the absence of calcium and without the need for cell firing. An exchange-diffusion process, in which the amphetamine binds to a transporter on the outside of the cell, is probably the release mechanism for dopamine in the presence of amphetamine. Chronic use of amphetamines may lead to symptoms that are indistinguishable from those of paranoid schizophrenia.

34–5.   **Answer: 2.** Antipsychotic drugs are highly lipid soluble, more than 90% protein bound, and readily absorbed. They undergo first-pass metabolism, and very little of the drug is excreted unchanged in the urine.

34–6.   **Answer: 3.** The defining characteristic for an atypical antipsychotic medication is efficacy at least equal to that of traditional antipsychotic medications and fewer extrapyramidal side effects. Improved efficacy in treating negative symptoms (e.g., social withdrawal, flat affect) or disorganization is not required for an antipsychotic to be considered atypical. Only possessing efficacy clearly superior to that of traditional antipsychotics is not sufficient. Demonstrating lower risk of tardive dyskinesia is not required for an antipsychotic to be considered atypical.

34–7.   **Answer: 2.** Chlorpromazine, a phenothiazine, was initially used as a presurgical anesthetic. Postoperatively, it is still used to ameliorate nausea, vomiting, and hiccups caused by vagal stimulation. Reserpine, a rauwolfia alkaloid, was developed as an antihypertensive. Chlorpromazine is associated with orthostatic hypotension.

34–8.   Muscarinic: **b, f**

34–9.   Cholinergic: **c, e** (central effects), **h, k** (parotitis secondary to dry mouth), **l, m, n** (diarrhea caused by cholinergic stimulation and constipation due to anticholinergic effects)

34–10.   Adrenergic: **b, f**

34–11.   Endocrine: **a, g, j** (edema and gynecomastia also due to secretion of hypothalamic hormones and prolactin)

34–12.   **Answer: C (2 and 4).** The hypothesis that schizophrenia is related to a relative excess of central dopaminergic system activity in the mesolimbic system is supported by the following principles: 1) traditional antipsychotic medications block dopamine receptors, and their affinity for being an antagonist of the D_2 receptor correlates with the clinical potency; 2) drugs that increase dopaminergic activity and/or dopamine release, such as amphetamine, cocaine, and L-dopa, may produce symptoms indistinguishable from those of schizophrenia; and 3) some studies have reported an increase in levels of the dopamine metabolite homovanillic acid. The hypothesis of the exclusive role of dopamine in the etiology of symptoms consistent with those of schizophrenia is challenged by the following findings: 1) the clinical response follows the initial dopaminergic blockage by weeks; 2) 30% of schizophrenic patients fail to respond to traditional antipsychotic medications; 3) dissociation occurs between D_2 receptor blockade and at least one atypical antipsychotic, clozapine; 4) an inverse relationship exists between dopamine function in the mesocortical system and the mesolimbic brain areas, such that decreased cortical dopamine activity may contribute to increased subcortical limbic dopamine transmission (decreased dopaminergic activity in the frontal cortex may be related to negative symptoms); and 5) increasing evidence points to the likelihood that the neurotransmitter systems are related in complex networks.

34–13.   **Answer: B (1 and 3).** The soma of long-length dopaminergic systems are located in the ventral mesencephalon and are composed of A8, A9, and A10 cell body groups with extensive projections into the ventral putamen, entorhinal cortex, nucleus accumbens, amygdala (A8), caudate-putamen (A9), and mesolimbic and mesocortical systems (A10). A dysfunction of the A9 nigrostriatal system is involved in the symptoms of Parkinson's disease. The A10 mesocortical system is related to the performance of cognitive tasks. Intermediate-length dopaminergic systems (A12, A13, and A14) have their soma located in the hypothalamus. These systems are responsible for dopaminergic modulation of beta-endorphin, melanocyte-stimulating hormone, vasopressin, and oxytocin release from the posterior pituitary and prolactin from the median eminence. The ultrashort dopaminergic systems are highly specific connections between the amacrine cells of the retina and the periglomerular neurons in the olfactory bulb.

34–14. **Answer: D (Only 4).** Tryptophan is the precursor for serotonin. Tyrosine is the precursor for dopamine and norepinephrine.

34–15. **E (All).** Tyrosine hydroxylase is the rate-limiting step in the synthesis of dopamine and norepinephrine. The second enzyme in the synthesis is dihydroxyphenylalanine (dopa) decarboxylase. Gamma-aminobutyric acid (GABA) and glutamate are both inhibitory neurotransmitters that may modulate the synthesis and release of dopamine. Serotonin, D_2 autoreceptors, acetylcholine, opiates, and amphetamines can also modulate dopamine synthesis and/or release.

34–16. **Answer: D (Only 4).** Homovanillic acid is the major metabolite of dopamine in humans; it may be measured in the urine, plasma, and cerebrospinal fluid. Dihydroxyphenylacetic acid (DOPAC) is the primary metabolite found in the rodent brain. Catechol-O-methyltransferase (COMT) and monoamine oxidase (MAO) are the major enzymes involved in the metabolism of dopamine and norepinephrine.

34–17. **Answer: A (1, 2, and 3).** Clozapine and other atypical antipsychotics have numerous effects on the serotonergic system. The $5-HT_{2A}$ receptor may be involved in perception, motor control, mood regulation, and regulation of the release of dopamine.

34–18. **Answer: D (Only 4).** Dopamine receptor D_1 increases cAMP, D_2 either has little effect on cAMP levels or is coupled to an inhibitory G-protein that inhibits cAMP formation, and D_3 and D_4 have no effect on cAMP.

34–19. **Answer: A (1, 2, and 3).** The D_2 receptor is the target of traditional antipsychotic agents. The receptors are distributed to the nigrostriatal, mesolimbic, and mesocortical areas. The receptors in the mesolimbic and nigrostriatal areas do not possess autoreceptors. The D_3 and D_4 receptors are predominantly located in the limbic areas. The D_4 receptor is speculated to be the site at which clozapine acts.

CHAPTER 35

━━━━━━━━━━━━━━━━━━■━━━━━━━━━━━━━━━━━━

Clinical Psychopharmacology of Schizophrenia

■ **DIRECTIONS: For questions 35–1 through 35–5, select the single best answer.**

35–1. Several classes of antipsychotic drugs are now at the disposal of the treating psychiatrist. What criterion should most strongly influence the choice of antipsychotic?

1. Low-potency, highly sedating antipsychotics should be given to agitated patients.

2. High doses of high-potency antipsychotics (e.g., > 20 mg haloperidol) should be given initially.

3. Positive past response to an antipsychotic is the most useful predictor.

4. Atypical antipsychotics with lower risks of extrapyramidal side effects should be the first line of treatment for newly diagnosed patients with schizophrenia.

35–2. Mr. N. is a 23-year-old who presents to the emergency room acutely agitated and talking about a "sparrow hawk that has invaded my insides." With threatening gestures, he demands that the "sparrow hawk" be removed. He is alone and refuses to answer any questions, stating that "they will do me harm if I speak." His medical records reveal a diagnosis of schizophrenia, undifferentiated. What would be an initial treatment plan?

1. Assessment of vital signs as soon as possible, urine drug screen, and rapid tranquilization with intramuscular haloperidol

2. Assessment of vital signs as soon as possible, urine drug screen, and rapid tranquilization with intramuscular clozapine

3. Assessment of vital signs as soon as possible, no urine drug screen, intramuscular diazepam, and intramuscular haloperidol 2–5 mg

4. Assessment of vital signs as soon as possible, urine drug screen, lorazepam 1–4 mg, and intramuscular haloperidol 2–5 mg

35–3. For patients who have persistent aggressive behavior, which of the following is helpful in controlling the outbursts?

1. Propranolol

2. Clonidine hydrochloride

    3. Amoxapine

    4. Lorazepam

35–4. What is the incidence of agranulocytosis with clozapine?

    1. 0.05%

    2. 0.1%

    3. 0.8%

    4. 1.6%

35–5. Which of the following antipsychotics is associated with pigmentary retinopathy?

    1. Clozapine

    2. Haloperidol

    3. Thioridazine

    4. Risperidone

■ **DIRECTIONS: For questions 35–6 through 35–12, match the medication with the appropriate response(s). Each response may be used once, more than once, or not at all.**

35–6.   Haloperidol

35–7.   Chlorpromazine

35–8.   Risperidone

35–9.   Clozapine

35–10. Thioridazine

35–11. Fluphenazine

35–12. Benztropine

a. There are no documented cases of tardive dyskinesia associated with the use of this medication.

b. Acute treatment may require doses of 10–20 mg/day.

c. The dose should be titrated over 3 days.

d. Cholestatic jaundice may occur.

e. The seizure threshold is lowered.

f. Four weeks may be needed to demonstrate a response.

g. There is an affinity for D_2 receptors.

h. This medication may be used in patients with severe tardive dyskinesia.

i. There is an affinity for serotonin (5-HT) receptors.

j. This medication is associated with extrapyramidal side effects.

k. Postural hypotension may occur.

l. The average dose is 6–8 mg/day.

m. Insomnia is the most common side effect.

n. Weight gain may occur.

o. There is an affinity for D_4 receptors.

p. This medication is used to treat acute extrapyramidal side effects.

q. There is an association with photosensitization.

■ **DIRECTIONS: For questions 35–13 through 35–16, indicate**

    A if answers 1, 2, and 3 are correct.

    B if answers 1 and 3 are correct.

    C if answers 2 and 4 are correct.

    D if only answer 4 is correct.

    E if all are correct.

35–13. In the United States, which antipsychotics are available in decanoate form?

    1. Haloperidol

    2. Thioridazine

    3. Fluphenazine

    4. Chlorpromazine

35–14. Intermittent medication has been advocated for some patients to improve compliance and permit better social adaptation. Which of the following statements are **true** regarding intermittent medication treatment?

    1. Prodromal signs are predictive of relapse.

    2. The rationale for this form of treatment is based, in part, on the fact that many patients will not relapse for several months after discontinuing antipsychotics.

    3. This is an excellent form of pharmacotherapy, with improvement in social outcome and subjective well-being.

    4. The goal of this therapy is to reduce adverse effects of medications.

35–15. Prospective studies have indicated a 5% annual incidence of tardive dyskinesia from neuroleptic exposure in young adults. What are the risk factors for developing tardive dyskinesia?

    1. Being older than 50 years of age

    2. Discontinuing long-standing neuroleptic treatment abruptly

    3. Being female

    4. Being treated with clozapine

35–16. What type of treatment regimen is the most efficacious in preventing relapses for patients with chronic schizophrenia?

    1. Intermittent medications

    2. Depot medications given every 2–4 weeks

    3. Crisis management

    4. Maintenance oral medications with doses titrated for the individual patient

■ **ANSWERS:**

35–1. **Answer: 3.** There is no evidence that highly sedating antipsychotics are more efficacious in the treatment of agitated patients. Treatment with high doses of high-potency antipsychotics is a controversial issue. Positive past response to an antipsychotic is the best indicator for the initial choice in antipsychotic treatment. Currently, clozapine and other atypical antipsychotic medications generally are reserved for treatment of patients who are unresponsive to traditional antipsychotic medications.

35–2. **Answer: 4.** Despite the patient's diagnosis of schizophrenia, the presence or absence of any street drug or prescription drug must be ascertained. Substance abuse is not an infrequent diagnosis in patients with schizophrenia. Rapid tranquilization with high- or low-dose antipsychotics will usually result only in an increased frequency of complicating side effects, such as acute dystonia, akathisia, blurred vision, dry mouth, or even exacerbation of psychosis by anticholinergic effects on the central nervous system. Diazepam (Valium) is not well absorbed intramuscularly, but lorazepam (Ativan) is well absorbed and is short acting.

35–3. **Answer: 1.** Propranolol has some efficacy with aggressive patients. Clonidine hydrochloride is a centrally and peripherally acting alpha-adrenergic antagonist that is used to decrease impulsivity and improve attention in children with attention-deficit/hyperactivity disorder (ADHD). Amoxapine is an antipsychotic without any special qualifications with regard to aggression. Lorazepam is a short-acting benzodiazepine.

35–4. **Answer: 3.** The incidence of agranulocytosis with clozapine is between 0.8% and 1.0%, even with close monitoring of complete blood counts. Chlorpromazine (Thorazine) has less than 0.05% incidence of agranulocytosis. Despite the low incidence of agranulocytosis, life-threatening complications must be kept in mind, because chronically ill patients may not be able to report the signs and symptoms of an illness that may herald this rare agranulocytosis.

35–5. **Answer: 3.** In doses greater than 800 mg/day, thioridazine (Mellaril) may cause irreversible degenerative changes. Pigmentation of the lens, cornea, conjunctiva, and retina (associated with skin pigmentation) can occur with the use of low-potency antipsychotics.

35–6. Haloperidol: **b, e, f, g, j, n, q**

35–7. Chlorpromazine: **d, e, f, g, j, k, n, q**

35–8. Risperidone: **a, c, g, j, l, n, q**

35–9. Clozapine: **a, e, f, h, i, k, m, n, o**

35–10. Thioridazine: **e, f, g, j, n, q**

35–11. Fluphenazine: **e, f, g, j, n, q**

35–12. Benztropine: **p**

35–13. **Answer: B (1 and 3).** Haloperidol (Haldol) and fluphenazine (Prolixin) are available in decanoate preparations that are administered at an interval of every 2 to 4 weeks. Thioridazine (Mellaril) is not available in any parenteral form. Chlorpromazine (Thorazine) is available in parenteral form.

35–14. **Answer: C (2 and 4).** The rationale for intermittent medication treatment is that many patients will not relapse for several months after discontinuing antipsychotics. The goals of the therapy are to reduce adverse effects and improve social well-being. Several studies have found no improvement in relapse rate, social outcome, or subjective well-being with intermittent medication treatment.

35–15. **Answer: A (1, 2, and 3).** The older the patient, the greater the risk of developing tardive dyskinesia. Antipsychotics may mask the symptoms and signs of tardive dyskinesia, and abrupt discontinuation of the antipsychotic may unmask or exacerbate tardive dyskinesia. There is some evidence that females are at increased risk for tardive dyskinesia.

35–16. **Answer: C (2 and 4).** Although medications cannot cure schizophrenia, relapses can be at least partially alleviated with maintenance medications, administered either orally or parenterally.

CHAPTER 36

━━━━━━━━━━━━━━━━━━■━━━━━━━━━━━━━━━━━━

Psychosocial Therapies of Schizophrenia: Individual, Group, and Family

■ **DIRECTIONS: For questions 36–1 through 36–9, indicate**

A if answers 1, 2, and 3 are correct.

B if answers 1 and 3 are correct.

C if answers 2 and 4 are correct.

D if only answer 4 is correct.

E if all are correct.

36–1. Flexible psychotherapy for schizophrenia is based on the vulnerability-stress model. What are the biomedical determinants of vulnerability for schizophrenia?

1. Genetic predisposition
2. Peripartum birth trauma
3. Viral infections of the central nervous system
4. Deficits in information processing

36–2. In a discussion of the pathogenesis of schizophrenia with family members, which of the following statements may be constructive?

1. The biomedical, psychophysiological, and behavioral determinants of schizophrenia are ubiquitous among individuals with schizophrenia.
2. Vulnerability to this disorder is not shaped by the environment.
3. The genetic transmission of schizophrenia is well documented and fully conceptualized.
4. There is an association between stressful life events, the emotional quality of the environment, and the onset and course of schizophrenia.

36–3. Patients with schizophrenia may be particularly anxious or suspicious about their first therapy appointment. What modifications in technique are helpful?

1. The patient should always be seen with his or her primary support person.
2. Coffee may be offered.
3. The interviewer should assume a nondirective and completely neutral stance.
4. Patterning the interview with a specific set of questions may be necessary.

36–4. Which of the following statements are **accurate** regarding the involvement of the family or significant others in the treatment of patients with schizophrenia?

1. The family should never be involved because such involvement would break the confidentiality with the patient.

2. Families should be encouraged to contact the therapist should they have concerns.

3. The family should be seen only by the family therapist.

4. At the initiation of the treatment process, the frequency of contact with the family and the conditions under which the family will be notified are outlined for the patient and family.

36–5. The quality of the therapeutic relationship between the patient and the therapist is central to a successful treatment outcome. The patient with schizophrenia may be beset with suspiciousness, withdrawal, and ambivalence about any type of relationship with another person. The clinical literature supports which of the following as characteristics of psychotherapy with patients with schizophrenia?

1. A consistent and straightforward style of relating

2. A capacity to tolerate intense affects and ambiguous communication

3. Availability on an "after hours" basis

4. An expectation that the patient will regularly attend sessions

36–6. Patients with schizophrenia are at high risk for suicide. Which of the following statements are **true**?

1. Patients with paranoid schizophrenia are at the highest risk.

2. The completed suicide rate is approximately 10%.

3. Comorbid depression increases the risk of suicide.

4. Immediately following discharge from the hospital, patients are at a higher risk for suicide.

36–7. Group therapy was developed to enhance self-esteem and to offer corrective experiences in a supportive environment. Group therapy involves 6–12 patients and 1–2 therapists. What are the goals of group therapy?

1. To provide psychoeducation about the disease process and medications

2. To facilitate insight into unconscious processes

3. To help the patient improve social skills

4. To confront the patient's substance abuse

36–8. Deinstitutionalization has left many families to care for their chronically mentally ill members. Expressed emotion (EE) is an operational measure of family criticism and emotional overinvolvement. Which of the following are **true** regarding the attitudes and behavior of high-EE families?

1. Schizophrenia is not viewed as a disease process, and symptoms are regarded as under the patient's conscious control.

2. Family members are willing and able to engage in problem-solving discussions.

3. Family members may have extensive and protracted conversations with the patient that are analogous to monologues.

4. Family members may neglect the patient at particular times.

36–9. Ms. N. is a 45-year-old woman with chronic schizophrenia. She has never married, and her last employment was 20 years ago. Her elderly parents have been in family therapy and a variety of support groups for 10 years. Despite her parents' efforts and several attempts by her to leave their home, Ms. N. still resides with her parents. Ms. N. was hospitalized for the fifteenth time in a psychiatric unit, where she and her family feel confident with the hospital staff. What may be the parents' and patient's reactions when they are told that she must leave after 2 days?

1. They may be outraged, feeling rejected by the "system" and burdened by the continued care required by their adult daughter.

2. They may not fully understand what has happened to their child and are afraid of losing her forever.

3. The patient may be fearful of leaving the hospital.

4. The reactions would be minimal because patients with schizophrenia do not form relationships with hospital staff.

■ **DIRECTIONS: For questions 36–10 through 36–15, select the single best response.**

36–10. In reviewing the history of Mr. D., you note that he has several ritualized behaviors that he must perform a certain number of times per day and that he drinks 10 to 12 beers per day. Mr. D. was diagnosed with schizophrenia in his mid-20s. What can be said about Mr. D.'s prognosis?

1. There is no relationship between prognosis and comorbid symptoms.

2. The absence of schizotypal features improves his prognosis.

3. The presence of borderline features improves his prognosis.

4. The presence of obsessive-compulsive symptoms worsens his prognosis.

36–11. In the model of flexible psychotherapy, which of the following statements is **true** regarding the therapist who is best able to integrate the assessments and treatment interventions at various points in the patient's illness?

1. The therapist may be a paraprofessional, because these individuals tend to focus on the health of the patient rather than the pathology.

2. The therapist may be a social worker, because these individuals will have the best training in family dynamics.

3. The therapist may be a psychiatrist, because these individuals may be the best trained in the integration of psychodynamic and biological treatment modalities.

4. A case manager who is closely identified with the patient is the best therapist.

36–12. Insight-oriented psychotherapy arose in the 1930s from psychoanalytic theory. Which of the following is **true** regarding the suitability of patients with schizophrenia for this type of psychotherapy in combination with pharmacotherapy?

1. No patient with schizophrenia should be treated with insight-oriented psychotherapy.

2. Outpatients who have had good premorbid functioning, have had minimal residual deficits, and have retained the capacity for self-observation and humor would benefit.

3. Patients who have failed to respond to long-term hospitalization may benefit from intensive outpatient therapy.

4. Patients who experienced onset of the illness in adolescence would benefit.

36–13. How much time should elapse after an acute exacerbation or initial psychotic break before complex psychoeducational and rehabilitative elements are implemented?

1. None—there is no clinically justifiable reason to delay any elements of treatment

2. Several years

3. Six to 12 months

4. Twelve to 15 months

36–14. Which of the following can substantially enhance the therapeutic relationship?

1. Allowing patients to self-regulate medication dosages

2. Maintaining strict neutrality

3. Supporting the belief that medication is a sign of weakness

4. Focusing only on dosing regimens and medication levels

36–15. Which of the following will decrease the possibility of discharge against medical advice?

1. Allowing the patients' families to ventilate their feelings and educating them about the illness

2. Allowing unlimited access by the patient to the family, even when a family member has stated that a respite is needed

3. Supporting the family's notion that schizophrenia is "caused" by the afflicted person's choice of friends

4. Requesting that the family refrain from visiting

■ ANSWERS:

36–1. **Answer: A (1, 2, and 3).** Posited biomedical determinants of schizophrenia include genetic predisposition; intrauterine, peri-, or postpartum neurological trauma; and viral infections of the central nervous system. Psychophysiological determinants include deficits in information processing, inability to maintain consistent attention, and deficient sensory inhibition and autonomic responsivity. Behavioral determinants are impairments in social competence, a tendency toward cognitive slippage, disorganization, perceptual distortions, and poor coping skills.

36–2. **Answer: D (Only 4).** The biomedical, psychophysiological, and behavioral determinants of schizophrenia are *not* ubiquitous among individuals with schizophrenia. The genetic transmission of schizophrenia is not well conceptualized. The majority of individuals with schizophrenia have a negative family history of the disorder. Vulnerability to this disorder is influenced by the environment. Stressful life events, cultural milieu, social class, social network, and the emotional quality of the living environment all are involved in the pathogenesis of schizophrenia.

36–3. **Answer: C (2 and 4).** If the patient arrives with his or her primary support, after introductions, the patient may be seen alone. After the interview with the patient, the accompanying individuals may be interviewed alone. This sequence of interviews allows the patient to have a modicum of privacy and establishes a relationship between therapist and patient while acknowledging and integrating the family or other significant others into the process. The interviewer should express warmth but should maintain a low level of expressed emotion. The interviewer should outline what will be reviewed; a structured set of inquiries may be helpful. Offering coffee and pointing out places to sit are useful in lowering the anxiety of the patient.

36–4. **Answer: C (2 and 4).** The importance of support by the family and/or significant others cannot be overestimated. At the initiation of therapy, the family should be encouraged to contact the physician whenever they have concerns, and regular contact with the support system should be prearranged. Circumstances such as suicidal ideation, imminent relapse, and other serious concerns should prompt contact with the support system.

36–5. **Answer: A (1, 2, and 3).** A consistent and straightforward overall demeanor without an authoritarian or rigid posture is best suited to creating a therapeutic alliance with patients with schizophrenia. Excessive therapeutic zeal and expectations of dramatic improvement will disappoint the therapist and alienate the patient. Patients with schizophrenia may have idiosyncratic, ambiguous styles of communication, in conjunction with little to no affect or strongly inappropriate affect that must be tolerated by the therapist. Individuals with chronic mental illness experience more crises than do the general population, so the therapist must arrange for consistent "after hours" coverage. An expectation of regular and prompt attendance is a goal of treatment, not an initial expectation.

36–6. **Answer: E (All).** Patients with paranoid schizophrenia have the best prognosis. These individuals, compared with individuals with deficit schizophrenia, experience onset of the illness later in life and have better premorbid functioning. Ironically, however, this places them at a higher risk for suicide. They tend to recognize the severity and chronicity of their illness, retaining the capacity to reflect on their life situation. The rate of completed suicide is 10%–13%, with an attempt rate of 50%–60%. Actuarial risks include being single, divorced, young, or male and having fewer social supports, comorbid depression, a past history of attempts, and recent loss. The risk of suicide is increased in the period of time immediately following discharge from the hospital.

36–7. **Answer: A (1, 2, and 3).** Group therapy may involve patients with schizophrenia, the patients and their families, or families alone. Groups may be supportive, using a professional facilitator, or psychoeducational, with or without a specific didactic format. Skills in communication, social relations, and problem solving may be addressed in a group format. To counter the prevailing view that group therapy is less desirable than other forms of therapy, the use of group therapy to enhance survival skills for independent living and improved understanding of the illness should be emphasized. Confrontation, with its concomitant high level of expressed emotion, is poorly tolerated by patients with schizophrenia.

36–8. **Answer: B (1 and 3).** Relatives in families with high EE may view the symptoms and signs of schizophrenia as reflective of lack of moral development or laziness. They may engage in protracted conversations in which they use peculiar language patterns that have two or more meanings. These conversations tend to be negative and one-sided, with the patient's viewpoint negated. Families with high EE show overconcern for the patient, whereas families with very low EE may actually neglect the patient. Problem-solving discussions, with use of clear language that is emotionally neutral, characterize families with low EE.

36–9. **Answer: B (1 and 3).** Families whose child or spouse has been ill for a protracted period may feel despairing and helpless, angry at a system that has been unable to ameliorate their relative's illness and relieve their relative's or their own suffering. Hospital admissions may be the family's only respite from the unrelenting illness of their relative, and they may be outraged if an early discharge is planned or forced by third parties. This patient has been ill for at least two decades, so a time-limited transitional living approach will not be suitable. Thoughtful planning with the parents about their adult child's future is in the best interest of the patient and her family.

36–10. **Answer: 4.** The relationship between individual personality traits and the course of schizophrenia is poorly understood. The presence of obsessive-compulsive symptoms or obsessive-compulsive disorder significantly worsens the prognosis. Comorbid schizotypal or borderline features predict better long-term outcome. Approximately 47% of all schizophrenic patients have comorbid substance abuse, and this significantly complicates treatment and prognosis.

36–11. **Answer: 3.** The treatment of a patient with schizophrenia requires a thorough grounding in psychopharmacology; biological aspects of the disease process; psychodynamics of the onset and course; and knowledge of social programs, legal issues of social entitlement programs, and available medical facilities. A well-trained psychiatrist is best suited to integrate the treatment of the patient with schizophrenia.

36–12. **Answer: 2.** Although the majority of patients with schizophrenia will benefit from some form of psychotherapy, insight-oriented psychotherapy is reserved for those patients who have above-average intelligence, had good premorbid functioning, have had minimal residual deficits, and have retained the capacity for self-observation, curiosity, frustration tolerance, and humor.

36–13. **Answer: 3.** To minimize stresses and avoid relapse, in the first 6 to 12 months after a psychotic episode, only acute medical stabilization, mobilization of social support, and establishment of supportive, ongoing treatment should be attempted. Complex psychoeducational and rehabilitative elements may be initiated after this period.

36–14. **Answer: 1.** During periods of clinical stability, allowing patients to self-regulate medications within agreed-on parameters will enhance the therapeutic relationship and facilitate compliance with medications. Some communities, treaters, and cultures believe that schizophrenia is not really an illness and that taking medications is a sign of weakness. Education and supportive measures for patients and their families regarding the pathogenesis of schizophrenia are indicated. Maintaining strict neutrality is not usually helpful in dealing with patients who have concerns about their reality testing and perceptions of the environment. Likewise, a strictly pharmacological interaction with patients is not helpful in building trust and facilitating an understanding of their world.

36–15. **Answer: 1.** Discharges against medical advice occur more commonly when families 1) believe that their relative is not really ill, 2) cannot tolerate the separation imposed by hospitalization, or 3) feel excessively guilty. Barring the family from the patient's care may increase the risk of suicide.

CHAPTER 37

Psychiatric Rehabilitation

■ **DIRECTIONS: For questions 37–1 through 37–5, indicate**

    A if answers 1, 2, and 3 are correct.

    B if answers 1 and 3 are correct.

    C if answers 2 and 4 are correct.

    D if only answer 4 is correct.

    E if all are correct.

37–1. Impairments in which aspects of basic cognitive processing may interfere with rehabilitation efforts in patients with schizophrenia?

    1. Selective attention

    2. Concept formation

    3. Cognitive flexibility

    4. Impulsivity

37–2. What are the central components of psychosocial rehabilitation?

    1. Identifying cognitive impairments

    2. Assessing current life skills

    3. Mobilizing the individual's and societal resources

    4. Modifying the individual's environment

37–3. Job clubs were originally developed to train non–mentally ill individuals to help them locate and secure jobs. This concept has been adapted to individuals with severe mental illness. What factors are related to success in this form of rehabilitation?

    1. Having been employed before the onset of the illness

    2. Receiving social security or other benefits

    3. Having good job interview skills

    4. Having a diagnosis of schizophrenia

37–4. Vocational rehabilitation has several features that may need to be reevaluated in rehabilitation work with the individual with schizophrenia. Which of the following must be considered specifically regarding this population?

    1. Clients need a time-limited amount of support.

2. Clients need an indefinite period of support.

3. The need for support fades in a linear model.

4. The need for support will wax and wane with the course of the illness.

37–5. Which of the following skills can be taught in a training environment and transferred to another environment?

1. Self-administration of medications

2. Personal grooming

3. Engagement in recreation and leisure activities

4. Ability to monitor symptoms

■ **DIRECTIONS: For questions 37–6 through 37–8, select the single best answer.**

37–6. Which of the following treatment approaches resulted in the lowest rate of relapse after 2 years in individuals with schizophrenia?

1. Medication management

2. Medication management and skills training

3. Medication management, skills training, and family psychoeducation

4. There is no difference in relapse rates.

37–7. Case managers monitor the quality of services being delivered and coordinate relationships with various agencies. The case manager is a focal point of accessibility and accountability. What is known about case management for patients with schizophrenia?

1. It is relatively ineffective.

2. It is cost-effective.

3. Case managers are professionals.

4. Relapse rates are significantly lower in patients who receive case management compared with those who do not.

37–8. What is a major predictor of success in competitive employment?

1. The absence of cognitive impairments

2. The absence of any positive symptoms

3. The ability to relate to peers and supervisors

4. The ability to perform the task required at the time the individual is hired

■ **DIRECTIONS: For questions 37–9 through 37–13, match the instrument with what it measures or predicts. Each answer may be used once, more than once, or not at all.**

37–9. Degraded Stimulus Continuous Performance Test   a. Semantic memory

37–10. Digit Span Distractibility Test   b. Processing of visual information

37–11.	Rey Auditory Verbal Learning Test	c.	Social skills
37–12.	Forced-Choice Span of Apprehension Test	d.	Occupational functioning
37–13.	Wechsler Memory Scale		

■ ANSWERS:

37–1.   **Answer: A (1, 2, and 3).** Patients with schizophrenia have impairments in sustained attention, selective attention, readiness to respond, efficiency of initial storage and readout of information, short- and long-term memory recall, concept formation, and cognitive flexibility. Impulsivity is characteristic of attention-deficit disorder, oppositional defiant disorder, and borderline personality disorder.

37–2.   **Answer E (All).** The components of psychosocial rehabilitation are 1) identifying short- and long-term living, learning, and working roles and environments to which the individual aspires; 2) identifying, and as far as possible, ameliorating cognitive impairments; 3) listing skills necessary to function in the new environment; 4) modifying the environment; 5) comparing present skill level with that required by the new situation; and 6) listing and mobilizing the individual's and societal resources.

37–3.   **Answer: B (1 and 3).** Individuals who were employed before the onset of their illness and have good job interview skills have the best results with job clubs. Individuals who receive Social Security Insurance, Social Security Disability Insurance, or other benefits are less successful in job clubs. Patients who have a diagnosis of schizophrenia are less successful than patients with affective or substance use disorders.

37–4.   **Answer: C (2 and 4).** Two standard assumptions of vocational rehabilitation are time-limited interventions and a linear model of decreasing support. The very nature of schizophrenia, with its course of exacerbations, remissions, and chronicity, argues for an indefinite period of support and for varying the intensity of services in rehabilitation work with individuals with this disorder.

37–5.   **Answer: E (All).** Patients can be taught how to administer their own medications, to groom and attend to personal hygiene, to engage in recreational activities, and to self-monitor symptoms. These skills do transfer to other environments, although they are not performed as smoothly in the new environment.

37–6.   **Answer: 3.** Relapse rates are significantly lower for those patients who receive medication management, skills training, and family psychoeducation (25%), compared with those who receive medication management alone (62%) or medication management and skills training (50%).

37–7.   **Answer: 1.** Case managers are generally paraprofessionals. Case management appears to be effective in work with physically challenged individuals. In patients with schizophrenia, however, case management has not reduced the relapse rate or enhanced rehabilitation.

37–8.   **Answer: 3.** The major predictor for being able to transition successfully from "training" or transitional jobs to competitive jobs is an ability to "get along" with peers and supervisors.

37–9.   Degraded Stimulus Continuous Performance Test: **b, c, d**

37–10. Digit Span Distractibility Test: **a, c**

37–11. Rey Auditory Verbal Learning Test: **a, c**

37–12. Forced-Choice Span of Apprehension Test: **b, c, d**

37–13. Wechsler Memory Scale: **a, c**

CHAPTER 38

■

Schizophrenia-Related Disorders and Dual Diagnosis

■ **DIRECTIONS: For questions 38–1 through 38–13, indicate**

A if answers 1, 2, and 3 are correct.

B if answers 1 and 3 are correct.

C if answers 2 and 4 are correct.

D if only answer 4 is correct.

E if all are correct.

38–1. The relationship of psychotic disorders to each other is beginning to be understood as patients are carefully followed through the course of the initial disorder. Which of the following statements are **true** regarding the progression of each disorder?

1. Approximately 50% of patients with brief psychotic disorder will progress to a more chronic course of schizophrenia and bipolar disorder.

2. Approximately 50% of patients with postpartum psychosis will progress to bipolar disorder.

3. Approximately 66% of patients with schizophreniform disorder will progress to schizophrenia.

4. Approximately 66% of patients with drug-induced psychosis will progress to schizophrenia.

38–2. What should the medical evaluation entail for an initial psychotic episode?

1. Urine drug screen

2. Electroencephalogram (EEG)

3. Magnetic resonance imaging (MRI) scan of the brain

4. Human immunodeficiency virus (HIV) screen

38–3. Treatment of brief psychotic disorder involves which of the following?

1. Containment in a safe, secure environment

2. Interviewing and supporting family and significant others

3. Haloperidol

4. Diazepam

38–4. After years of ill repute, electroconvulsive therapy (ECT) is regaining popularity as a treatment for several disorders. Which of the following disorders may be treated with ECT?

1. Brief reactive psychosis
2. Schizophrenia, acute exacerbation
3. Schizoaffective disorder
4. Delusional disorder

38–5. Ms. K. is a 33-year-old woman with a history of social withdrawal and vivid auditory hallucinations, but she has maintained her job as a county clerk. According to her husband of 6 years, she does not drink, smoke, or use any illicit drugs. Her symptoms arose abruptly 2 months before presenting to the community mental health clinic. What would be included in the differential diagnosis?

1. Postpartum psychosis
2. Drug-induced psychosis
3. Schizophreniform disorder
4. Brief psychotic disorder

38–6. Which of the following disorders are found more often in men?

1. Schizophreniform disorder
2. Schizophrenia
3. Schizoaffective disorder
4. Drug-induced psychosis

38–7. In the treatment of refractory schizoaffective disorder that is currently being managed with carbamazepine and thiothixene, what should be considered?

1. Carbamazepine level may be low due to autoinduction of the cytochrome P450 system.
2. An adjunctive medication such as lithium may be beneficial.
3. The patient may need an additional neuroleptic.
4. The patient may not be taking the medications.

38–8. The cardinal feature of delusional disorder is the presence of one or more nonbizarre delusions for at least 1 month. Which of the following can be stated about the treatment of delusional disorder?

1. There are no studies on the efficacy of *any* type of treatment.
2. Supportive, nonconfrontive psychotherapy may be acceptable to many patients.
3. Fluoxetine may be useful.
4. Pimozide may be used.

38–9. In what areas are there differences in the treatment of schizophreniform disorder and schizoaffective disorder?

1. Involvement of the family in supportive therapy
2. Neuroleptic treatment

3. Individual treatment with supportive psychotherapy

4. Mood-stabilizing agents

38–10. Stimulant-induced psychosis is characterized by what type of neuroleptic treatment or reactions to treatment?

1. Autonomic instability

2. High-potency neuroleptic treatment

3. Seizures

4. Neuroleptics are not used to treat this disorder.

38–11. In treating patients who have received a dual diagnosis of substance abuse and schizophrenia, what modalities must be used?

1. Modified Alcoholics Anonymous or Narcotics Anonymous program

2. Regular involvement of the patient's social support network

3. Neuroleptic medications

4. Confrontation and intense exploration of denial

38–12. What adjunctive therapies are useful in the treatment of patients who have received a dual diagnosis of substance abuse and schizophrenia?

1. Methadone maintenance for opioid addiction

2. Benzodiazepines for alcohol withdrawal

3. Tricyclic antidepressants for cocaine abuse

4. Disulfiram for chronic alcoholism

38–13. Lysergic acid diethylamide (LSD) ingestion is associated with vivid visual hallucinations, euphoria, and dissociative states. If supportive contact, "talking down," and benzodiazepines are not alleviating symptoms of persistent psychosis, then which antipsychotics should be considered?

1. Chlorpromazine

2. Thioridazine

3. Clozapine

4. Thiothixene

◼ **DIRECTIONS: For questions 38–14 through 38–20, select the single best answer.**

38–14. Ms. B. is a 58-year-old who underwent emergency exploratory laparotomy and resection of the head of the pancreas for carcinoma of the pancreas. Preoperatively, she was on imipramine 250 mg/day for a persistent depression, and she was taking diphenhydramine for a "head cold." Postoperatively, she has received a total of 80 mg of chlorpromazine for severe hiccups. In the ICU, she is agitated, confused, and "talking to people who aren't there." Her vital signs are BP 120/75 on no inotropic supports, P 78 beats per minute, and Temp 36.8°C, and her PaO_2 is 85% on 21% oxygen. What are the diagnosis and treatment?

1. Atropine psychosis, and treatment consists of holding all anticholinergic medications and possibly administration of physostigmine.

2. "ICU" psychosis, and treatment consists of low-dose haloperidol.

3. Atropine psychosis, and treatment consists of giving anticholinergic medications.

4. Neuroleptic malignant syndrome, and treatment consists of sodium dantrolene.

38–15. What is the treatment of choice for shared psychotic disorder?

1. High-potency antipsychotics
2. Low-potency antipsychotics
3. Antidepressants
4. Separation of the dyadic partners

38–16. How long must psychosis persist in psychostimulant-induced psychosis before treatment with a neuroleptic is initiated?

1. Treatment is initiated immediately.
2. The psychosis must persist for more than 24 hours.
3. The psychosis must persist for more than 36 hours.
4. Treatment with a neuroleptic is never warranted.

38–17. Alcoholic psychotic disorder generally arises how long after the last intake of alcohol or significant reduction in intake?

1. 8 hours
2. 16 hours
3. 24 hours
4. 48 hours

38–18. What is the treatment of choice for the persecutory delusions, emotional lability, depersonalization, and amnesia associated with cannabis-induced psychosis?

1. Lorazepam
2. Supportive environment
3. Clonazepam
4. Clonidine hydrochloride

38–19. What percentage of patients with schizophrenia abuse drugs or alcohol?

1. 25%
2. 50%
3. 75%
4. 10%

38–20. Mr. K. is a 35-year-old with auditory hallucinations, social withdrawal, poor personal hygiene, and persistent ego-dystonic intrusive thoughts who exhibits several rituals involving counting. He currently is receiving clozapine after failure to respond to eight different treatment regimens. What additional medication may be added?

1. Haloperidol
2. Lorazepam
3. Fluoxetine
4. Imipramine

■ **ANSWERS:**

38–1. **Answer: B (1 and 3).** Approximately 50% of patients with brief psychotic disorder and 66% of patients with schizophreniform disorder will go on to develop schizophrenia. The presence of postpartum psychosis is more common in women with a history of bipolar disorder. The exact percentage of women who develop bipolar disorder after experiencing a postpartum psychosis is not known. Approximately 50% of women who have one episode of postpartum psychosis will experience psychosis after subsequent deliveries. The number of patients with a drug-induced psychosis who develop secondary psychotic or affective disorders is difficult to ascertain because frequently it is difficult to determine which disorder was the initial one.

38–2. **Answer: E (All).** Urine drug screens should be routinely obtained from patients who present with an initial episode of psychosis and, based on clinical judgment, from patients experiencing an apparent exacerbation of an existing psychotic disorder. Electroencephalograms (EEGs) may be helpful in ruling in a seizure disorder. A seizure disorder may exist even in the presence of a normal EEG. Nasopharyngeal leads are usually necessary to ascertain the presence of temporal lobe conduction abnormalities. Anatomic imaging, such as MRI or computed tomography (CT) scans, will help determine the presence of space-occupying lesions. Tertiary syphilis was nearly eradicated by the late 1960s but has once again presented itself as a cause of psychosis, so a VDRL should be obtained. An HIV test should be obtained if the clinical history is suggestive of risk factors such as unprotected sexual intercourse or intravenous drug use.

38–3. **Answer: E (All).** Brief psychotic disorder is associated with an increased incidence of suicide compared with in the general population. The first step in treatment of a patient with this disorder is containment in a safe and secure environment, which does not, however, necessarily imply an inpatient psychiatric unit. Interviewing the family and significant others in the patient's life is important in gaining historical information concerning the patient and in determining what factors could be precipitating the psychosis. Educating and strengthening the patient's support system are also critical. Benzodiazepines, such as diazepam (Valium), may resolve symptoms associated with acute stress-related psychosis. As with other new-onset psychoses, brief psychotic disorder may respond quite well to a low dose of antipsychotic medication such as haloperidol (Haldol).

38–4. **Answer: E (All).** Treatment-resistant brief reactive psychosis may be treated with ECT, as may schizoaffective disorder, depressed type, and treatment-resistant schizophrenia. In the case of schizophrenia, an acute exacerbation with psychotic symptoms of less than 6 months offers the best prognosis for treatment with ECT. Delusional disorder is not generally responsive to treatment with ECT; however, when there is a strong family history of affective disorder and/or many depressive symptoms, this treatment may be considered.

38–5. **Answer: A (1, 2, and 3).** The patient does not meet the criteria for a brief psychotic disorder because her symptoms have lasted for more than 1 month. Schizophreniform disorder is a possibility, because the psychotic symptoms have lasted for more than 1 month and less than 6 months at the time of evaluation and because the patient has maintained her marriage and employment.

Deterioration in social or vocational function is not a requirement for the diagnosis of schizophreniform disorder. The history is inadequate to rule out postpartum psychosis. Drug-induced psychosis is a diagnosis of exclusion. A thorough history and a negative urine drug screen are required. Even over-the-counter and prescription drugs used appropriately may induce a psychosis in some vulnerable individuals.

38–6. **Answer: D (Only 4).** Drug-induced psychosis has a male-to-female diagnostic ratio of 4 to 1. Schizophrenia, schizoaffective disorder, and schizophreniform disorder all have equal gender distributions.

38–7. **Answer: E (All).** For all medical disorders, the number one reason for poor efficacy for a proven modality is patient noncompliance. Carbamazepine autoinduces its metabolism by the hepatic cytochrome P450 system. There is some evidence that carbamazepine may also lower neuroleptic levels, necessitating an increase in the neuroleptic. Lithium and the anticonvulsants appear to work through different patterns of efficacy, and switching or combining mood stabilizers may reduce psychosis and cycling between affective states.

38–8. **Answer: E (All).** Individuals with delusional disorder rarely come into treatment and may only do so if coerced by family members, employers, or, especially in erotomania or pathological jealousy, by the legal system. The manner in which these patients arrive for treatment and their reluctance to be treated have contributed to the absence of any efficacy studies. Many of these patients may feel overwhelmed by other aspects of their environments or isolated and lonely. Supportive, life-issue–oriented psychotherapy with a well-trained, empathic psychotherapist may alleviate some of the secondary legal and social difficulties. Case reports of success with pimozide for the treatment of erotomania and pathological jealousy have emerged in the literature. Low-dose antipsychotics may also be helpful for the tactile hallucinations that occasionally accompany this disorder. In some cases, body dysmorphic disorder may be indistinguishable from delusional disorder, somatic type, and may respond to serotonin reuptake inhibitors.

38–9. **Answer: D (Only 4).** Neuroleptic treatment is the hallmark of pharmacotherapeutic treatment of schizophreniform disorder, and a neuroleptic with the addition of lithium, carbamazepine, valproic acid, and/or antidepressant medication is the pharmacological treatment of choice for schizoaffective disorder. Unlike the adjustment-related mood disorders of schizophrenia, the affective component of schizoaffective disorder is relatively unresponsive to psychotherapy. The use of individual and family therapy in both schizophreniform disorder and schizoaffective disorder improves the overall outcome.

38–10. **Answer: A (1, 2, and 3).** Patients who have stimulant-induced psychosis are particularly vulnerable to the autonomic instability of neuroleptic malignant syndrome and seizures. Low doses of high-potency neuroleptics are used to treat psychosis that persists for longer than 24 hours.

38–11. **Answer: A (1, 2, and 3).** Patients with schizophrenia are not able to tolerate the traditional confrontational approach to drug and alcohol treatment. They are likely to leave treatment or experience an exacerbation of their psychosis. The treatment must be long-term and continuous despite the patient's intermittent contact and alliance. Locating the appropriate Alcoholics Anonymous or

Narcotics Anonymous group can be essential in the treatment of the dually diagnosed patient. The patient's social support can be enlisted to help maintain both sobriety and neuroleptic therapy. The longer these patients are sober, the more likely contact with their social support will be positively reinforcing. Treatment with neuroleptics should be continued.

38–12. **Answer: E (All).** Patients with schizophrenia and substance abuse or dependence must receive treatment for the substance abuse or dependence in addition to treatment for their schizophrenia. The treatments outlined are standard therapies.

38–13. **Answer: A (1, 2, and 3).** The serotonergic hallucinogens are thought to produce their psychotic effects by stimulating the 5-HT$_2$ receptor. Low-potency neuroleptics such as chlorpromazine, thioridazine, and clozapine are highly effective in blocking the 5-HT$_2$ receptor. Chlorpromazine is the most widely used of this group of antipsychotics.

38–14. **Answer: 1.** This patient presents with a typical history for atropine-induced psychosis. She has received or ingested at least three different anticholinergic compounds—imipramine, diphenhydramine, and chlorpromazine—in a brief period of time and has experienced the somatic stress of a major surgical procedure. (She may also have received atropine preoperatively to decrease secretions and vomiting, an approach that is used when a patient who has ingested food recently is undergoing an emergent procedure.) Treatment consists of withdrawing the anticholinergic medications, and if her symptoms persist, she may need physostigmine 1–4 mg intravenously. Sodium dantrolene is a treatment for neuroleptic malignant syndrome, and this patient is not exhibiting muscle rigidity or autonomic instability associated with neuroleptic malignant syndrome. The patient is at risk for developing a brief reactive psychosis in her present condition and environment.

38–15. **Answer: 4.** Shared psychotic disorder usually occurs in a socially isolated couple when the dominant member has a significant psychiatric disorder that usually involves some thought or perceptual disturbance. The treatment of the disorder involves treating the dominant individual's disorder and separation of the dyad. In the case of parents and children, this may involve hospitalizing one or both individuals or foster care for the child.

38–16. **Answer: 2.** When psychosis has extended beyond 24 hours and no response to benzodiazepines has occurred, then neuroleptics may be indicated.

38–17. **Answer: 4.** Alcoholic withdrawal may begin with tremor and lightheadedness within 8 hours after the last intake of alcohol or reduction in the blood alcohol level below that usually experienced by the patient. Alcoholic psychosis, characterized by a high frequency of visual hallucinations, generally arises within 48 hours after the last drink or decrease in intake.

38–18. **Answer: 2.** In general, no pharmacological supports are required for the persecutory delusions, emotional lability, depersonalization, and amnesia associated with cannabis-induced psychosis, and this disorder will remit following the cessation of drug use.

38–19. **Answer: 2.** Approximately 47% to 50% of patients with schizophrenia abuse at least one substance. The most commonly abused substance is alcohol.

38–20. **Answer: 3.** The patient described has mixed features of schizophrenia and obsessive-compulsive disorder, known as "schizo-obsessive." The prognosis is poorer than that for schizophrenia. Treatment is usually difficult. The addition of fluoxetine (Prozac) may lessen the counting rituals.

CHAPTER 39

Treatment Settings: Providing a Continuum of Care for Patients With Schizophrenia and Related Disorders

■ **DIRECTIONS: For questions 39–1 through 39–3, select the single best answer.**

39–1. Modern treatment of schizophrenia involves which modality?

1. Moral treatment
2. Mental Hygiene Movement
3. Medical management
4. Medical management in combination with flexible psychotherapy, skills training, and family therapy

39–2. Which of the following conditions or symptoms warrants long-term hospitalization?

1. Cycling in and out of hospitals for brief hospitalizations
2. Severe antisocial behaviors
3. A previous long-term hospitalization
4. Significantly below-average intelligence

39–3. What are the goals of long-term hospitalization?

1. To control persistent, treatment-resistant psychotic states
2. To "break through" extreme denial of illness and treatment resistance
3. To understand symptoms relative to the individual's environment and self
4. For rapid neuroleptization of agitated patients

■ **ANSWERS:**

39–1. **Answer: 4.** Moral treatment was practiced in the 19th century and focused on the humanitarian approach to patients and their environment. The social system of treatment continued in the United States with Dorothea Dix and the

Mental Hygiene Movement. Medical management and institutional care were emphasized in the 1940s to the 1960s. In the 1960s, deinstitutionalization was initiated, and today the majority of patients with schizophrenia are treated as outpatients with a combination of medical management, flexible psychotherapy, skills training, and family therapy.

39–2.   **Answer: 1.** Severe antisocial behaviors, substance abuse, organically based psychopathology, significantly below–average intelligence, and a previous long-term hospitalization argue against a long-term hospitalization. Patients who are chronically suicidal, who cycle in and out of the hospital for brief admissions, who cannot negotiate the discharge phase of a brief hospitalization, who demonstrate persistent outpatient noncompliance, or who have a significant characterological disorder may benefit from long-term hospitalization.

39–3.   **Answer: 3.** The goals of long-term hospitalization are more nebulous than those of brief or emergent hospitalization. Patients who manifest extreme violence or denial of illness and treatment resistance are probably not suited to long-term hospitalization and are better treated in a custodial setting. Rapid neuroleptization is rarely used in this era. In an emergency situation, a neuroleptic in combination with a benzodiazepine is usually used to decrease psychotic agitation. Long-term hospitalization provides an opportunity to find and titrate medications, work with comorbid symptoms such as affective and characterological disorders, and establish a therapeutic alliance in which these patients can come to a better understanding of their symptoms in the context of the environment and their inner world.

SECTION 6

Mood Disorders

CHAPTER 40

Antidepressant and Antimanic Medications

◼ **DIRECTIONS: For questions 40–1 through 40–7, select the single best answer.**

40–1. Which of the following statements is **true** regarding antidepressant medications?

    1. Antidepressant medications restore function without altering the pathological state.

    2. Antidepressant medications have a profound effect on the pathological state.

    3. Antidepressant medications will treat the etiology of the depression.

    4. Antidepressant medications may significantly alter the patient's internal world.

40–2. When should antidepressant medication be immediately used?

    1. When the patient is most reluctant to take medication

    2. When there is a strong family history of mood disorder

    3. When there is minimal suicide risk

    4. When the patient is an adolescent

40–3. The acute treatment phase includes making a diagnosis and a decision to treat with medications, psychotherapy, and/or other therapeutic modalities. What is the usual length of the acute treatment phase?

    1. 1 to 3 weeks

    2. 4 to 12 weeks

    3. 13 to 36 weeks

    4. Approximately 4 months

40–4. What percentage of patients with a major depressive episode respond to medication treatment?

    1. 25%

    2. 45%–60%

    3. 75%–80%

    4. > 90%

40–5.   Monoamine oxidase inhibitors (MAOIs) are among the oldest of the antidepressant medications. The initial enthusiasm following their discovery in the late 1950s was tempered by reports of serious side effects—specifically, interactions with foods and drugs. Which of the following drugs or foods will interact with an MAOI to produce a delirium?

    1. Bacon

    2. Chianti wine

    3. Meperidine

    4. Fluoxetine

40–6.   Monoamine oxidase inhibitors inhibit the primary enzyme responsible for extracellular degradation of monoamines, resulting in increased levels of neurotransmitters available at the synapses. There are two forms of the MAOI receptors in the central nervous sytem: type A and type B. Which of the following MAOIs are type-A receptor inhibitors?

    1. Phenelzine

    2. Deprenyl

    3. Moclobemide

    4. Isocarboxazid

40–7.   Antidepressant medications require a period of time before they may be effective in an individual patient. The patient can be told to expect a response how long after a full dose has been achieved?

    1. Immediately

    2. Up to 6 weeks

    3. 5 to 10 days

    4. 10 to 21 days

■ DIRECTIONS: For questions 40–8 through 40–22, indicate

    A if answers 1, 2, and 3 are correct.

    B if answers 1 and 3 are correct.

    C if answers 2 and 4 are correct.

    D if only answer 4 is correct.

    E if all are correct.

40–8.   The majority of the antidepressant medications are metabolized through the hepatic microsomal systems. Which of the following hepatic enzymes are found in individuals who are slow metabolizers of medications?

    1. P450 IIA3

    2. P450 IIC

    3. P450 IIA4

    4. P450 IID6

40–9.   Ms. J. is a 65-year-old woman who has been diagnosed with major depressive disorder, recurrent. She also has a history of having fractured her left hip. Which of the medications would you **not** want to use with this woman?

1. Imipramine
2. Nortriptyline
3. Desipramine
4. Sertraline

40–10. Which of the following statements are **true** regarding the use of amoxapine in the treatment of major depressive disorder?

1. Amoxapine is a tricyclic antidepressant.
2. Amoxapine is reported to cause extrapyramidal reactions.
3. Amoxapine is a norepinephrine reuptake inhibitor.
4. Amoxapine is associated with a high frequency of seizures.

40–11. Which of the following medications have been approved by the Food and Drug Administration (FDA) for the treatment of bipolar disorder?

1. Carbamazepine
2. Valproic acid
3. Clonidine hydrochloride
4. Lithium

40–12. Ms. S. presents with a 48-hour history of acute agitation, auditory and visual hallucinations, psychomotor agitation, and poor sleep habits. She has been awake for the past 96 hours and has had little appetite. Ms. S. is running about the emergency room, dumping over gurneys and talking about being the mother of Mary and the son of Christ. Which of the following laboratory and physiological signs and symptoms would be necessary before treatment of this woman?

1. Urine drug screen
2. Electrocardiogram
3. Serum electrolytes, blood urea nitrogen, and creatinine levels
4. She cannot be treated because she is not currently able to give consent for medications.

40–13. The teratogenic effects of medications are always a concern to physicians and their patients. Which of the following medications has documented teratogenic effects?

1. Carbamazepine
2. Lithium
3. Valproic acid
4. Imipramine

40–14. A young woman who is currently being treated with carbamazepine and lithium for rapid-cycling bipolar disorder presents with bullous skin lesions covering her entire body. The lesions began on her trunk and quickly spread. Her temperature is now 101°F. Which of the following statements would explain this clinical description?

1. She has been shooting up heroin.

    2. This disorder is unrelated to her current drug consumption.

    3. She may have gotten hold of some "bad street drugs."

    4. She has Stevens-Johnson syndrome.

40–15. Major depressive episodes are now considered to be chronic illnesses subject to recurrences and relapses. Which of the following statements are **false** regarding maintenance therapy?

    1. The most studied medication in maintenance management of major depressive episodes is imipramine.

    2. Maintenance dosage should be the same as that used in the acute treatment phase.

    3. Maintenance doses should be continued for a minimum of 6 months.

    4. Rates of depressive relapse appear to be higher when antidepressant drugs are discontinued rapidly compared with when these drugs are slowly tapered.

40–16. Which of the following statements are **true** regarding norepinephrine reuptake blockade?

    1. Nausea occurs because of norepinephrine reuptake blockade.

    2. Tremor occurs secondary to norepinephrine reuptake blockade.

    3. Extreme sedation may occur secondary to norepinephrine reuptake blockade.

    4. Tachycardia may occur secondary to norepinephrine reuptake blockade.

40–17. Plasma drug level monitoring is most important when

    1. Clinical signs of toxicity are present.

    2. There are a higher-than-expected number of side effects.

    3. The patient is not responding.

    4. The patient is suspected of noncompliance.

40–18. Late-occurring side effects of the antidepressant and antimanic medications include which of the following?

    1. Weight gain

    2. Sexual dysfunction

    3. Myoclonus

    4. Orthostatic hypotension

40–19. A patient presents with the following conditions: He has acute gastrointestinal distress and a severe headache. He is highly agitated and moving rapidly about the emergency room. His temperature is 103°F, heart rate is 125 beats per minute, respiratory rate is 18 breaths per minute, and blood pressure is 80/60. Which of the following statements are **true** regarding this patient?

    1. This syndrome may progress to convulsions and coma.

    2. This patient is at no risk of further sequelae.

    3. This patient may have been taking an MAOI as well as fluoxetine.

    4. This syndrome is not potentially lethal.

40–20. Cardiovascular effects may be the most lethal of all the effects seen with a tricyclic antidepressant. What type of electrocardiogram findings are consistent with use of a tricyclic antidepressant?

1. Heart rate greater than 100 beats per minute
2. PR interval greater than 0.2 msec
3. Widening of the QRS
4. Appearance of a Q prime wave

40–21. Which of the following medications have therapeutic windows associated with their efficacy?

1. Carbamazepine
2. Nortriptyline
3. Valproic acid
4. Imipramine

40–22. Therapeutic levels of lithium range from 0.5 to 1.5 nmol/L. Which of the following statements are **valid** regarding lithium levels?

1. Patients maintained with lithium levels between 0.4 and 0.6 nmol/L are at least three times more likely to have recurrences of mania.
2. Therapeutic lithium levels should always be maintained between 0.8 and 1.0 nmol/L.
3. Side effects may occur at therapeutic lithium levels between 1.0 and 1.3 nmol/L.
4. Any lithium level between 0.5 and 1.5 nmol/L is considered acceptable for the treatment of acute mania.

■ **ANSWERS:**

40–1. **Answer: 1.** Antidepressant medications simply restore function without altering the pathological state, analogously to the nonspecific anti-inflammatory effects of corticosteroids and the effects of insulin in the treatment of other medical conditions. The internal world and intrapsychic issues are not dealt with by the use of antidepressant medications. The medications do not make permanent alterations in the neuroanatomy of the patient.

40–2. **Answer: 2.** Those patients who have a strong family history of mood disorders should be treated immediately with an antidepressant medication to prevent a deepening of the depressive disorder. Furthermore, when a patient's symptoms are very mild or the patient feels very strongly against the use of the medication, the medication should be postponed. There are limited data to support the use of antidepressant medications in the adolescent population.

40–3. **Answer: 2.** The acute treatment phase generally lasts 4 to 12 weeks.

40–4. **Answer: 2.** Approximately 45%–60% of all patients treated with antidepressants will have at least a partial response to medications.

40–5.   **Answer: 3.** When an MAOI is combined with meperidine, a delirium will result that may be life-threatening. Less severe interactions have been reported with other opioid agonists such as morphine and partial agonists such as buprenorphine, butorphanol, and pentazocine.

40–6.   **Answer: 3.** Agents constituting a new category of selective reversible inhibitors of MAO-A are being developed. Moclobemide and brofaromine are examples of such agents currently under consideration for FDA approval. Selective MAO-B inhibitors, such as deprenyl, which is used to treat Parkinson's disease, are relatively ineffective for the treatment of depression. The original MAOIs (i.e., phenelzine, tranylcypromine, and isocarboxazid) are all irreversible inhibitors of both the MAO-A and MAO-B receptors.

40–7.   **Answer: 4.** A period of approximately 10–21 days of antidepressant medications after full dose has been achieved is required before the patient will experience beneficial signs and symptoms.

40–8.   **Answer: D (Only 4).** Cytochrome P450 IID6 has been shown to have two subtypes (isoenzymes) as a result of a genetic polymorphism. One subtype of P450 IID6 causes slow metabolization of the antidepressant medications, resulting in higher plasma concentrations. This increase in plasma levels is especially apparent with serotonin reuptake inhibitor medications, most of which are potent inhibitors of the P450 IID6 system.

40–9.   **Answer: B (1 and 3).** Nortriptyline, a tricyclic antidepressant, has a well-deserved reputation for being better tolerated in the elderly, with much less orthostatic hypotension, leading to a decreased risk of falls. Sertraline is a selective serotonin reuptake inhibitor (SSRI) that causes virtually no orthostatic hypotension. Both imipramine and desipramine are secondary amines with orthostatic hypotension as a major side effect, and this would be a limiting feature in the use of these medications in an older woman, especially after she has suffered a hip fracture. Hip fractures are a significant cause of mortality and morbidity in the older female population.

40–10.   **Answer: E (All).** Amoxapine is a tricyclic antidepressant. Studies have shown that it has the same efficacy as a combination of a traditional tricyclic antidepressant and an antipsychotic drug in the treatment of major depressive disorder with psychotic features. Amoxapine is a potent dopaminergic type-2 receptor blocker. It has been reported to cause extrapyramidal reactions and tardive dyskinesia, a finding that is consistent with its dopaminergic properties. It also is associated with a high frequency of seizures, and it is lethal in overdose. The maximum dose of amoxapine is 650 mg/day.

40–11.   **Answer: D (Only 4).** Lithium is currently the only drug approved by the FDA for the acute- or maintenance-phase treatment of bipolar disorder.

40–12.   **Answer: A (1, 2, and 3).** The patient presented in this vignette may be having a drug intoxication or withdrawal disorder or an acute psychosis secondary to schizophrenia. She might also be experiencing a manic psychosis secondary to a bipolar disorder, a psychotic disorder not otherwise specified, or a brief reactive psychosis of unspecified etiology. Drug reactions such as reactions to phencyclidine (PCP) and ketamine should not be treated with lithium, carbamazepine, or valproic acid. Such interactions may be treated by talking the patient down; providing a quiet, secluded room; and administering benzodiazepines.

This patient also may be experiencing a delirium secondary to a renal failure of acute or chronic onset. There is not enough history provided in this vignette to rule out any of these disorders.

40–13. **Answer: A (1, 2, and 3).** Both carbamazepine and valproic acid are associated with spina bifida (an incidence of 1%), low birth weight, and small head circumference. Lithium is associated with Ebstein's cardiac malformation. Imipramine has no known teratogenic effects but is not recommended for use during pregnancy.

40–14. **Answer: D (Only 4).** The clinical description provided is of Stevens-Johnson syndrome, a relatively rare but life-threatening dermatological reaction. Patients with this syndrome must be admitted to a burn unit, where they can receive appropriate treatment.

40–15. **Answer: E (All).** The most studied medication in the maintenance treatment of major depressive episodes is imipramine, although there have been anecdotal reports and small clinical studies on the use of the other tricyclic antidepressants as well as the serotonin reuptake inhibitors for this purpose. Maintenance medication should be continued at the full antidepressant level. It has been shown that the relapse rate is 20%–30%, whereas the relapse rate for placebo approaches 80% over 1 to 3 years of treatment. The relapse rate for depressive disorder appears to be much higher when antidepressant medications are discontinued rapidly compared with when a slow (3- to 4-week) taper is effected.

40–16. **Answer: C (2 and 4).** Norepinephrine reuptake blockade can cause tremor, tachycardia, and erectile and ejaculatory dysfunction. Serotonin reuptake inhibition can cause nausea, anxiety, or sedation.

40–17. **Answer: E (All).** Plasma drug levels are most important when assessment is being made of the reasons for lack of response, including noncompliance. Patients who experience multiple side effects may have higher-than-anticipated serum levels at a given dose of medication. When toxicity is suspected, a level should be obtained.

40–18. **Answer: A (1, 2, and 3).** Orthostatic hypotension may be seen after the first dose of antidepressant or antimanic medication. This is especially common with a tricyclic antidepressant that has a higher anticholinergic effect. Weight gain is more common with tertiary tricyclic antidepressants than with MAOIs, but it may be seen with SSRIs after long-term treatment. Myoclonus or tremors can occur with SSRIs, MAOIs, and tricyclics but is most common with the use of lithium. Sexual dysfunction may be reported most often as a late effect, because at that point patients are generally having fewer signs and symptoms of a major depressive disorder and, consequently, less inhibition of sexual desire.

40–19. **Answer: B (1 and 3).** This clinical picture is known as the *serotonin syndrome*, a hypermetabolic state that consists of gastrointestinal distress, headache, agitation, hyperpyrexia, increased heart rate, increased respiratory rate, hypotension or hypertension, muscular rigidity, myoclonus, convulsions, coma, and possibly death. Two weeks should elapse between discontinuation of a serotonin reuptake inhibitor and initiation of an MAOI, except in the case of fluoxetine, with which a 6-week interval is required between discontinuation of the fluoxetine and initiation of the MAOI.

40–20. **Answer: A (1, 2, and 3).** With tricyclic antidepressants, there is dose-related increase in heart rate and prolongation of ventricular conduction (increase in PR to greater than 0.2 msec, increase in QRS). In addition, orthostatic hypotension and ventriculo-arrhythmia may be seen. A Q prime wave is seen in Wolff-Parkinson-White syndrome.

40–21. **Answer: A (1, 2, and 3).** Nortriptyline has a therapeutic window with plasma levels between 50 and 150 ng/mL. Carbamazepine has a therapeutic window of 4–12 µg/mL, and valproic acid has a therapeutic window of 50–100 µg/mL. The therapeutic level of imipramine, desipramine, and amitriptyline is at least 150 ng/mL. Plasma levels of desipramine, imipramine, and amitriptyline above 300 ng/mL are associated with risk of potentially lethal side effects such as cardiac conduction abnormalities or seizures.

40–22. **Answer: E (All).** Lithium levels are related to both the rate of relapse and the extent of side effects. Those patients who are maintained on relatively high lithium levels of 0.8–1.0 nmol/L had a significantly lower (i.e., three times lower) rate of recurrence of mania than did those maintained on levels between 0.4 and 0.6 nmol/L. However, lithium levels are related to the number of side effects: the higher the level, the more side effects. For the maintenance treatment of acute mania, a lithium level between 0.8 and 1.0 nmol/L is recommended.

CHAPTER 41

Reeducative Psychotherapies

■ **DIRECTIONS: For questions 41–1 through 41–11, select the single best answer.**

41–1. What is the usual length of time used in reeducative models of psychotherapy?

　　1. 4–8 weeks

　　2. 8–16 weeks

　　3. 16–32 weeks

　　4. There is no time limit.

41–2. Who is credited with providing the basis for the development of interpersonal psychotherapy?

　　1. Sigmund Freud

　　2. Aaron T. Beck

　　3. B. F. Skinner

　　4. Adolph Meyer

41–3. Which of the following does **not** apply to behavior therapy?

　　1. Social learning theory

　　2. Social casework

　　3. Operant conditioning

　　4. Classical conditioning

41–4. Which of the following therapies emphasizes the overall role of depressed persons within their nuclear family and environment?

　　1. Behavior therapy

　　2. Cognitive therapy

　　3. Interpersonal psychotherapy

　　4. None of the above

41–5. Interactions between therapist and patient are central to which of the following modalities?

　　1. Cognitive therapy

　　2. Analytic therapy

    3. Behavior therapy

    4. Interpersonal psychotherapy

41–6. Behavior therapy emphasizes the reciprocity between the depressed patient's behavior and the environment. Which of the following occurs in the relationships of the depressed patient?

    1. Significant others are empathic.

    2. Significant others avoid the patient.

    3. Significant others become overinvolved.

    4. Significant others become highly supportive.

41–7. Unconscious patterns are important in which of the following therapeutic modalities?

    1. Behavior therapy

    2. Interpersonal psychotherapy

    3. Cognitive therapy

    4. None of the above

41–8. Which of the following are used to assess quality of cognitive therapy sessions?

    1. Mood chart

    2. Daily record of dysfunctional thoughts

    3. Structured clinical interview

    4. Cognitive Therapy Scale

41–9. In general, a Hamilton Rating Scale for Depression score of what level will predict a poor response to psychotherapy as the sole treatment for depression?

    1. 5

    2. 10

    3. 15

    4. 20

41–10. How many sessions should be allotted to a time-limited cognitive therapy?

    1. 8

    2. 16

    3. 24

    4. There is no predetermined number.

41–11. Which of the following is the best-studied psychological treatment for depression?

    1. Cognitive therapy

    2. Group therapy

    3. Interpersonal psychotherapy

    4. Behavior therapy

DIRECTIONS: For questions 41–12 through 41–19, indicate

    A if answers 1, 2, and 3 are correct.

    B if answers 1 and 3 are correct.

    C if answers 2 and 4 are correct.

    D if only answer 4 is correct.

    E if all are correct.

41–12. What are the usual themes in interpersonal psychotherapy?

    1. Unresolved grief

    2. Social role disputes

    3. Interpersonal deficits

    4. Deficient social reinforcement

41–13. Relaxation training is widely used to deal with which of the following symptoms?

    1. Anxiety

    2. Sadness

    3. Insomnia

    4. Poor concentration

41–14. Which of the following patients would be suitable for psychotherapy as a first-line treatment for depression?

    1. A 17-year-old gifted high-school senior who is vehemently opposed to "putting any impurities in my system" and who has met the criteria for mild major depression for the past 4 weeks

    2. A 55-year-old woman who has been intermittently depressed for the past 5 years

    3. A 26-year-old married graduate student who has been moderately depressed for 1 week

    4. A 28-year-old single high-school dropout who has been depressed for 1 week and attempted suicide 2 days before presenting to the clinic

41–15. According to the theory underlying behavior therapy, the neurobehavioral disturbances experienced by depressed individuals are consequences of which of the following?

    1. Thinking gloomy unpleasant thoughts about themselves, their world, and their future

    2. Experiencing prolonged unresolvable stress

    3. Having state-dependent errors in information processing

    4. Developing hopeless/helpless beliefs

41–16. What attributes in the therapist are associated with better outcomes?

    1. Having technical competence in structuring therapy

    2. Having years of therapeutic experience

    3. Having high levels of core skills

    4. Being a sympathetic person

41–17. Which of the following conditions argue against a positive outcome in cognitive therapy?

1. Having a personality disorder
2. Being male
3. Being unmarried
4. Having a single episode of depression

41–18. Which of the following have been specifically modified to treat hospitalized depressed patients?

1. Expressive therapy
2. Behavior therapy
3. Interpersonal psychotherapy
4. Cognitive therapy

41–19. Compared with pharmacotherapy, psychological treatments offer which advantages?

1. A more rapid amelioration of symptoms
2. No exposure to cardiac, gastrointestinal, or central nervous system side effects
3. Better efficacy if there is evidence of a pretreatment electroencephalographic sleep architecture abnormality
4. Better amelioration of vocational and interpersonal aspects of depression

■ ANSWERS:

41–1. **Answer: 2.** Reeducative psychotherapies such as behavior therapy, cognitive therapy, and interpersonal psychotherapy are time limited, lasting 8 to 16 weeks. The goal of each therapy is to achieve relief of symptoms.

41–2. **Answer: 4.** Sigmund Freud is credited with developing psychoanalysis. Aaron T. Beck created cognitive-behavior therapy (CBT). B. F. Skinner is well known for his work with behavioral investigations. Adolph Meyer provided the basis for the development of interpersonal psychotherapy.

41–3. **Answer: 2.** Interpersonal psychotherapy draws heavily on social casework, whereas behavior therapy is rooted in social learning theory, operant conditioning, and classical conditioning.

41–4. **Answer: 3.** Interpersonal psychotherapy addresses the role of depressed persons within their nuclear family, social relationships, and workplace. Behavior therapy focuses on how individuals manage their behavior. Cognitive therapy deals with the impact of negative cognitions on those relationships.

41–5. **Answer: 2.** Transference/countertransference and other aspects of the patient-therapist relationship are central to psychoanalytic therapy. The ability to competently conduct interpersonal psychotherapy is correlated with the ability to establish a working alliance and to provide empathy and genuineness. In behavior therapy, the relationship between therapist and patient is not directly addressed. Cognitive therapists, like those using interpersonal psychotherapy, establish a working alliance.

41–6. **Answer: 2.** Acute changes in mood evoke sympathy and support from significant others. Sustained contact with a depressed person results in withdrawal and avoidance of family members and peers.

41–7. **Answer: 3.** According to cognitive theory, pathological schemas are unconscious, nonobservable constructs that arise from adverse early experiences.

41–8. **Answer: 4.** The mood chart is a daily charting of affect, medications, sleep, psychotic symptoms, and work impairment. The daily record of dysfunctional thoughts is used to teach patients about their negative cognitions. The structured clinical interview is a diagnostic interview. The Cognitive Therapy Scale is used to assess the technical fidelity and quality of the cognitive therapy sessions.

41–9. **Answer: 4.** Patients scoring 20 or higher on the Hamilton Rating Scale for Depression do not respond as well to psychotherapy as those with a score below 20. In fact, psychotherapy alone was as effective as treatment with pharmacotherapy combined with psychotherapy in those patients with a score of less than 20.

41–10. **Answer: 4.** The exact number of sessions for a time-limited therapy process should be based on clinical information. In one study, only 10% of patients who terminated their individual cognitive therapy after achieving Hamilton scores of ≤ 6 for 8 weeks had relapsed at 1-year follow-up, compared with 50% of patients who had terminated without meeting this clinical criterion.

41–11. **Answer: 1.** Cognitive therapy is the most studied psychological treatment modality for depression.

41–12. **Answer: A (1, 2, and 3).** Interpersonal psychotherapists focus on unresolved grief, social role disputes, interpersonal deficits, and social role transitions. Behavior therapists address deficient social reinforcement, poor social skills, and inefficient problem-solving strategies.

41–13. **Answer: B (1 and 3).** Anxiety and insomnia are the primary symptoms dealt with in relaxation training. This technique may have mild antidepressant effects.

41–14. **Answer: B (1 and 3).** Reeducative psychotherapies are most effective as a single modality in those patients whose depression is not melancholic, severe, or recurrent. Sufficient social support and psychological mindedness are important prognostic factors. There is some evidence to support that younger patients may have more symptom relief with interpersonal psychotherapy than with pharmacotherapy or CBT. Patient preference should be considered in decisions regarding treatment modalities.

41–15. **Answer: C (2 and 4).** Neurobehavioral disturbances are due to prolonged unresolvable stress and/or the development of hopeless/helpless beliefs. CBT posits three types of problems that converge in the depressed person: 1) automatic negative thoughts about the self and the environment, 2) state-dependent errors in information processing, and 3) dysfunctional attitudes and depressogenic schemas.

41–16. **Answer: A (1, 2, and 3).** High levels of technical competence in structuring therapy, years of therapeutic experience, and, in some studies, high levels of core skills are correlated with positive treatment outcomes. Being a sympathetic person may complicate matters, whereas being able to establish a nonjudgmental and empathic atmosphere is helpful in forming a therapeutic alliance.

41–17. **Answer: B (1 and 3).** Negative outcomes and a high dropout rate in cognitive therapy are associated with unmarried status, high pretreatment levels of dysfunctional attitudes, chronicity of symptoms, and comorbid personality disorder. The last-mentioned condition has not been thoroughly investigated, because most studies specifically exclude individuals with an Axis II diagnosis. Men and women are equally responsive to cognitive therapy. Positive correlates include having high levels of learned resourcefulness, being optimistic, being motivated, and having had no previous episodes of depression.

41–18. **Answer: D (Only 4).** Cognitive therapy is the only form of individual psychological treatment to have been specifically modified for treatment of hospitalized depressed patients.

41–19. **Answer: C (2 and 4).** Psychological treatments do not carry the risk of cardiac, gastrointestinal, or central nervous system effects compared with pharmacological treatments. Pharmacological treatments alone more rapidly ameliorate symptoms of depression compared with interpersonal psychotherapy, cognitive therapy, or behavior therapy alone. Combination treatments of pharmacotherapy and psychotherapy have revealed enhanced response rates in some studies. There is some evidence that individuals with an abnormal electroencephalogram (EEG) may not respond as well to interpersonal psychotherapy as those with no EEG abnormality. Psychological therapies are especially useful in ameliorating vocational and interpersonal aspects of depression.

CHAPTER 42

Psychodynamic Psychotherapies

■ **DIRECTIONS: For questions 42–1 through 42–4, indicate**

A if 1, 2, and 3 are correct.

B if 1 and 3 are correct.

C if 2 and 4 are correct.

D if only answer 4 is correct.

E if all are correct.

42–1. Systematic studies on the efficacy of extended dynamic psychotherapy and psychoanalysis with depressed patients

1. Have demonstrated positive response to these modalities.
2. Have demonstrated negative response to these modalities.
3. Have shown mixed results.
4. Have not been conducted.

42–2. The current thinking about the indications for extended dynamic psychotherapy and psychoanalysis include which of the following?

1. Some patients who have failed to respond fully to pharmacotherapy or reeducative psychotherapies
2. Highly perfectionistic and self-critical patients
3. Patients with significant Axis II pathology in addition to major depressive episodes
4. Patients with uncomplicated major depression in the acute phase of treatment

42–3. Which of the following statements are **true** regarding dynamic pharmacotherapy/dynamic clinical management?

1. The core psychodynamic principles of transference, countertransference, and resistance apply to the prescribing of medication in much the same way as they do to psychotherapy.
2. Transference is generally involved when the doctor insists in an authoritarian way that the patient must comply with the doctor's prescribed medication.

3. One form of resistance is manifested by patients who refuse to take the medication because they are convinced that they deserve to be punished for their perceived sins and transgressions.

4. Countertransference is the patient's attribution to the doctor of qualities that belong to a person in the patient's past.

42–4. Dynamic therapy as a modality in the continuation and maintenance phases of the treatment of depression

1. Has been rigorously studied.

2. Is highly effective.

3. Is ineffective.

4. Has not been rigorously studied.

■ **DIRECTIONS: For questions 42–5 through 42–10, match the individual with the psychodynamic theme found in depression as proposed by that individual.**

42–5.	Freud	a.	Concern that internalized representations of parents have been destroyed by one's own destructiveness and greed
42–6.	Klein	b.	Tension between ideals and reality
42–7.	Bibring	c.	Self-fragmentation and response to the failure of parents and other significant persons to provide the patient's self with responses necessary for growth
42–8.	Jacobson	d.	Anger turned inward
42–9.	Arieti	e.	The patient's ego becoming victimized by a cruel superego
42–10.	Kohut	f.	A preexisting ideology that involves living for someone else rather than for oneself

■ **DIRECTIONS: For questions 42–11 through 42–13, select the single best answer.**

42–11. The therapist's interventions in dynamic psychotherapy reside on an expressive-supportive continuum. At the expressive end of the continuum, which of the following is the intervention most associated with exploratory and uncovering strategies?

1. Interpretation

2. Advice

3. Praise

4. Affirmation

42–12. In the prediction study of female-female twin pairs by Kendler and co-workers (1993), what was the most important and influential predictor of a major depressive episode?

1. Neuroticism

2. Genetic factors

     3. Interpersonal relations

     4. Recent stressful events

42–13. Which of the following unconscious meanings is associated with suicidal behavior?

     1. The wish to kill others

     2. The wish for a magical reunion with an idealized and unconditionally loving parental figure

     3. The wish to appease an internalized sadistic tormentor

     4. All of the above

■ ANSWERS:

42–1.   **Answer: D (Only 4).** Whereas limited data are available on brief dynamic psychotherapy, so far no systematic studies of either psychoanalysis or extended dynamic therapy with depressed patients have been conducted. Although these modalities are generally *not* indicated as the exclusive treatment for acute-phase patients with major depression, their efficacy has not been established either way.

42–2.   **Answer: A (1, 2, and 3).** A reanalysis of the data from the National Institute of Mental Health Treatment of Depression Collaborative Research Program suggested that highly perfectionistic and self-critical patients were not likely to respond to either brief pharmacological or brief psychological treatments. For this subgroup of depressed patients, extended psychodynamic approaches may be particularly suited. Patients who fail to respond fully to pharmacotherapy or brief reeducative psychotherapies may also benefit from more extended dynamically oriented treatment. Finally, patients who have significant Axis II pathology in addition to major depressive episodes may require psychoanalysis or extended psychodynamic psychotherapy. A growing body of literature demonstrates that personality disorders complicate the treatment of depression and lead to poorer outcomes with greater residual depressive symptoms as compared with absence of personality disorders.

42–3.   **Answer: B (1 and 3).** Dynamic pharmacotherapy or dynamic clinical management is based on the premise that psychodynamic principles like transference, countertransference, and resistance apply to the prescribing of medication in the same manner as they do to psychotherapy. Transference—not countertransference—involves the patient's attribution to the doctor of qualities that belong to a person in the patient's past. Countertransference involves the tendency of the doctor to experience the patient as someone from the doctor's past. These unconscious attributions of past qualities to the present may affect compliance in the patient as well as the interpersonal manner of the doctor. For example, if the doctor becomes frustrated with the patient for not complying with the prescribed medication, he or she may become increasingly authoritarian. This form of countertransference may, in part, reflect the doctor's experiencing the situation as he or she did a similar event in the past. Resistance to medication may indicate that the patient is highly ambivalent about getting better. Depressed patients, in particular, may feel that they deserve to be punished for their perceived sins and transgressions and therefore do not comply with the prescribed medication.

42–4. **Answer: D (Only 4).** The Depression Guideline Panel (1993) concluded that current studies of the prophylactic effects following acute-phase brief dynamic therapy are too methodologically problematic to allow for any definitive conclusions. No studies on the continuation effects of acute-phase dynamic therapy have been reported. Published reports on the efficacy of maintenance brief dynamic therapy are not sufficiently rigorous to determine whether the modality is useful in that phase.

42–5. Freud: **d**

42–6. Klein: **a**

42–7. Bibring: **b**

42–8. Jacobson: **e**

42–9. Arieti: **f**

42–10. Kohut: **c**

42–11. **Answer: 1.** The expressive-supportive continuum in dynamic psychotherapy is largely defined by the nature of the therapist's interventions and the goals. At the expressive end of the continuum, the therapist seeks to uncover previously unconscious wishes and conflicts. Interpretation is the most expressive intervention designed to make the unconscious issues conscious. Other expressive interventions include confrontation and clarification. At the supportive end of the continuum, the therapist seeks to support the patient's strength and bolster adaptive defenses so that the patient's functioning will improve. Interventions at the supportive end of the continuum include advice, praise, empathic validation, encouragement to elaborate, and affirmation.

42–12. **Answer: 4.** Kendler and co-workers studied 680 female-female twin pairs of known zygosity, and this enabled them to construct a complex and integrated etiological model of depression. Recent stressful events appeared to be the most important and influential predictor of a major depressive episode. Other significant elements were interpersonal relations, genetic factors, and neuroticism.

42–13. **Answer: 4.** Suicidal wishes, in part determined by biological factors, also have psychological meanings for the patient that may be largely unconscious. The patient may experience an internal struggle with a sadistic tormentor and feel that the only solution is to appease the tormentor by committing suicide. Karl Menninger noted that the wish to die is often accompanied by the wish to kill, and the aggression inherent in the act of suicide is readily apparent to survivors left behind. Family members may feel that they were the target of the suicide and that the patient seemed to want to destroy their lives by the act. A common fantasy in suicidal patients is that somewhere an unconditionally loving parent exists who will take care of them. Suicide may have the meaning of a reunion with that idealized and unconditionally loving parent.

CHAPTER 43

Combined Medication and Psychotherapy

■ **DIRECTIONS: For questions 43–1 through 43–9,
indicate whether the statement is true or false.**

43–1. _____ Successful treatment with pharmacotherapy confers a measure of immunity to future depressions.

43–2. _____ Psychotherapy enhances the stability of the patient's response to treatment.

43–3. _____ Cognitive therapy is the best studied of the psychotherapies.

43–4. _____ Patients who receive psychotherapy are more willing to tolerate medication side effects.

43–5. _____ The optimal timing for combining pharmacotherapy and psychotherapy is well studied.

43–6. _____ Severity of depression predicts responsivity to medications.

43–7. _____ Chronicity of depression predicts responsivity to psychotherapy.

43–8. _____ Psychotherapy produces more lasting effects than pharmacotherapy.

43–9. _____ Marital therapy is effective in improving the overall quality of the marital relationship.

■ **DIRECTIONS: For questions 43–10 through 43–14,
select the single best answer.**

43–10. The indication for combined treatment with psychotherapy and medications is

  1. Chronic depression with multiple interpersonal conflicts.

  2. A high level of psychological mindedness regardless of the diagnosis.

  3. A poor response to medications.

  4. Poorly delineated at this time.

43–11. What percentage of individuals with affective disorders will experience multiple episodes during their lifetime?

  1. 90%

  2. 75%

3. 50%

4. 10%

43–12. A study of psychoeducational family therapy with patients who have unipolar or bipolar disorder revealed which of the following results?

1. There was no improvement in symptoms.

2. The results were too complicated to be analyzed.

3. The women with bipolar disorder fared better than the men with bipolar disorder.

4. The men with bipolar disorder fared better than the women with bipolar disorder.

43–13. In general, what have been the effects of combined treatment utilizing interpersonal psychotherapy or behavior therapy and pharmacotherapy?

1. There were no differences between the combined therapeutic modalities.

2. The use of combined therapy produced faster symptom relief.

3. Relapse rates were unaffected by the use of psychotherapy.

4. There was no effect on interpersonal relationships or social skills.

43–14. Which statement is **true** regarding cognitive therapy and relapse rates for depression?

1. The relapse rate for patients treated with cognitive therapy is equal to that of patients maintained on pharmacological agents as assessed at 2-year follow-up.

2. There is no difference in relapse rates for patients treated with pharmacotherapy alone and those treated with psychotherapy alone.

3. The relapse rates for patients treated with psychotherapy are higher than those for patients treated with pharmacotherapy.

4. The relapse rates for patients treated with psychotherapy are significantly lower than those for patients treated with pharmacotherapy.

■ ANSWERS:

43–1. **False** Successful treatment with pharmacotherapy predicts another successful treatment in a future depression but does not confer any immunity.

43–2. **True** Psychotherapy may solidify the response to treatment.

43–3. **True** Cognitive therapy is the best studied of all the psychotherapies.

43–4. **True** Patients who are engaged in psychotherapy tolerate side effects from pharmacotherapy better than do those who are not engaged.

43–5. **False** There are few studies of combined psychotherapy and pharmacotherapy.

43–6. **True** The more severe depressions seem to be the most responsive to pharmacotherapy.

43–7. **False** There is no correlation between chronicity of depression and response to psychotherapy.

43–8. **True** Effects from psychotherapy are longer lasting than effects from pharmacotherapy.

43–9. **True** Marital therapy improves the overall quality of the marital relationship.

43–10. **Answer: 4.** Neither indications nor contraindications for combined treatment are well documented.

43–11. **Answer: 1.** At one time it was believed that 50% of all depressions would be limited to a single episode. New research indicates that up to 90% of individuals will experience multiple episodes.

43–12. **Answer: 3.** The findings of this study suggest a complex interaction between psychopathology, gender, and the type of marital/family therapy utilized. The women with bipolar disorder had improvements in social functioning and symptoms relative to the other groups.

43–13. **Answer: 2.** Despite the numerous methodological difficulties in the study of efficacy of combined therapy, the data suggest that there appears to be some benefit to combined therapies. There is a faster reduction in symptoms, and some studies report a lower rate of relapse at 1- and 2-year follow-up. There also appears to be improvement in social skills and interpersonal relationships.

43–14. **Answer: 1.** The relapse rate for patients who were treated with cognitive therapy is equal to that of patients maintained on antidepressants as assessed at 2-year follow-up.

CHAPTER 44

■

Electroconvulsive Therapy

■ **DIRECTIONS: For questions 44–1 through 44–9, select the single best answer.**

44–1. Which age group may have the best response to electroconvulsive therapy (ECT)?

1. Children aged 12 years or younger

2. Adolescents aged 13 to 19 years

3. Adults aged 20 to 60 years

4. Adults older than 60 years

44–2. American Psychiatric Association (APA) guidelines recommend which of the following for ECT administered to children who are younger than 12 years of age?

1. ECT may be administered based on the same recommendations as for adults.

2. A second opinion should be obtained from an independent psychiatrist who has experience in treating children and adolescents.

3. Two independent opinions must be obtained from psychiatrists who have experience in treating children and adolescents.

4. ECT may not be administered to children, regardless of clinical indications.

44–3. What is the mortality rate with ECT?

1. 1 per 100 patients

2. 1 per 1,000 patients

3. 1 per 10,000 patients

4. 1 per 100,000 patients

44–4. Which of the following statements is **true** regarding ECT relative to other treatments for major depression?

1. ECT has a slower onset of action than fluoxetine.

2. ECT is less efficacious than psychotherapy.

3. ECT is less efficacious than imipramine.

4. ECT is more efficacious than bupropion.

44–5. Which of the following affective disorders is associated with the highest likelihood of success with ECT?

    1. Severe nonmelancholic depression

    2. Depression with psychotic features

    3. Severe melancholic depression

    4. Major depression that is resistant to medication

44–6. What percentage of patients with mania will experience a remission when treated with ECT?

    1. 20%

    2. 40%

    3. 60%

    4. 80%

44–7. Prophylactic ECT for depressive disorders is used in the same manner as other prophylactic treatments. How long should prophylactic ECT be continued after the signs and symptoms of depression remit?

    1. Prophylactic ECT is never indicated.

    2. 3 to 6 months

    3. 6 to 12 months

    4. 12 to 18 months

44–8. Which of the following conditions represents an absolute contraindication to ECT?

    1. Recent myocardial infarction

    2. Space-occupying intracerebral lesions

    3. Pheochromocytoma

    4. None of the above

44–9. What is the usual number of ECT treatments?

    1. 3 to 5

    2. 6 to 12

    3. 12 to 18

    4. There is no usual number of treatments.

■ **DIRECTIONS: For questions 44–10 through 44–15, indicate**

    A if answers 1, 2, and 3 are correct.

    B if answers 1 and 3 are correct.

    C if answers 2 and 4 are correct.

    D if only answer 4 is correct.

    E if all are correct.

44–10. Although randomized controlled trials have not been conducted for continuation/maintenance ECT, this treatment is indicated in which of the following circumstances?

1. Mr. G. has had five episodes of major depression in the past 7 years, all of which were successfully treated with ECT.

2. Ms. S. is a 25-year-old who has had three episodes of major depression with psychotic features in the past 4 years. Each episode was successfully treated with ECT. She appears to relapse when she decides to stop her medication because of the intolerable side effects.

3. Mrs. K. is a 40-year-old who has had four episodes of major depression in the past 6 years. The last episode was associated with psychotic features and was particularly distressing to Mrs. K. The major depressive episodes have recurred despite appropriate psychotherapy and compliance with three classes of antidepressants. Her preference is to continue with ECT.

4. Mr. P. is a 16-year-old who was treated with ECT for major depression with psychotic features that did not respond to medications. He has had no other episodes of major depression.

44–11. ECT may have a role in treating which of the following disorders?

1. Schizoaffective disorder

2. Schizophrenia

3. Schizophreniform disorder

4. Parkinson's disease

44–12. Which of the following are common side effects of ECT?

1. Transient hypertension

2. Body fractures

3. Muscle pain

4. Structural central nervous system changes

44–13. Which of the following statements are **true** regarding cognitive functioning and ECT?

1. The individual may lose information learned during the time of the treatments and during the 6 months prior to treatment.

2. The individual's cognitive functioning may improve dramatically.

3. The individual may have difficulty in retaining newly learned information.

4. The individual may lose all cognitive abilities.

44–14. Patients receiving ECT may have other underlying disorders or be on psychotropic medications. Which of the following statements are **true**?

1. Tranylcypromine must be discontinued 2 weeks prior to initiation of ECT.

2. A theophylline level of 18 mg/L (within a range of 10–20 mg/L) is acceptable prior to initiation of ECT.

3. Lithium must be discontinued prior to initiation of ECT.

4. A valproic acid level of 55 mg/L (within a range of 50–100 mg/L) would probably not have an appreciable effect on the ECT.

44–15. The minimal stimulus required to produce a seizure is the *seizure threshold*. What factors increase the seizure threshold?

    1. Being male

    2. Having ECT administered with right unilateral electrode placement

    3. Having a history of multiple treatments with ECT

    4. Being younger than 18 years of age

■ **DIRECTIONS: For questions 44–16 through 44–26, match the medication or treatment with the correct statement(s). Each statement may be used once, more than once, or not at all.**

44–16.	Glycopyrrolate	a.	Is associated with more substantial cognitive deficits.
44–17.	Labetalol	b.	Obtain serum electrolytes prior to administration.
44–18.	Bilateral ECT	c.	Is a short half-life barbiturate.
44–19.	Atropine	d.	Obtain electrocardiogram prior to administration.
44–20.	Esmolol	e.	Is an anticholinergic agent.
44–21.	Multiple monitored ECT	f.	Two to more than 10 seizures are produced for each treatment.
44–22.	Ketamine	g.	Is less likely to cross the blood-brain barrier.
44–23.	Propofol	h.	Antidepressant effect is more rapid and pronounced.
44–24.	Right unilateral ECT	i.	Is used for patients with high seizure threshold.
44–25.	Succinylcholine	j.	May be safely administered during pregnancy.
44–26.	Caffeine sodium benzoate	k.	May produce psychosis.
		l.	Is a beta-blocking agent used to treat hypertension.
		m.	Increases duration of seizures.
		n.	Cannot be used in patients with pseudocholinesterase deficiency.
		o.	May shorten seizure duration.
		p.	Is more efficacious in some types of depression than in other types.
		q.	Intubation is required.
		r.	Is administered two to three times per week.

■ **ANSWERS:**

44–1. **Answer: 4.** There is evidence that older adults may be more responsive to treatment with ECT than younger age groups.

44–2. **Answer: 3.** APA guidelines recommend one second opinion from an independent psychiatrist for children aged 13 to 17 years and opinions of two independent psychiatrists for children younger than 12 years of age. The psychiatrists must have experience in treatment of children and adolescents. Some states have minimum age requirements for ECT (e.g., in Texas, at the time of this writing, the minimum age is 16 years).

44–3. **Answer: 3.** The rate of mortality from ECT is comparable to that expected from brief anesthetic (i.e., 1 per 10,000).

44–4. **Answer: 4.** ECT is the most efficacious and has the most rapid onset of action of *all* the treatment modalities available for major depression.

44–5. **Answer: 2.** Both melancholic and nonmelancholic depression are responsive to treatment with ECT, as are manic states. Depressed patients who have not responded to treatment with antidepressant medications are *less* responsive to treatment with ECT. Psychotic depression, particularly if mood-congruent delusions are present, is associated with an increased likelihood of response to ECT.

44–6. **Answer: 4.** ECT is highly effective in the treatment of acute mania, with 80% of patients experiencing remission.

44–7. **Answer: 3.** The recommended duration of prophylactic ECT is similar to that of medication prophylaxis (i.e., 6 to 12 months).

44–8. **Answer: 4.** There are no absolute contraindications to ECT. Relative contraindications include recent myocardial infarction, space-occupying intracerebral lesions, pheochromocytoma, unstable vascular aneurysms, intracerebral hemorrhage, acute or impending retinal detachment, or increased intracranial pressure.

44–9. **Answer: 2.** The usual number of treatments is 6 to 12. There is no clinical reason to continue treatment with ECT after a plateau of symptom response has been achieved. There is no lifetime maximum number of treatments.

44–10. **Answer: A (1, 2, and 3).** Specific indications for continuation/maintenance ECT include 1) history of recurrent episodes responsive to ECT, 2) ineffectiveness of prophylactic pharmacotherapy, or 3) patient preference for ECT and past favorable response to ECT.

44–11. **Answer: E (All).** Patients with schizoaffective disorder or schizophreniform disorder appear to respond more readily to ECT than do those with schizophrenia. However, a number of studies have established that when the patient is in a distinct acute episode of psychosis, ECT in addition to a neuroleptic is more effective than either modality alone. ECT may produce transient improvement (i.e., lasting weeks to months) in Parkinson's disease.

44–12. **Answer: B (1 and 3).** During ECT, parasympathetic and sympathetic discharges occur, resulting in transient tachycardia and hypertension. Headache, muscle pain, and nausea are also associated with these discharges. Prolonged apnea, status epilepticus, or fractures are not usually associated with ECT in this era of musculoskeletal relaxation and anesthesia. Available evidence does not support any structural changes in the central nervous system after treatment with ECT.

44–13. **Answer: A (1, 2, and 3).** *Retrograde amnesia,* a difficulty in remembering information learned before the course of ECT, may occur. Generally, the losses dissipate over several weeks, except for information learned and memory of events that took place during the 6 months preceding ECT and around the time of the treatments. *Anterograde amnesia* refers to difficulty learning new information. This difficulty typically remits within days to weeks following completion of ECT treatment. Some patients with severe depression may actually present with cognitive deficits so severe as to give the clinical impression of dementia, a condition known as *pseudodementia.* In this population, cognitive processing may improve. The loss of all cognitive abilities would be extremely unlikely to occur as a result of ECT.

44–14. **Answer: D (Only 4).** Theoretically, it is best to have the patient medication free for several days prior to initiating ECT, but this may not be clinically feasible. The combination of lithium and ECT has historically been reputed to lower the efficacy of ECT and increase cerebral toxicity, but these points are not consistently validated in the literature. Likewise, discontinuation of monoamine oxidase inhibitors (MAOIs), such as tranylcypromine, is now considered unnecessary. Benzodiazepines should at least be tapered prior to ECT because they raise the seizure threshold. Theophylline is epileptogenic, and the dose should be kept to a minimum, with a level at the lower part of the range. Similarly, anticonvulsants, such as valproic acid, should be at minimum levels.

44–15. **Answer: B (1 and 3).** Seizure threshold is *increased* for men, for patients when bilateral electrode placement is used, for patients with a history of multiple treatments with ECT, and for patients with advancing age.

44–16. Glycopyrrolate: **e, g**

44–17. Labetalol: **d, e**

44–18. Bilateral ECT: **a, b, d, h, i, j, p, r**

44–19. Atropine: **d, e, k**

44–20. Esmolol: **d, e**

44–21. Multiple monitored ECT: **a, b, d, f, h, i, j, p, r,**

44–22. Ketamine: **i, k**

44–23. Propofol: **c, o**

44–24. Right unilateral ECT: **b, d, j, r**

44–25. Succinylcholine: **n**

44–26. Caffeine sodium benzoate: **m**

CHAPTER 45

Light Therapy

■ **DIRECTIONS: For questions 45–1 through 45–6, indicate**

   A if answers 1, 2, and 3 are correct.
   B if answers 1 and 3 are correct.
   C if answers 2 and 4 are correct.
   D if only answer 4 is correct.
   E if all are correct.

45–1.   Caution is required when light therapy is used for which of the following patients?

   1. Patients receiving chlorpromazine
   2. Patients with a history of bipolar disorder
   3. Patients with systemic lupus erythematosus (SLE)
   4. Patients receiving risperidone

45–2.   Which of the following are **true** statements regarding light therapy?

   1. More intense light sources are superior to less intense sources.
   2. Skin exposure is more effective than eye exposure to light.
   3. Green light is superior to red light.
   4. Red light is superior to green light.

45–3.   Which of the following parameters are associated with the most efficacy?

   1. 2,500-lux intensity
   2. 10,000-lux intensity
   3. 2 hours of therapy
   4. 30 minutes of therapy

45–4.   Which of the following predict a **good** response to light therapy?

   1. A history of improved mood following trips to southern latitudes during winter months
   2. A craving for sweets during the afternoon
   3. A history of hypersomnia
   4. A history of anorexia and weight loss

45–5.   Which of the following are side effects of light therapy?

    1. Eye strain

    2. Overactivation

    3. Headache

    4. Fatigue

45–6.   For which of the following disorders is there unequivocal evidence for light therapy?

    1. Advanced sleep-phase syndrome

    2. Seasonal affective disorder

    3. Delayed sleep-phase syndrome

    4. Nonseasonal depression

■ **DIRECTIONS: For questions 45–7 through 45–13, indicate whether the statement is true or false.**

45–7. _____ Light therapy can be effectively combined with antidepressants.

45–8. _____ Dawn simulation therapy simulates a summer dawn and may increase compliance.

45–9. _____ Tanning salons are as efficacious as light box therapy for the treatment of seasonal affective disorder.

45–10. _____ There is an increased prevalence of eye problems in patients who have received light therapy for several years.

45–11. _____ Sunscreen agents are important adjunctive medications when light therapy is used.

45–12. _____ There are numerous long-term studies documenting the efficacy of light therapy.

45–13. _____ Light therapy may be used at any point in the day that is convenient for the patient.

■ **ANSWERS:**

45–1.   **Answer: E (All).** There are no absolute contraindications to light therapy. Patients whose eyes or skin is photosensitive should be given special consideration. Chlorpromazine and probably risperidone cause photosensitivity. Patients with SLE are particularly vulnerable to exposure to light. Patients who have a history of mania may shift into a manic episode when treated with light therapy.

45–2.   **Answer: B (1 and 3).** Several studies have found more intense light superior to less intense, eye exposure more efficacious than skin exposure, and green light superior to red light.

45–3.   **Answer: C (2 and 4).** The original light boxes used a 2,500-lux intensity and required at least 2 hours of treatment per day. Light boxes that provide 10,000-lux intensity require only 30 minutes per day of treatment and are more efficacious.

45–4.   **Answer: A (1, 2, and 3).** Predictors of a good response to light therapy include a history of hypersomnia, craving sweets in the afternoon, and a preponderance of atypical vegetative symptoms. Improved mood following vacations in southern latitudes during winter months also predicts a good response to light therapy.

45–5.   **Answer: E (All).** Side effects of light therapy include eye strain, headaches, insomnia, fatigue, and overactivation.

45–6.   **Answer: A (1, 2, and 3).** Advanced sleep-phase syndrome, seasonal affective disorder, and delayed sleep-phase syndrome have all been successfully treated with light therapy. Nonseasonal depression is occasionally responsive to light therapy.

45–7.   **True**   Light therapy and pharmacotherapy may be combined.

45–8.   **True**   A more naturalistic approach such as dawn stimulation may enhance compliance.

45–9.   **False**   Tanning salons do *not* provide appropriate intensity or wavelength of light.

45–10. **False**   There is no evidence of permanent eye damage in patients who have received light therapy for several years.

45–11. **True**   Sunscreens may protect the skin from unwanted light during treatment.

45–12. **False**   There are no long-term studies documenting the efficacy of light therapy.

45–13. **True**   Light therapy may be timed at the patient's convenience.

CHAPTER 46

───────────────■───────────────

Treatment-Resistant
Mood Disorders

■ **DIRECTIONS: For questions 46–1 through 46–13,
select the single best answer.**

46–1.   What percentage of patients who initially responded to treatment for depression will relapse within the first year?

　　1.　5%–10%

　　2.　10%–25%

　　3.　25%–50%

　　4.　50%–75%

46–2.   What percentage of patients will **not** respond to standard treatment for depression?

　　1.　10%

　　2.　20%

　　3.　30%

　　4.　40%

46–3.   If a patient is diagnosed with bipolar disorder in adolescence, how many episodes of either mania, depression, or mixed affective disorder may he or she experience in his or her lifetime?

　　1.　The patient may expect to have only the initial episode if he or she is compliant with prophylaxis.

　　2.　The patient may expect to have only two or three more episodes during his or her lifetime.

　　3.　The patient may have 5 to 10 episodes during his or her lifetime.

　　4.　The patient may have 10 or more episodes during his or her lifetime.

46–4.   Which of the following statements is **false** regarding atypical depression?

　　1.　Mood reactivity is present.

　　2.　Chronic oversensitivity to rejection is present.

　　3.　Atypical depression is more responsive to tricyclic antidepressants.

　　4.　There is no weight loss.

46–5. Which of the following medications is the most efficacious solo treatment for psychotic depression?

    1. Imipramine

    2. Desipramine

    3. Amoxapine

    4. Nortriptyline

46–6. Mr. D. is a 21-year-old college student who presents with early-morning waking, poor appetite, decreased concentration, anhedonia, and irritability that have lasted for 3 weeks. He reports improvement in all symptoms except concentration after 2 weeks of fluoxetine. On further questioning, he states that he had difficulty with out-of-seat behaviors in grade school and high school and had experienced poor peer relationships and difficulties with concentration. What adjunctive medication may be indicated?

    1. Augmenting with lithium

    2. Augmenting with levothyroxine

    3. Switching to imipramine

    4. Adding methylphenidate

46–7. Anger attacks are present in approximately 40% of all depressed outpatients. Which of the following medications is most effective in the treatment of this subpopulation of depressed patients?

    1. Imipramine

    2. Desipramine and lithium

    3. Fluoxetine

    4. Amoxapine

46–8. Psychotherapy is **not** helpful for which of the following disorders?

    1. Lithium-resistant bipolar disorder

    2. Double depression

    3. Major depression, in maintenance-treatment phase

    4. None of the above

46–9. What percentage of patients with bipolar disorder fail to respond to lithium as a monotherapy?

    1. 30%

    2. 50%

    3. 70%

    4. 90%

46–10. Which of the following statements is **true** regarding the use of neuroleptic medications for bipolar disorder?

    1. There are no studies reporting an advantage for maintenance therapy with neuroleptics in patients with bipolar disorder.

    2. Clozapine should be used as a first-line neuroleptic because it has no risk of tardive dyskinesia.

3. Mania or psychosis does not occur frequently when a neuroleptic is tapered.

4. Depression is less common in patients treated with a neuroleptic and lithium.

46–11. Which of the following medications are **not** used as mood-stabilizing agents?

1. Verapamil

2. Phenytoin

3. Carbamazepine

4. Valproic acid

46–12. Which of the following antidepressants may be **less** likely to induce mania?

1. Sertraline

2. Protriptyline

3. Trazodone

4. Bupropion

46–13. Which type of patients responds best to thyroid augmentation for major depression?

1. There are no significant treatment predictors.

2. Patients with a family history of Hashimoto's disease

3. Female patients

4. Patients with a history of alcoholism

■ **DIRECTIONS: For questions 46–14 through 46–23, indicate**

A if answers 1, 2, and 3 are correct.

B if answers 1 and 3 are correct.

C if answers 2 and 4 are correct.

D if only answer 4 is correct.

E if all are correct.

46–14. Which of the following describe patients who are **less** likely to respond to treatment for a depressive disorder?

1. Mr. K. has a history of severe, recurrent peptic ulcer disease.

2. Ms. M. has virtually no contact with her family and few friends.

3. Ms. L. is a single mother of three children younger than 6 years of age and is estranged from her family.

4. Mrs. P. has recently lost her husband of 45 years and her only child.

46–15. Which of the following symptoms, patient characteristics, or comorbid disorders predict a poor response to lithium augmentation for unipolar depression?

1. Weight gain with overeating

2. Weight loss with anorexia

3. Hypersomnia

4. Insomnia

46–16. Which of the following describe patients who may be unresponsive to lithium maintenance therapy?

    1. Kim is an 11-year-old who has had three documented episodes of mania and one episode of major depression in the past year.

    2. Mr. P. is a 45-year-old who was diagnosed with bipolar disorder when he was 23 and alcohol dependence when he was 24.

    3. Ms. S. has had 15 episodes of mania, depression, and mixed affective disorder in the past year. She was also diagnosed with bulimia in the past month.

    4. Mr. Z. is a 40-year-old who was diagnosed with bipolar disorder when he was 23. He has had one episode each of mania and major depression. His mother was diagnosed with major depression when Mr. Z. was 7 years of age.

46–17. Which of the following comorbid diagnoses predict a **poorer** response to antidepressants?

    1. Generalized anxiety disorder

    2. Panic disorder

    3. Alcohol dependence

    4. Borderline personality disorder

46–18. Lithium therapy is the first line of treatment in bipolar disorder and is an adjunctive therapy in the treatment of unipolar depression. Which of the following statements are **true**?

    1. There is a linear relationship between lithium blood level and augmentation response.

    2. In clinical practice, 12 weeks of nonresponse to antidepressant should elapse before augmentation with lithium is attempted.

    3. Lithium should be continued for at least 12 weeks before lack of efficacy is assumed.

    4. Lithium should be initiated at 600 mg/day.

46–19. What are the most common causes of mixed episodes in patients with bipolar disorder?

    1. Systemic lupus erythematosus (SLE)

    2. Graves' disease

    3. Multiple sclerosis (MS)

    4. Möbius' syndrome

46–20. Interventions to decrease rapid cycling include discontinuation of which of the following medications?

    1. Imipramine

    2. Risperidone

    3. Pemoline

    4. Albuterol

46–21. Anxiety is a frequent complication of bipolar disorder. In general, anxiolytic therapy should be tapered if patients are stable through the continuation phase of treatment. Which of the following may be safely and effectively used to treat anxiety in patients with bipolar disorder?

1. Lorazepam
2. Clonidine hydrochloride
3. Clonazepam
4. Propranolol

46–22. Mrs. G. is a 63-year-old who smokes three packs of cigarettes per day and has treatment-resistant major depressive disorder. What considerations should be made prior to initiation of thyroid augmentation?

1. Osteoporosis may occur with long-term treatment with thyroid.
2. Cardiac disease may be present.
3. T3 would be more appropriate than T4 as a supplement.
4. A response should be seen within days of initiating treatment.

46–23. Which of the following statements are **true** regarding the combination or switching of medications for the treatment of major depression?

1. Fluoxetine can be safely added to isocarboxazid.
2. No adjustment in fluoxetine dose is required when fluoxetine and desipramine are being combined.
3. A washout period of 24 hours is required when switching from imipramine to deprenyl.
4. Clomipramine and isocarboxazid should not be used in combination.

■ **ANSWERS:**

46–1. **Answer: 2.** Approximately 10%–25% of patients who initially responded to treatment for depression will relapse within the first year.

46–2. **Answer: 3.** Approximately 30% of patients diagnosed with a major depressive disorder will fail to respond to treatment.

46–3. **Answer: 4.** Bipolar disorder is characterized by recurrence rather than remission, even with prophylactic treatment for recurrences. Individuals who receive a diagnosis during their adolescence may have 10 or more episodes of mood disorder during their lifetime.

46–4. **Answer: 3.** Atypical depression is found more commonly in outpatient settings compared with endogenous or melancholic depression. In contrast to melancholic depression, atypical depression is characterized by mood reactivity, overeating, oversleeping or extreme fatigue when depressed, and chronic oversensitivity to rejection. Monoamine oxidase inhibitors (MAOIs) and selective serotonin reuptake inhibitors (SSRIs) were found to be more efficacious in the treatment of atypical depression than were tricyclic antidepressants.

46–5. **Answer: 3.** In general, patients with a psychotic depression respond best to an antidepressant and a neuroleptic medication. Among the tricyclic antidepressants, amoxapine is metabolized to a neuroleptic and is variably successful as the sole medication in the treatment of psychotic depression.

46–6.   **Answer: 4.** This patient gives a past history and present symptom of poor concentration consistent with attention-deficit/hyperactivity disorder (ADHD). Systematic research on the treatment of patients with depression and ADHD has not been conducted. Adjunctive treatment with stimulants, such as methylphenidate (Ritalin), has proved beneficial for some patients with depression without concomitant ADHD.

46–7.   **Answer: 3.** Fluoxetine (Prozac) appears more efficacious than tricyclic antidepressants in the treatment of the subpopulation of depressed patients who have anger attacks.

46–8.   **Answer: 4.** Psychotherapy is helpful for augmenting the prophylactic benefit of lithium and alleviating the social and interpersonal effects of depression. It may be useful also in decreasing the risk of relapse in the maintenance phase of the treatment of major depression.

46–9.   **Answer: 3.** Approximately 30% of patients with bipolar disorder can be maintained on lithium alone. The other 70% require adjunctive treatment.

46–10. **Answer: 1.** There are no studies that report an advantage for maintenance therapy with a neuroleptic for patients with bipolar disorder. The frequent clinical finding of resurgence of symptoms consistent with mania and/or psychosis when the neuroleptic is tapered is clinical justification for the continued use of neuroleptic therapy. Clozapine is a promising therapy in treatment-resistant patients, but it is not a first-line antipsychotic. Depression is more common in patients treated with a neuroleptic and lithium.

46–11. **Answer: 2.** Phenytoin (Dilantin) is an anticonvulsant that is not used as a mood-stabilizing agent. Carbamazepine and valproic acid are both anticonvulsants that have proven efficacy as mood-stabilizing agents. Verapamil is a calcium channel–blocking agent that may have mood-stabilizing properties.

46–12. **Answer: 4.** Bupropion (Wellbutrin) is a novel antidepressant that may be less likely to induce hypomania/mania.

46–13. **Answer: 1.** Only one study has attempted to determine patient characteristics and response to treatment with thyroid augmentation for unipolar depression. In that study, there were no significant predictors.

46–14. **Answer: E (All).** Unrecognized and recognized medical conditions significantly lower the rate of responsiveness to treatment. In one study, only 40% of patients with a medical condition responded to antidepressant therapy. Unrecognized medical illness was found to have either caused or exacerbated psychiatric symptoms in approximately 50% of patients in another study. The presence of severe family conflicts and the relative absence of family support may predict poor outcome for depressed patients. Multiple losses through death of family members are significantly correlated with chronicity in depression.

46–15. **Answer: C (2 and 4).** Patients who do not respond to lithium augmentation for unipolar depression tend to be more severely depressed and to have more insomnia and weight loss.

46–16. **Answer: A (1, 2, and 3).** Nonresponse to prophylactic lithium treatment is predicted by several clinical factors, including 1) onset before 18 years, 2) mixed affective episodes (dysphoric mania, depressive mania), 3) more than three exacerbations of the disorder, 4) rapid cycling (traditionally defined as four or more episodes per year, but may be redefined as 12 or more episodes per year), 5) substance abuse (60% of patients with bipolar disorder meet the criteria for substance abuse), 6) ADHD, 7) anxiety disorders, 8) comorbid medical disorders, 9) bulimia, and 10) no family history of affective disorders.

46–17. **Answer: A (1, 2, and 3).** Patients with anxiety disorders may have hypochondriacal concerns and sensitivity to somatic cues that contribute to poor tolerance of side effects. In general, patients with panic attacks have been reported to have poorer response to treatment for depression. Patients with concomitant substance abuse or dependence have poorer response to antidepressants. Patients meeting the criteria for Cluster B personality disorders (i.e., histrionic, borderline, antisocial, and narcissistic) actually have a significantly better response to medications (SSRIs) than do patients who do not meet those criteria.

46–18. **Answer: D (Only 4).** Despite the numerous studies of lithium levels and dosing in the treatment of bipolar disorder, few have studied lithium augmentation for unipolar depression. In the studies conducted thus far, there appears to be no relationship between lithium dose/blood level and augmentation response. Research trials have waited 12 weeks before initiating lithium augmentation, but in clinical practice, 4 weeks of nonresponse to an antidepressant is sufficient. A lithium trial is conducted for 4 to 6 weeks prior to declaring a nonresponse. The most efficacious starting dose for augmentation is 600 mg/day.

46–19. **Answer: A (1, 2, and 3).** Mixed mood disorders are a frequent cause of nonresponse to lithium and are frequently due to autoimmune diseases such as SLE or MS or to thyroid disease (Graves' disease and Hashimoto's disease), nonparoxysmal electroencephalogram (EEG) abnormalities, ADHD, bulimia, migraine headaches, and substance abuse.

46–20. **Answer: E (All).** Antidepressants (e.g., imipramine), neuroleptics (e.g., risperidone), stimulants (e.g., pemoline, caffeine), and bronchodilators (albuterol, theophylline) may increase the frequency of the rapid cycling.

46–21. **Answer: E (All).** Benzodiazepines (lorazepam and clonazepam) and adrenergic receptor–blocking agents (clonidine hydrochloride and propranolol) may be used to treat anxiety associated with bipolar disorder. Clonidine hydrochloride also may be a mood stabilizer.

46–22. **Answer: A (1, 2, and 3).** The patient in this case, because of her age and smoking history, is at risk for cardiac disease. Thyroid supplementation is associated with increased atrial irritability and increased ventricular function, leading to high-output cardiac failure. Long-term use of thyroid hormone is associated with osteoporosis, a condition also linked to smoking, female gender, and age. In one study, 53% of patients responded to T3, whereas only 19% responded to T4. Dopaminergic agents are effective within days, whereas lithium and thyroid augmentation effects may not be seen for 3 to 6 weeks. Occasionally, dopaminergic agents are used to augment antidepressant medication.

46–23. **Answer: C (2 and 4).** The combination of tricyclic antidepressants (except clomipramine) and MAOIs can be safely and effectively used. MAOIs are not compatible with SSRIs. Starting a TCA and an MAOI together at low doses is the most effective method. A washout period of at least 1 week for TCAs (except protriptyline, for which a period of 3 weeks is necessary) and 2 weeks for SSRIs (except fluoxetine, for which a period of at least 5 weeks is necessary) is required prior to initiation of an MAOI. Fluoxetine, like all SSRIs, induces the cytochrome P450 IID6 system and *increases* the level of TCAs. A downward adjustment of the TCA is required when combining a TCA and an SSRI.

CHAPTER 47

Mood Disorders and
General Medical Illness

■ DIRECTIONS: For questions 47–1 through 47–6, select the single best answer.

47–1. What is the incidence of affective disorders in patients with general medical conditions?

1. 10%
2. 20%
3. 30%
4. 50%

47–2. What percentage of patients in the general medical setting have their mood disorders correctly diagnosed?

1. 95%
2. 75%
3. 50%
4. 25%

47–3. Ms. K. is a 23-year-old with a history of bulimia, brittle juvenile-onset diabetes, and partial complex seizure disorder. For the past 3 weeks she has been experiencing lethargy, dysphoria with suicidal ideation, early-morning waking, and decreased appetite. Which medication would be safest in this patient?

1. Bupropion
2. Imipramine
3. Tranylcypromine
4. Sertraline

47–4. You have made a decision to use a selective serotonin reuptake inhibitor (SSRI) in a patient with the following transaminase levels: SGOT 150 (14–50 U/L) and SGPT 250 (21–72 U/L). Which of the following SSRIs causes the most significant inhibition of the cytochrome P450 system?

1. Sertraline
2. Fluoxetine

3. Paroxetine

4. There is no difference in the degree of inhibition among the various SSRIs.

47–5. You have been asked to consult on a 23-year-old who was involved in a motor vehicle accident and has multiple fractures and internal injuries but no central nervous system injuries and no loss of consciousness. The patient has developed stress ulcers and appears quite depressed. What antidepressant would effectively treat the stress ulcers and the depression?

1. Nortriptyline

2. Fluoxetine

3. Bupropion

4. Tranylcypromine

47–6. Which of the following is **not** implicated as a precipitating agent of depressive disorders?

1. Clonidine hydrochloride

2. Reserpine

3. Glucocorticoids

4. Anabolic steroids

■ **DIRECTIONS: Using the following clinical vignette, for questions 47–7 through 47–11, indicate**

A if answers 1, 2, and 3 are correct.

B if answers 1 and 3 are correct.

C if answers 2 and 4 are correct.

D if only answer 4 is correct.

E if all are correct.

Mr. K. is a 65-year-old with chronic obstructive pulmonary disease, four-vessel coronary artery disease, adult-onset diabetes, obesity, and poorly controlled hypertension, and yet he continues to smoke three packs of cigarettes per day. His past psychiatric history is positive for bipolar disorder and alcoholism. According to Mr. K., his medications include furosemide, theophylline, captopril, digoxin, insulin, albuterol inhalers, and sublingual nitroglycerin. Mr. K. reports early morning waking and difficulty falling asleep, extreme nervousness and sadness, loss of interest in activities, and thoughts of killing himself. His wife and internist report that he has not slept for several days; that he has struck his wife, screaming that she was a witch out to "do him in"; and that he has emptied their savings account in the past 24 hours to buy various defunct stocks, because he knew that he could "turn the market around." His internist has managed to get Mr. K. to consent to a psychiatric consultation.

47–7. What should be included in the evaluation of Mr. K.?

1. Electrolyte levels, blood urea nitrogen, and creatinine

2. Urine drug screen

3. Liver transaminase levels

4. Arterial blood gas

47–8. Which of the following medications could complicate the patient's hypertension?

1. Bupropion

2. Imipramine

3. Venlafaxine

4. Sertraline

47–9. This patient may benefit from a mood-stabilizing agent. Which of the following must be considered in selecting the agent?

1. Potassium levels

2. Ammonia levels

3. Creatinine levels

4. Transaminase levels

47–10. Mr. K.'s psychiatric symptoms may be due to which of the following?

1. Bipolar disorder

2. Theophylline toxicity

3. Alcoholic encephalitis

4. Alzheimer's disease

47–11. Which of the following attitudes, if adopted by the clinician, may inhibit Mr. K. from being appropriately diagnosed and treated?

1. Attributing all of his symptoms to his cardiovascular or pulmonary diseases

2. Attributing all of his symptoms to a psychiatric disorder

3. Believing that Mr. K. deserves to have all of his affective symptoms because his diseases are so life-threatening

4. Believing an integrated approach between medical specialties is best

■ ANSWERS:

47–1. **Answer: 3.** Prevalence of affective disorders in patients with general medical conditions approaches 30%, whereas in the general population it is 6%–10%.

47–2. **Answer: 3.** Only half of patients with a mood disorder are correctly diagnosed in the general medical setting.

47–3. **Answer: 4.** Bupropion (Wellbutrin) is an atypical antidepressant with a seizure rate of 0.4% even when used in doses of less than the maximum recommended dose of 450 mg/day. The frequency of seizures may increase 10-fold if this dose is exceeded. The high rate of seizures with bupropion was originally noted in patients with eating disorders. Imipramine is a tricyclic antidepressant that is potentially lethal in overdose situations and lowers the seizure threshold. Tranylcypromine, a monoamine oxidase inhibitor (MAOI), potentiates hypoglycemic insulin reactions. Sertraline (Zoloft), an SSRI, is the safest choice of the listed antidepressants; it has no known cardiovascular effects, will not lower the seizure threshold, is not lethal in overdose situations, and has no effect on blood glucose levels.

47–4.   **Answer: 3.** Paroxetine is the most significant inhibitor of the cytochrome P450 system, and sertraline is the least.

47–5.   **Answer: 1.** The tricyclic antidepressants (amitriptyline, nortriptyline, imipramine, desipramine, and amoxapine) are as efficacious as H_2 blockers (cimetidine and ranitidine) in the treatment of ulcers.

47–6.   **Answer: 1.** Reserpine, glucocorticoids, and anabolic steroids are strongly implicated as precipitating agents of depressive disorders. Clonidine hydrochloride was previously thought to cause depression, but recent evidence has refuted this idea.

47–7.   **Answer: E (All).** This patient may be experiencing an exacerbation of his bipolar disorder, a drug interaction, a recurrence of alcoholism, an electrolyte imbalance, episodes of hypoxia, renal or hepatic failure secondary to his cardiovascular disease, or pulmonary disease. One or more of these conditions could account for his psychiatric symptoms.

47–8.   **Answer: A (1, 2, and 3).** Bupropion and venlafaxine may produce hypertension in previously unaffected patients and complicate the treatment of patients receiving antihypertensive medications. Imipramine, like most tricyclic antidepressants (nortriptyline [Pamelor] is a notable exception), may produce significant orthostatic hypotension. Sertraline is an SSRI with minimal effects on blood pressure.

47–9.   **Answer: E (All).** This patient is taking furosemide (Lasix), a potent diuretic, without taking a potassium supplement, and this may lead to hypokalemia. Hypokalemia will exacerbate digoxin levels, leading to digoxin toxicity and lithium toxicity. Both digoxin toxicity and lithium toxicity can contribute to atrial and ventricular conduction abnormalities. In the presence of renal insufficiency, elevated creatine levels or decreased creatinine clearance can lead to elevated lithium levels. Valproic acid may cause an increase in serum ammonia levels and should be avoided in patients with hepatic insufficiency. Carbamazepine inhibits the cytochrome P450 system, leading to an increase in medications such as theophylline. In patients with hepatic insufficiency, carbamazepine toxicity is easily induced because of the inability of the cytochrome system to metabolize the drug.

47–10.   **Answer: E (All).** The patient's symptoms of sleep instability, grandiose beliefs about money, and affective states of irritability and sadness are indicative of a dysphoric manic state, depression with psychotic features, or early dementia. Theophylline toxicity is associated with manic symptoms. Alzheimer's disease may present with depression in 50% of cases. Alcoholic encephalitis may be accompanied by manic symptoms. These symptoms may also represent an exacerbation of the patient's bipolar disorder.

47–11.   **Answer: A (1, 2, and 3).** A thoughtful, empathic, and knowledgeable approach that takes into account all of the possible signs and symptoms of the patient's multiple disease processes will allow the best possible treatment and diagnosis.

CHAPTER 48

Strategies and Tactics in the Treatment of Depression

■ DIRECTIONS: For questions 48–1 through 48–3, match the phase of treatment with the associated statement(s). Each statement may be used once, more than once, or not at all.

48–1. Acute

48–2. Continuation

48–3. Maintenance

a. One goal of this phase is prevention of relapse.

b. Medications are utilized in this phase.

c. 45%–55% of patients will respond in this phase.

d. One goal of this phase is restoration of psychosocial functioning.

e. This phase may last the patient's lifetime.

f. Electroconvulsive therapy (ECT) may be used.

g. One goal of this phase is prevention of a new episode.

h. Medication and psychotherapy may be used together.

i. Symptom remission is achieved.

j. Medication trial should last 6 to 8 weeks.

k. Adjunctive medications are not usually used in this phase.

l. The choice of drugs during this phase is not influenced by side effects.

m. Treatment lasts 4 to 9 months in this phase.

n. Psychotherapy alone may be used.

■ DIRECTIONS: For questions 48–4 through 48–8, indicate

A if answers 1, 2, and 3 are correct.

B if answers 1 and 3 are correct.

C if answers 2 and 4 are correct.

D if only answer 4 is correct.

E if all are correct.

265

48–4.   Psychiatrists should see which of the following patients?

     1. Patients who have failed therapeutic intervention with nonpsychiatrists

     2. Patients with recurrent or chronic affective disorders

     3. Patients with psychotic disorders

     4. Patients who prefer to be seen by a psychiatrist

48–5.   Characterological disorders may complicate depressive disorders. Which of the following statements are **true** regarding Axis II disorders and depression?

     1. The diagnosis must remain tentative in the midst of a major depressive disorder.

     2. The diagnosis may be easily made because these disorders are pervasive.

     3. The presence of an Axis II disorder may delay or prevent a response during the acute treatment phase.

     4. The presence of an Axis II disorder has no bearing on the long-term prognosis.

48–6.   Which of the following disorders have a 15%–25% rate of depression associated with them?

     1. Myocardial infarction

     2. Diabetes mellitus

     3. Cerebral vascular accidents

     4. Asthma

48–7.   What are the reasons for initial treatment failures?

     1. Poor adherence to treatment, whether pharmacotherapy, psychotherapy, or a combined approach

     2. Failure to select the appropriate treatment

     3. Presence of an Axis II disorder

     4. Failure to utilize combined treatment on a regular basis

48–8.   Which of the following factors influence in a **positive** manner or are predictive of better adherence to treatment?

     1. More frequent sessions

     2. Once-a-day dosing of medication

     3. Past history of compliance with treatment

     4. A high socioeconomic status

■ ANSWERS:

48–1.   Acute: **b, c, f, h, i, j, k, l, n**

48–2.   Continuation: **a, b, f, h, m, n**

48–3.   Maintenance: **b, e, f, g, h, n**

48–4.   **Answer: E (All).** Patients who should be seen by a psychiatrist include those with psychotic disorders or recurrent or chronic affective disorders, those with conditions that have been difficult to diagnose, and those who have failed to respond to one or two (at the most) therapeutic interventions with nonpsychiatrists. Patient preference should also be considered.

48–5.   **Answer: B (1 and 3).** Axis II disorders affect both strategic planning and the prognosis. The long-term management of patients with Axis II disorders may exact a toll on the therapeutic skills of the clinician. The presence of an Axis II disorder is associated with a slower and perhaps less complete response to medications as well as to time-limited psychotherapies.

48–6.   **Answer: A (1, 2, and 3).** One year following a myocardial infarction or cerebral vascular accident, 15%–25% of patients will develop a major depressive disorder. In addition, 15%–25% of patients with diabetes mellitus or cancer will develop a major depression.

48–7.   **Answer: A (1, 2, and 3).** Poor adherence to the selected and agreed-on treatment modality is probably the single most common reason for treatment failure. The presence of an Axis II disorder is a predictor of poor response to several types of treatment. Failure to select the correct treatment modality, whether medication or psychotherapy or some combination, may account for some treatment failures. The routine combination of psychotherapy and medications remains under investigation.

48–8.   **Answer: A (1, 2, and 3).** More frequent sessions early in the treatment process, simplified dosing of medications, and a past history of compliance argue for compliance with treatment. Adherence is *not* related to gender, educational level, or socioeconomic status.

Anxiety Disorders, Dissociative Disorders, and Adjustment Disorders

CHAPTER 49

Panic Disorder and Agoraphobia

DIRECTIONS: For questions 49–1 through 49–14, select the single best answer.

49–1. In the treatment of panic disorder, which is the **least** studied selective serotonin reuptake inhibitor (SSRI)?

1. Fluoxetine
2. Sertraline
3. Paroxetine
4. Fluvoxamine

49–2. Patients with panic disorder may be more sensitive to side effects of SSRIs. Which side effect creates the most difficulty for patients with panic disorder who are treated with fluoxetine?

1. Sexual impotence
2. Jitteriness
3. Headache
4. Nausea

49–3. Anticonvulsants may be useful in the treatment of complicated cases of patients with panic disorder, mood disorders, and coexisting alcoholism. Which of the following anticonvulsants has proven efficacy for such patients?

1. Phenobarbital
2. Carbamazepine
3. Ethosuximide
4. Valproate

49–4. What percentage of children are born with overreactivity to unfamiliar people and situations that predisposes them to anxiety disorders?

1. 5%
2. 10%
3. 15%
4. 20%

49–5. Superior combined effects in the treatment of panic disorder are found for which of the following combinations of therapeutic modalities?

1. Imipramine and behavior therapy
2. Clonazepam and behavior therapy
3. Alprazolam and behavior therapy
4. Lorazepam and behavior therapy

49–6. The extensive outcome data on behavioral and cognitive-behavioral treatment of panic disorder with and without agoraphobia indicate what overall range of effectiveness for these treatment modalities?

1. 20%–30%
2. 40%–50%
3. 60%–70%
4. 80%–90%

49–7. Therapist-assisted exposure to decrease anxiety during anxiety-provoking situations is no more effective than self-exposure instructions plus daily homework assignments in all of the following disorders **except**

1. Agoraphobia.
2. Social phobia.
3. Specific phobia.
4. Panic disorder.

49–8. Antidepressants exert their antipanic effects how many weeks after their initiation?

1. 1 to 3 weeks
2. 3 to 6 weeks
3. 6 to 9 weeks
4. 9 to 12 weeks

49–9. Which benzodiazepine is most frequently associated with "clock watching" in anticipation of the next scheduled dose?

1. Lorazepam
2. Diazepam
3. Clonazepam
4. Alprazolam

49–10. Of the following medications with proven efficacy in the treatment of panic disorder, which is relatively safe in an overdose?

1. Paroxetine
2. Tranylcypromine
3. Amitriptyline
4. Phenelzine

49–11. What side effect do imipramine and phenelzine share that is frequently bothersome to patients with panic disorder who need long-term pharmacotherapy?

1. Dry mouth

    2. Blurred vision

    3. Weight gain

    4. Constipation

49–12. All of the following statements are **true** regarding patients who have both panic disorder and major depression **except**

    1. The risk of attempted suicide is not increased relative to the risk for either panic disorder or major depression.

    2. These patients require more intensive psychiatric treatment.

    3. These patients may remain ill for an extended period of time.

    4. The odds ratio of an individual with major depression having panic disorder at some time is approximately 18:8.

49–13. Which of the following statements is **false** regarding benzodiazepine use in the treatment of panic disorder?

    1. Daily benzodiazepine use is not highly predictive of withdrawal symptoms in patients who are being tapered off their medications.

    2. Moderate alcohol use in patients being treated with benzodiazepines is indicative of a difficult withdrawal from benzodiazepines.

    3. Chronic, long-term use of benzodiazepines in the treatment of panic disorder is contraindicated.

    4. The majority of withdrawal symptoms occur during the last half of a scheduled tapering off of benzodiazepines.

49–14. What is the optimal dose of alprazolam in patients with panic disorder?

    1. 2 mg/day

    2. A plasma level must be obtained to determine the optimal dose.

    3. 2 mg to 4 mg/day

    4. Alprazolam is highly addictive and should not be used in the treatment of panic disorder.

■ ANSWERS:

49–1. **Answer: 2.** The most extensively studied SSRIs in the treatment of panic disorder are fluoxetine, paroxetine, and fluvoxamine.

49–2. **Answer: 2.** All of the problems listed (sexual impotence, jitteriness, headache, and nausea) are side effects of fluoxetine. Jitteriness during initiation of the medication is the main problem seen in patients with panic disorder.

49–3. **Answer: 4.** Valproate and carbamazepine have been compared in the treatment of panic disorder, and only valproate was found efficacious in reducing the frequency of panic attacks. Phenobarbital and ethosuximide are not used in the treatment of panic attacks or affective disorders.

49–4. **Answer: 2.** Approximately 10% of children are born with behavioral inhibition. These children are fearful and shy and develop a disproportionate number of anxiety disorders in later childhood.

49–5. **Answer: 1.** Combined treatment with an antidepressant and behavior therapy has been shown to have more efficacy than either treatment alone. Benzodiazepines (clonazepam, alprazolam, and lorazepam) are associated with state-dependent learning and do not produce superior results when combined with behavior therapy.

49–6. **Answer: 3.** Behavioral and cognitive-behavioral treatment are highly effective, with a 60%–70% response rate and only a 10% relapse rate.

49–7. **Answer: 2.** Individuals with social phobia benefit the most from therapist-accompanied exposure.

49–8. **Answer: 2.** As with their antidepressant effects, antidepressants exert their anti-panic effects after 3 to 6 weeks. Six to 12 weeks of medications are required for substantial symptomatic improvement for most patients.

49–9. **Answer: 4.** Short-acting benzodiazepines, such as alprazolam, are associated with "clock watching" as the patient anticipates the next dose. Alprazolam is usually administered three to four times a day.

49–10. **Answer: 1.** Tricyclic antidepressants (amitriptyline) and monoamine oxidase inhibitors (tranylcypromine and phenelzine) are potentially lethal in overdose situations. Paroxetine, an SSRI, is relatively safe in overdose situations.

49–11. **Answer: 3.** The anticholinergic effects of dry mouth, blurred vision, and constipation are seen with both imipramine and phenelzine, but many patients will accommodate to these effects. However, the untoward effect of weight gain is not well tolerated.

49–12. **Answer: 1.** The risk of suicide attempts in patients with combined panic disorder and major depression is approximately twice as great as that in patients with either disorder alone.

49–13. **Answer: 3.** There is no evidence to support the concern that long-term treatment of panic disorder with benzodiazepines is associated with a pattern of progressively increasing dosage requirements. Panic disorder is one of the conditions for which long-term benzodiazepine therapy is indicated.

49–14. **Answer: 3.** A plasma level of alprazolam between 20 ng/mL and 60 ng/mL is effective for many patients. In clinical practice, this corresponds to a dose between 2 mg and 4 mg/day of alprazolam. A plasma level may be required to determine if a patient is a "rapid metabolizer" who requires more medication to achieve a therapeutic level. Alprazolam is potentially addictive, but it is efficacious in the treatment of patients with panic disorder. This medication should be avoided in the treatment of patients who have coexisting alcoholism or abuse illicit substances.

CHAPTER 50

Social Phobia and Specific Phobias

■ **DIRECTIONS: For questions 50–1 through 50–11, indicate**

    A if answers 1, 2, and 3 are correct.

    B if answers 1 and 3 are correct.

    C if answers 2 and 4 are correct.

    D if only answer 4 is correct.

    E if all are correct.

50–1. The application of social skills training is based on the assumption that individuals with social phobia experience a deficiency in which of the following areas?

    1. Culturally normative eye contact

    2. Speech content

    3. Social gestures appropriate to the culture

    4. Thought content

50–2. Applied relaxation techniques provide the patient with social phobia a means of coping with anxiety. Which of the following statements are **true** regarding applied relaxation?

    1. Patients learn to recognize the physiological signs of anxiety.

    2. Patients learn to relax for 20 to 30 seconds.

    3. Progressive muscle relaxation is a key component.

    4. Relaxation is maintained during anxiety-provoking social situations.

50–3. Which of the following medications have documented efficacy in the treatment of social phobia?

    1. Phenelzine

    2. Imipramine

    3. Moclobemide

    4. Desipramine

50–4. Dietary restrictions (including restrictions against cured meats, mozzarella cheese, Chianti wine) and avoidance of many of the over-the-counter cold preparations containing pseudoephedrine are required for all of the following MAOIs **except**

1. Phenelzine.
2. Brofaromine.
3. Isocarboxazid.
4. Moclobemide.

50–5. Substantial overlap exists between social phobia and which of the following personality disorders?

1. Obsessive-compulsive
2. Dependent
3. Paranoid
4. Avoidant

50–6. Beta-adrenergic blockers have received increased attention for treatment of psychiatric disorders in the past decade. Which of the following statements are true?

1. Atenolol is more effective than cognitive therapy for treatment of social phobia.
2. Performance anxiety is successfully treated with propranolol.
3. Propranolol is superior to placebo for the treatment of social phobia.
4. Diabetes mellitus is a relative contraindication for the use of beta-blockers.

50–7. Sustained gains in the treatment of social phobia are achieved by which of the following treatment modalities?

1. In vivo exposure therapy
2. Cognitive therapy
3. Pharmacotherapy
4. Exposure therapy and cognitive therapy

50–8. What are the components of cognitive-behavioral group therapy for social phobia?

1. Patient training in identification and disruption of problematic cognitions
2. Homework assignments for exposure to real-life situations
3. Cognitive restructuring procedures to teach patients to control their maladaptive thinking
4. Exposure to simulations of anxiety-provoking situations during the group therapy sessions

50–9. Specific phobias are an excessive or unreasonable fear of circumscribed objects or situations. Which of the following statements are **true** regarding specific phobias?

1. Most individuals with specific phobias are severely impaired by their phobia.
2. No behavioral treatment should ever be undertaken without a thorough analysis to identify potential antecedents and consequences of the phobia.
3. Pharmacotherapy is a mainstay of treatment.
4. Addressing the underlying conflict is not generally necessary for remission of symptoms.

50–10. Both social phobia and specific phobias respond to which of the following medications?

1. Phenelzine
2. Fluoxetine
3. Moclobemide
4. Diazepam

50–11. Which of the following therapies are nearly equivalent in efficacy in the treatment of specific phobias?

1. Nondirective supportive psychotherapy
2. Cognitive therapy
3. Systematic hierarchical desensitization
4. Interpersonal psychotherapy

■ **DIRECTIONS: For questions 50–12 through 50–14, select the single best answer.**

50–12. What percentage of patients with specific phobias prematurely discontinue treatment?

1. 10%–25%
2. 25%–50%
3. 50%–75%
4. None of the above

50–13. Patients who are distressed by the tachycardia and shortness of breath that they experience when their specific stimulus is encountered resemble which other group of patients?

1. Patients with avoidant personality disorder
2. Patients with depression
3. Patients with panic disorder
4. Patients with generalized anxiety disorder

50–14. Which of the following is **true** regarding flooding?

1. There is a systematic hierarchical progression from the least anxiety-provoking stimulus to the most anxiety-provoking stimulus.
2. Patients initially observe the therapist as he or she makes contact with the feared stimulus.
3. The patient is exposed to a highly feared stimulus for a prolonged period.
4. The patient is exposed by images or pictures to a highly feared stimulus for a prolonged period of time.

■ **ANSWERS:**

50–1. **Answer: A (1, 2, and 3).** Anxiety reactions in individuals with social phobia are secondary to deficiencies in appropriate verbal (speech content) and nonverbal (eye contact, gestures, posture) behaviors. The goal of social skills training is to correct these deficiencies. Thought content distortions or deficits are applicable to individuals with psychosis or cognitive dysfunction.

50–2. **Answer: E (All).** There are four steps in applied relaxation: 1) recognizing early the physiological signs of anxiety, 2) learning progressive muscle relaxation, 3) maintaining the relaxation through a variety of physical activities, and 4) maintaining relaxation during anxiety-provoking social situations. Relaxation is maintained for 20 to 30 seconds.

50–3. **Answer: B (1 and 3).** Phenelzine, an irreversible monoamine oxidase inhibitor (MAOI), is the most efficacious agent in the treatment of social phobia. Moclobemide, a reversible MAOI, also is efficacious in the treatment of social phobia. Imipramine and desipramine, both of which are tricyclic antidepressants, are not efficacious in the treatment of social phobia.

50–4. **Answer: C (2 and 4).** Moclobemide and brofaromine are selective A isoenzyme (MAO-A) monoamine oxidase inhibitors that bind reversibly to MAO. There is less need for dietary caution with these medications.

50–5. **Answer: D (Only 4).** Substantial overlap exists between avoidant personality disorder and social phobia.

50–6. **Answer: C (2 and 4).** Atenolol is less effective than cognitive therapy for the treatment of social phobia and is not superior to placebo. Propranolol is not superior to placebo in the treatment of social phobia. Diabetes mellitus and asthma are relative contraindications for the use of beta-blockers. Atenolol and propranolol are efficacious for mild to moderate performance anxiety.

50–7. **Answer: D (Only 4).** Exposure therapy is efficacious for the treatment of social phobia, as are cognitive therapy and pharmacotherapy. Sustained gains are associated with a combination of exposure therapy and cognitive therapy.

50–8. **Answer: E (All).** Cognitive-behavioral group therapy consists of 1) developing patients' cognitive-behavioral understanding of social phobia; 2) training patients in the skills of identification, analysis, and disputation of problematic cognitions through the use of structured exercises; 3) exposing patients to simulations of anxiety-provoking situations during group sessions; 4) using cognitive restructuring procedures to teach patients to control their maladaptive thinking before, during, and after exposure to anxiety-provoking situations; 5) assigning homework for exposure to real-life situations; and 6) assigning a self-administered cognitive restructuring routine.

50–9. **Answer: C (2 and 4).** Specific phobias are common, and most individuals with specific phobias are not so impaired that they seek treatment. Behavior therapy with in vivo exposure is the mainstay of treatment. No behavioral treatment should be undertaken without first addressing the possible primary and secondary gains of the phobia. Most phobias date from childhood, yet addressing the underlying conflict is generally not necessary for symptomatic improvement.

50–10. **Answer: D (Only 4).** Benzodiazepines, such as diazepam, have a role in the treatment of both social phobia and specific phobias.

50–11. **Answer: B (1 and 3).** Psychodynamic, nondirective supportive psychotherapy is as effective as systematic hierarchical desensitization in the treatment of specific phobias. Cognitive therapy and interpersonal psychotherapy are not generally used to treat specific phobias.

50–12. **Answer: 2.** Approximately 25%–50% of patients drop out of treatment for specific phobias.

50–13. **Answer: 3.** Patients with specific phobias who are more distressed by the bodily sensations (e.g., heart rate, rate of breathing, dizziness) than the consequences of an encounter with a feared object or situation resemble patients with panic disorder.

50–14. **Answer: 4.** A systematic hierarchical progression, either through imagination or in vivo, from the least to the most anxiety-provoking stimulus is known as *systematic desensitization. Participant modeling* is a technique in which the patient initially observes the therapist making contact with the feared stimulus. *Flooding* is in vivo exposure for a prolonged period of time with a highly feared stimulus. *Implosion* is prolonged exposure to the highly feared stimulus through images or pictures.

CHAPTER 51

Obsessive-Compulsive Disorder

DIRECTIONS: For questions 51–1 through 51–7, select the single best answer.

51–1. Which type of personality disorder is frequently found in patients with obsessive-compulsive disorder (OCD)?

1. Avoidant
2. Antisocial
3. Narcissistic
4. Obsessive-compulsive

51–2. How long, on average, after the first appearance of symptoms do patients with OCD wait to seek treatment?

1. < 1 year
2. 1 year
3. 5 years
4. 10 years

51–3. Most patients who engage in behavior therapy will have acute and sustained improvement in their symptoms. What percentage of patients with OCD will consent to behavior therapy?

1. 25%
2. 50%
3. 75%
4. 100%

51–4. Which of the following selective serotonin reuptake inhibitors (SSRIs) is the most efficacious in the treatment of OCD?

1. Sertraline
2. Fluoxetine
3. Fluvoxamine
4. They are all equally efficacious.

51–5. Side effects from clomipramine include all of the following **except**

1. Seizures.

2. Weight gain.

3. Orthostatic hypotension.

4. Watery eyes.

51–6. What percentage of patients experience a progressive, downward course of their OCD?

1. < 1%

2. 5%

3. 10%

4. 20%

51–7. A comorbid major depressive episode occurs in what percentage of OCD patients?

1. 30%

2. 60%

3. 90%

4. 100%

■ **DIRECTIONS: For questions 51–8 through 51–12, indicate**

A if answers 1, 2, and 3 are correct.

B if answers 1 and 3 are correct.

C if answers 2 and 4 are correct.

D if only answer 4 is correct.

E if all are correct.

51–8. Effective short-term treatment with which of the following reduces hypermetabolism in the right caudate nucleus?

1. Fluoxetine

2. Behavior therapy

3. Sertraline

4. Clomipramine

51–9. Effective behavior therapy for OCD encompasses which of the following?

1. In vivo exposure and response prevention

2. Relaxation

3. Establishment of a list of obsessions and rituals

4. Imaginary exposure and response prevention

51–10. Side effects are a common difficulty with clomipramine. Which of the following patient groups frequently discontinue their medications secondary to the untoward effects?

1. Patients with major depression

2. Patients with panic disorder

3. Patients with bipolar disorder, depressed type

4. Patients with OCD

51–11. Which of the following are reasonable augmentation strategies for patients who are unresponsive to treatment with a single agent?

1. Addition of haloperidol

2. Addition of buspirone

3. Addition of a second serotonin reuptake inhibitor

4. Addition of lithium

51–12. Consideration of neurosurgery is appropriate for approximately 1 in every 400 patients with OCD. What types of surgical procedures are used for OCD?

1. Frontal lobotomy

2. Anterior cingulotomy

3. Caudate tractotomy

4. Anterior capsulotomy

■ **DIRECTIONS: For questions 51–13 through 51–20, indicate whether the statement is true or false.**

51–13. _____ Psychodynamic therapy is never useful for patients with OCD.

51–14. _____ Personality changes associated with psychosurgery are usually positive.

51–15. _____ Children with OCD have a better rate of response to medication than do adults.

51–16. _____ With clomipramine, the side effects correlate with the plasma level.

51–17. _____ Clonazepam is more efficacious than diphenhydramine for the treatment of OCD.

51–18. _____ Therapists are more reluctant than their patients to use behavioral techniques for the treatment of OCD.

51–19. _____ Failure to maintain a written diary for exposure and response prevention is predictive of a poor response.

51–20. _____ There are no animal models for OCD.

■ **ANSWERS:**

51–1. **Answer: 1.** Avoidant personality disorder is much more commonly found in OCD than is narcissistic, antisocial, or obsessive-compulsive personality disorder.

51–2. **Answer: 4.** Patients wait, on average, a decade after the emergence of symptoms before seeking treatment.

51–3. **Answer: 3.** Approximately 75% of patients with OCD will engage in behavior therapy.

51–4. **Answer: 4.** A meta-analysis of multicenter controlled trials of fluoxetine, fluvoxamine, and sertraline found no differences in efficacy.

51–5. **Answer: 4.** Side effects of clomipramine include anticholinergic symptoms (e.g., dry eyes and mouth, constipation, blurred vision), antihistaminergic symptoms (e.g., somnolence and weight gain), and seizures.

51–6. **Answer: 3.** An unremitting downhill course will be experienced by 10% of patients with OCD.

51–7. **Answer: 2.** Approximately 60% of patients with OCD will experience a major depressive disorder at some point in their lives.

51–8. **Answer: A (1, 2, and 3).** Effective short-term treatment of OCD with an SSRI (fluoxetine or sertraline) or behavior therapy (exposure and response prevention) reduces hypermetabolism in the right caudate nucleus. Effective *long-term* treatment with clomipramine reduces hypermetabolism in the orbitofrontal cortex.

51–9. **Answer: B (1 and 3).** Effective behavior therapy for OCD consists of exposure in vivo and ritual or response prevention. Relaxation adds nothing to the effectiveness of treatment. Exposure in fantasy or imagination is not as effective as in vivo. An essential feature of all exposure and response prevention programs is the creation of a list of obsessions that engender anxiety, discomfort, distress, dysphoria, or disgust. A second list—that of rituals used to decrease unpleasant emotions and thoughts—should also be created.

51–10. **Answer: A (1, 2, and 3).** Unlike patients with major depression, bipolar disorder, or panic disorder, patients with OCD rarely discontinue clomipramine because of side effects.

51–11. **Answer: B (1 and 3).** The most promising augmentation strategy involves the addition of a neuroleptic to a potent serotonin reuptake inhibitor. Combining two potent serotonin reuptake inhibitors is a clinically feasible alternative. The addition of buspirone or lithium has not proven efficacious.

51–12. **Answer: C (2 and 4).** Currently, anterior cingulotomy, subcaudate tractotomy, a combination of these two techniques (referred to as "limbic leukotomy"), and anterior capsulotomy are all used for OCD.

51–13. **False** Psychodynamic therapy will not cure OCD. Patients may benefit from an exploration and better understanding of their noncompliance with medication, interpersonal functioning, and intrapsychic conflict.

51–14. **True** Despite the popular notion of "bad" traits arising from psychosurgery, personality changes associated with psychosurgery generally are positive.

51–15. **True** Children with OCD respond better to pharmacotherapy than do adults.

51–16. **False** With clomipramine, side effects correlate with the desmethylclomipramine level.

51–17. **False** Clonazepam is not more efficacious than diphenhydramine for the treatment of OCD.

51–18. **True** Patients are more likely than their therapists to be willing participants in behavior therapy for the treatment of OCD.

51–19. **True** Maintaining a written diary is essential for treatment with exposure and response prevention.

51–20. **False** Canine acral licking is an example of a possible animal model for OCD.

CHAPTER 52

Posttraumatic Stress Disorder

■ **DIRECTIONS: For questions 52–1 through 52–4,
select the single best answer.**

52–1. What percentage of the general population exhibit the full symptomatology
pattern of posttraumatic stress disorder (PTSD)?

    1. 1%

    2. 5%

    3. 9%

    4. 15%

52–2. Which of the following medications stimulates the locus coeruleus and induces
symptoms of PTSD?

    1. Tranylcypromine

    2. Sertraline

    3. Yohimbine

    4. Imipramine

52–3. Psychotherapy is commonly prescribed for treatment of PTSD. Which of the
following modalities has unequivocal documented efficacy in the treatment of
PTSD?

    1. Psychodynamic psychotherapy

    2. Cognitive-behavior therapy

    3. Systematic desensitization

    4. None of the above

52–4. The idea of fear as a cognitive structure contains all of the following elements
except

    1. Stimuli.

    2. Response to the stimuli.

    3. Conscious and unconscious meaning associated with the stimuli and re-
sponse.

    4. An inability to escape from the stimuli.

■ **DIRECTIONS: For questions 52–5 through 52–12, indicate**

    A if answers 1, 2, and 3 are correct.

    B if answers 1 and 3 are correct.

    C if answers 2 and 4 are correct.

    D if only answer 4 is correct.

    E if all are correct.

52–5. Which of the following medications can reverse conditioned avoidant responses characteristic of PTSD?

    1. Trazodone

    2. Imipramine

    3. Ritanserin

    4. Desipramine

52–6. Serotonin reuptake inhibitors have proven benefit in the treatment of which of the following symptoms of PTSD?

    1. Autonomic overarousal

    2. Impulse control

    3. Intrusive distressing recollections

    4. Affect regulation

52–7. Which of the following medications are clinically useful in the treatment of PTSD?

    1. Carbamazepine

    2. Propranolol

    3. Valproic acid

    4. Clonidine hydrochloride

52–8. Which of the following statements are **true** regarding pharmacotherapy in the treatment of PTSD?

    1. Pharmacotherapy should be instituted immediately.

    2. Pharmacotherapy alone is sufficient treatment of PTSD.

    3. A 4-week trial of tricyclic antidepressant or SSRI therapy is required to assess the effectiveness of treatment.

    4. Pharmacotherapy may be continued for years.

52–9. Difficulties with research on the efficacy of psychotherapy in the treatment of PTSD include which of the following?

    1. Inadequate control groups

    2. Poorly delineated treatments

    3. Vague or absent inclusion and exclusion criteria

    4. Lack of objective measures of target symptoms

52–10. Cognitive therapy and systematic desensitization may improve which of the following symptoms associated with PTSD?

    1. Unrealistic fears

    2. Depression

    3. Social adjustment

    4. Intrusive thoughts

52–11. Stress inoculation training includes which of the following techniques?

    1. Deep muscle relaxation

    2. Educational component

    3. Breathing control

    4. Thought stopping

52–12. Therapists who treat patients with PTSD may encounter which of the following complications?

    1. Patients may be reluctant to relinquish their symptoms when the symptoms are tied to receiving compensation.

    2. The embarrassing nature of the trauma may inhibit disclosure of the event.

    3. The symptoms may be chronically entrenched in the patient's characterological structure.

    4. The patient may have a comorbid Axis I diagnosis.

■ **DIRECTIONS: For questions 52–13 through 52–18, indicate whether the statement is true or false.**

52–13. _____ There is a direct relationship between plasma tricyclic levels and the therapeutic effect of the tricyclic in PTSD.

52–14. _____ Phenelzine may be useful in the treatment of highly refractory PTSD symptoms.

52–15. _____ The efficacy of sertraline for the treatment of PTSD has been documented in double-blind studies.

52–16. _____ The treatment goal for PTSD in many instances is to help patients master the symptoms and integrate the symptoms into their lives.

52–17. _____ Combination treatments of prolonged exposure, stress inoculation training, and supportive counseling are less effective than single-modality treatments for patients with PTSD.

52–18. _____ The effects of exposure on PTSD symptoms are more impressive for female rape victims than for Vietnam veterans.

■ **ANSWERS:**

52–1. **Answer: 3.** PTSD affects 9% of the general population. If subthreshold cases are added, then the combined prevalence in the general population is approximately 14%–15%.

52–2. **Answer: 3.** Tricyclic antidepressants, such as imipramine, and monoamine oxidase inhibitors (MAOIs), such as tranylcypromine, down-regulate the locus coeruleus. Selective serotonin reuptake inhibitors (SSRIs), such as sertraline, do not exert the majority of their effects on the noradrenergically rich region of the locus coeruleus. Yohimbine stimulates the locus coeruleus and may induce symptoms of PTSD in selective individuals.

52–3. **Answer: 4.** Mixed results have been obtained for psychodynamic, cognitive-behavioral, and systematic desensitization treatment of PTSD symptoms.

52–4. **Answer: 4.** The concept of fear as a cognitive structure involves three elements: stimuli, response, and the meaning associated with the stimuli and response. An inability to escape from the stimuli is part of the idea of *learned helplessness*.

52–5. **Answer: B (1 and 3).** 5-HT$_2$ antagonists such as trazodone and ritanserin can reverse conditioned avoidant responses.

52–6. **Answer: C (2 and 4).** Noradrenergically mediated symptoms include intrusive distressing recollections and autonomic overarousal. Serotonergically mediated symptoms, which are particularly helped by serotonin reuptake inhibitors, are impulse control and affect regulation.

52–7. **Answer: E (All).** The efficacy of anticonvulsant medications, such as carbamazepine and valproic acid, in the treatment of PTSD has not been validated with double-blind controlled studies. Clinically, these medications appear efficacious. Clonidine, which suppresses activity in the locus coeruleus, appears effective in decreasing symptoms. Beta-blockers, such as propranolol, appear clinically efficacious in the treatment of PTSD.

52–8. **Answer: D (Only 4).** Pharmacotherapy is indicated only after several weeks of persistent symptoms of PTSD. Generally, pharmacotherapy is combined with other treatment modalities. A minimum of 5 to 8 weeks is required to determine the efficacy of tricyclic and SSRI medications. Some individuals with chronic PTSD may require medications for several years.

52–9. **Answer: E (All).** Psychotherapy research in general is technically difficult and fraught with multiple problems, including inadequate or lack of control groups, poorly delineated treatments, vague or absent inclusion and exclusion criteria, absence of random assignment, and lack of objective measures of target symptoms.

52–10. **Answer: A (1, 2, and 3).** Outcome studies of cognitive-behavioral therapy and systematic desensitization reveal that ratings of unrealistic fears, anxiety, depression, and social adjustment may all improve. Intrusive thoughts are not generally affected by these treatments.

52–11. **Answer: E (All).** Stress inoculation training consists of two phases: an educational phase and a coping-skills phase. Elements of the coping-skills phase include deep muscle relaxation, breathing regulation, thought stopping, role-playing, covert modeling, and guided self-dialogue.

52–12. **Answer: E (All).** Patients may receive monetary compensations from social agencies or the legal system based on the intensity of their symptoms. For some patients, this may lead to a reluctance to relinquish their symptoms. The types of interpersonal traumas that may create PTSD are frequently intimate and embarrassing, inhibiting disclosure of the event. Many patients with PTSD may experience chronic trauma that has been interwoven into their character structure as they have matured. Comorbid Axis I diagnoses of depression and substance abuse are common complications in the treatment of patients with PTSD.

52–13. **False**   Unlike in the treatment of major depression, there is little to no correlation between plasma tricyclic antidepressant levels and response in the treatment of PTSD.

52–14. **True**   Phenelzine is efficacious in some patients with highly refractory PTSD symptoms.

52–15. **False**   There are no double-blind studies documenting the efficacy of sertraline in the treatment of PTSD.

52–16. **True**   PTSD may be a chronic disorder, and mastery and integration of symptoms may be a valid treatment goal.

52–17. **False**   Combinations of modalities are clinically more effective than single modalities in the treatment of PTSD.

52–18. **True**   PTSD symptoms in rape victims are particularly amenable to exposure treatment.

CHAPTER 53

■

Acute Stress Disorder

■ **DIRECTIONS: For questions 53–1 through 53–9, indicate**

A if answers 1, 2, and 3 are correct.

B if answers 1 and 3 are correct.

C if answers 2 and 4 are correct.

D if only answer 4 is correct.

E if all are correct.

53–1. What signs and symptoms immediately following a traumatic event are predictive of developing posttraumatic stress disorder (PTSD)?

1. Flashbacks

2. Detachment

3. Intense affective states

4. Numbing

53–2. When working with patients who have experienced an acute traumatic event, what are the initial objectives of treatment?

1. Getting to the memories

2. Understanding the unconscious conflicts surrounding the trauma

3. Working through the traumatic experience

4. Establishing a therapeutic alliance

53–3. Clonidine affects which of the following symptoms of acute stress disorder?

1. Impulsive behaviors

2. Affect numbing

3. Intrusive thoughts

4. Avoidance of situations

53–4. Propranolol is effective in reducing PTSD symptoms but is contraindicated when which conditions are present?

1. Asthma

2. Diabetes mellitus

3. Chronic obstructive pulmonary disease

4. Congestive heart failure

53–5. The overall orientation of psychotherapy for patients with acute stress disorder involves

    1. Working through developmental deficits.

    2. Understanding intrapsychic conflicts that have arisen in the remote past.

    3. Intensely analyzing personality factors.

    4. Working through the intrapsychic and interpersonal aftermath of the traumatic experience.

53–6. Diazepam is useful to treat which of the following symptoms of acute stress disorder?

    1. Hypervigilance

    2. Irritability

    3. Feelings of intense anxiety

    4. Affective numbing

53–7. In both group and individual therapy for patients with acute stress disorder, what would be examples of early interventions?

    1. Containment of intense affect

    2. Normalization of the patient's experience of and reactions to the event

    3. Use of active listening to enhance understanding

    4. Early establishment of a therapeutic relationship

53–8. A cognitive-behavioral approach to acute stress disorder involves which of the following techniques?

    1. Patients are deliberately exposed to reminders of the traumatic experience.

    2. The family members are made aware of the patient's level of tolerance to reminders of the event.

    3. Cognitive restructuring is used.

    4. The patient is seen at most once a week for 1 hour.

53–9. Front-line treatment was pioneered in World War I and resulted in lower levels of PTSD symptoms. What are the elements of front-line treatment in combat?

    1. Treatment occurs at the front lines.

    2. Treatment occurs immediately.

    3. There is an expectation that the soldier will return to battle.

    4. Physical needs such as food and sleep are critical elements.

■ ANSWERS:

53–1. **Answer: C (2 and 4).** "Psychic numbing" and detachment immediately following a traumatic event predict the development of PTSD.

53–2. **Answer: D (Only 4).** Establishing a therapeutic alliance with individuals who have recently experienced a trauma requires great sensitivity on the therapist's part and a here-and-now perspective, with current symptoms linked to the recent trauma.

53–3.   **Answer: B (1 and 3).** Clonidine is effective in decreasing impulsive behaviors and reducing intrusive thoughts.

53–4.   **Answer: E (All).** Propranolol, a nonselective beta-blocker, is contraindicated in patients who have asthma, diabetes mellitus, chronic obstructive pulmonary disease, congestive heart disease, and thyroid disease.

53–5.   **Answer: D (Only 4).** Long-term psychotherapy addresses developmental and personality issues as well as personality factors. The brief crisis-oriented therapy of acute stress disorder focuses on the consequences of the immediate trauma.

53–6.   **Answer: A (1, 2, and 3).** Benzodiazepines are useful for time-limited treatment of symptoms of hyperarousal and subjective anxiety. They do not ameliorate affective numbing.

53–7.   **Answer: E (All).** Group or individual initial psychotherapeutic interventions include normalization of the patient's experience of and reactions to the event within the context of a safe and secure environment where strong affects are contained and actively listened to. The interventions should be made as soon after the trauma as possible.

53–8.   **Answer: A (1, 2, and 3).** The cognitive-behavioral approach to the treatment of acute stress disorder involves 1 to 2 sessions per week lasting 1 to 2 hours at a time. In this therapy, patients are deliberately reminded of their traumatic experiences to facilitate cognitive restructuring. The patient's family or significant others may be involved in the therapy process.

53–9.   **Answer: E (All).** Essential elements of front-line treatment of soldiers are proximity, immediacy, and expectancy. Sleep, food, and shelter are provided to war-weary soldiers.

CHAPTER 54

━━━━━━━━━■━━━━━━━━━

Generalized Anxiety Disorder

■ **DIRECTIONS: For questions 54–1 through 54–8, match the medication with the most appropriate description(s). Each description may be used once, more than once, or not at all.**

54–1.   Diazepam
54–2.   Diphenhydramine
54–3.   Buspirone
54–4.   Propranolol
54–5.   Lorazepam
54–6.   Alprazolam
54–7.   Imipramine
54–8.   Fluoxetine

a.   Has abuse potential.
b.   Has immediate onset of action.
c.   Effects muscular relaxation.
d.   Decreases apprehension.
e.   Affects the autonomic system.
f.   Has half-life of 20–100 hours.
g.   Tolerance develops.
h.   Decreases apprehension.
i.   Is lethal in overdose.
j.   Is associated with weight gain.
k.   Electrocardiogram is required prior to administration.
l.   One of the most frequently prescribed medications for generalized anxiety disorder (GAD).
m.   Can cause sexual dysfunction.

■ **DIRECTIONS: For questions 54–9 through 54–17, select the single best answer.**

54–9.   Patients with GAD exhibit all of the following symptoms **except**

1. Hypervigilance.
2. Tachypnea.
3. Excessive worry.
4. Increased muscle tension.

295

54–10. Which of the following personality disorders is found more frequently in patients with GAD?

1. Avoidant personality disorder
2. Dependent personality disorder
3. Borderline personality disorder
4. None of the above

54–11. Progressive relaxation involves systematic tensing (for 5–7 seconds) and releasing of tension (for 30–45 seconds) for how many different muscle groups?

1. 4
2. 8
3. 12
4. 16

54–12. Which of the following is an example of *decatastrophizing,* a technique of cognitive therapy?

1. Ms. K. ruminates over her upcoming lecture.
2. Mr. P. says that what he fears most about public speaking is losing his lecture notes and having the audience laugh at his incompetence.
3. Mr. N. states that he has no idea why he worries about giving his lectures—he just wants "a pill so that it won't happen any longer."
4. None of the above

54–13. Which of the following statements does not apply to outcome for cognitive-behavioral approaches for the treatment of GAD?

1. The frequency of practicing new responses is not correlated with outcome.
2. The more chronic the GAD is, the more likely the patient will not respond to cognitive-behavioral approaches.
3. The presence of a depression does not affect the outcome of cognitive-behavior therapy for GAD.
4. The more that patients interpreted external situations as threatening prior to beginning therapy, the less improvement they experience.

54–14. Mr. L. receives diazepam 5 mg po tid for his GAD. Which of his symptoms is probably most relieved by this medication?

1. Hypersensitivity to interpersonal relationships
2. Hypervigilance
3. Ruminations
4. Catastrophization of daily events

54–15. Over the next several weeks, Mr. L. may develop a tolerance to all of the following effects of his medication **except**

1. Sedating.
2. Anticonvulsant.
3. Muscle-relaxant.
4. Autonomic.

54–16. Significant anterograde amnesia may be produced by which of the following medications?

  1. Triazolam

  2. Diazepam

  3. Clorazepate

  4. Chlordiazepoxide

54–17. Selective serotonin reuptake inhibitors (SSRIs) inhibit the cytochrome P450 system. Which of the following SSRIs has the least effect on this hepatic system?

  1. Fluvoxamine

  2. Paroxetine

  3. Sertraline

  4. Fluoxetine

■ **DIRECTIONS: For questions 54–18 through 54–22, indicate**

  A if answers 1, 2, and 3 are correct.

  B if answers 1 and 3 are correct.

  C if answers 2 and 4 are correct.

  D if only answer 4 is correct.

  E if all are correct.

54–18. Mr. Z. is on sertraline 100 mg po q day for his GAD. For which of the following symptoms may he report improvement?

  1. Muscle tension

  2. Feeling anxious

  3. Cardiac palpitations

  4. Ruminations

54–19. Even when psychological factors are prominent in the genesis of GAD in a specific patient, insight-oriented psychotherapy may not be indicated for which of the following reasons?

  1. The patient is incapable of forming meaningful human relationships.

  2. The patient is incapable of tolerating intense affects without experiencing a disruptive loss of control.

  3. The patient lacks the ability to reflect on inner psychological processes.

  4. The patient desires symptom relief rather than understanding.

54–20. Diminished physiological flexibility in patients with GAD is demonstrated by which of the following procedures?

  1. Electrocardiogram

  2. Electroencephalogram

  3. Electromyogram

  4. Brain-stem evoked potentials

54–21. Biofeedback methods of relaxation rely on expensive equipment that may not always be available. What other methods of relaxation are just as effective?

    1. Imagery techniques

    2. Meditation

    3. Paced diaphragmatic breathing

    4. Applied relaxation

54–22. Long-half-life benzodiazepines may accumulate in patients with slow hepatic clearance, such as in which of the following groups of patients?

    1. The elderly

    2. Those of Asian race

    3. Those with chronic alcoholism

    4. Adolescents

■ ANSWERS:

54–1. Diazepam: **a, b, c, d, e, f, g, l**

54–2. Diphenhydramine: **b, d**

54–3. Buspirone: **d**

54–4. Propranolol: **e, k, m**

54–5. Lorazepam: **a, b, c, d, e, g, l**

54–6. Alprazolam: **a, b, c, d, e, g, l**

54–7. Imipramine: **d, i, j, k**

54–8. Fluoxetine: **d, m**

54–9. **Answer: 2.** Unlike patients with panic disorder or posttraumatic stress disorder (PTSD), patients with GAD do not experience autonomic hyperactivity, such as tachypnea, tachycardia, or diaphoresis.

54–10. **Answer: 4.** No personality disorder is specifically associated with GAD. Patients with GAD do exhibit more maladaptive traits than nonanxious individuals.

54–11. **Answer: 4.** Progressive relaxation initially involves systematic tensing and relaxing of 16 different muscle groups. Over the course of the therapy process, the muscle groups are combined to shorten the procedure, and eventually the patient learns to produce a deeply relaxed state by focusing on the muscle groups.

54–12. **Answer: 2.** Decatastrophizing is a technique of cognitive therapy that involves taking a specific fear and helping the patient process what feared outcome is being predicted. Rarely have patients with GAD fully thought through to completion their fears about what exactly will happen.

54–13. **Answer: 2.** Chronicity of GAD is not a predictor of outcome for behavioral or cognitive-behavioral interventions.

54–14. **Answer: 2.** Hypervigilance and somatic manifestations are helped most by benzodiazepines, such as diazepam, whereas psychic symptoms are less affected.

54–15. **Answer: 4.** Tolerance may develop to the sedating, anticonvulsant, and muscle-relaxant properties of benzodiazepines. Tolerance to the autonomic effects of benzodiazepines will not develop.

54–16. **Answer: 1.** Longer-acting benzodiazepines, such as diazepam, clorazepate, and chlordiazepoxide, are least likely to induce amnesia.

54–17. **Answer: 3.** Sertraline, compared with other SSRIs, has the least inhibitory effect on the hepatic cytochrome P450 system.

54–18. **Answer: E (All).** Antidepressants exert minimal beneficial effects on the autonomic system and have no muscle-relaxant properties. Patients' subjective perception of bodily states may not correspond to their measured physiological states. Improvement in muscle tension and cardiovascular symptoms, as well as in psychic symptoms, may be reported by patients taking antidepressants for GAD.

54–19. **Answer: E (All).** Insight-oriented psychotherapy requires that the individual be motivated to seek psychological change and growth rather than symptom relief alone. The patient must be capable of forming meaningful human relationships. The patient also must be capable of tolerating intense affects without experiencing a disruptive loss of control. The patient must possess the ability to reflect on inner psychological processes.

54–20. **Answer: A (1, 2, and 3).** The electrocardiographic, electromyographic, and electroencephalographic responses of individuals with GAD appear more rigid and less adaptable to stressors than those of nonanxious individuals.

54–21. **Answer: E (All).** Imagery techniques, in which patients imagine a pleasant scene as if they were actually there, maximize the physiological and emotional relaxation response. Meditation provides a means of focusing on breathing while repeating a single word and directs the patient's attention away from worries. Paced diaphragmatic breathing involves the patient's shifting from shallow, rapid, thoracic breathing to slowed diaphragmatic breathing. In applied relaxation, the patient is taught to identify a variety of cues in his or her environment (e.g., ringing phone, doorbell, clock chime) that signal a reminder to pause, identify any anxious feelings or states, and relax until the detected anxiety is dissipated.

54–22. **Answer: A (1, 2, and 3).** Elderly patients, patients with chronic alcoholism (who are likely to have some hepatic insufficiency), and patients of Asian race may have delayed hepatic metabolism, which will lead to an accumulation of benzodiazepines.

CHAPTER 55

Dissociative Amnesia and Dissociative Fugue

■ **DIRECTIONS: For questions 55–1 through 55–11, indicate**

A if answers 1, 2, and 3 are correct.

B if answers 1 and 3 are correct.

C if answers 2 and 4 are correct.

D if only answer 4 is correct.

E if all are correct.

55–1. Which type of traumas are more likely to cause depersonalization disorder as opposed to an amnestic or fugue state?

1. Surviving a hurricane

2. Being raped

3. Having a car accident caused by a mechanical malfunction

4. Experiencing childhood abuse

55–2. What is the sequence for resolution of a trauma disorder?

1. Management of affect is addressed, then the physiological symptoms are managed.

2. Management of physiological symptoms is achieved, then feelings are addressed.

3. Self-esteem, damaged by the trauma, is restored, then a coherent narrative is developed.

4. A coherent narrative is developed from the memory of the traumatic event(s), then self-esteem, damaged by the trauma, is restored.

55–3. Patients coming to clinical attention after a dissociative fugue should be evaluated carefully for which of the following conditions?

1. Closed head injury

2. Sexually transmitted diseases

3. Fractures

4. Pregnancy

55–4. Patients with amnesia for personal identity may improve rapidly with which of the following treatments?

1. Thiothixene
2. Cognitive-behavior therapy
3. Lorazepam
4. Provision of a safe haven

55–5. Amnestic patients may present with a variety of self-harming behaviors. Which of the following are constructive responses to a patient who has presented with fresh and old scars from razor-blade slashing?

1. "I wonder if you were trying to understand a past traumatic experience?"
2. "You are a troublemaker who only comes to the emergency room to bother every new resident."
3. "Those slashes look painful. I wonder what is even more painful that you are trying to manage?"
4. "What are you doing? Don't you know that you could lose your arm if you keep this up?"

55–6. Dissociated memories are usually linked with overwhelming affects and cognitions. What factors constitute contraindications to uncovering dissociated memory material in a long-term psychotherapy process?

1. Ongoing substance abuse
2. Unstable therapeutic alliance
3. Severe primary alexithymia
4. Comorbid diagnosis

55–7. Grounding maneuvers consist of which of the following?

1. Orienting the patient to time and circumstances
2. Reminding the patient that the therapist is in the "here and now"
3. Telling the patient to open his or her eyes
4. Providing an interpretation of the experience

55–8. Under what circumstances will patients with dissociative fugue resist uncovering their actual identity?

1. The onset of the fugue is secondary to an acute trauma.
2. The patient has established a new identity, occupation, and social relationships.
3. The onset of the fugue is recent.
4. A matrix of family, sexual, and legal problems form the background of the fugue.

55–9. Amytal narcosynthesis is used to work with which type of patients?

1. Patients with conversion disorders
2. Patients who are not involved in legal proceedings
3. Patients with acute amnesias
4. Patients with chronic, lifelong history of abuse who have clear, conscious memories

55–10. Which of the following are dimensions of the traumatic experience that must be systematically accounted for?

 1. Sensory

 2. Affective

 3. Cognitive

 4. Behavioral

55–11. What are the goals in the final phase of treatment for dissociative disorders?

 1. Memories of traumatic experiences should have lost their special quality.

 2. The patient should have completely repressed all traumatic memories.

 3. There should no longer be involuntary intrusions of imagery, affect, or sensation.

 4. The patient should not meet the criteria for psychiatric disorder.

■ **DIRECTIONS: For questions 55–12 through 55–15, select the single best answer.**

55–12. Which pharmacological agent specifically targets dissociative amnesia or fugue states?

 1. Diazepam

 2. Fluoxetine

 3. Risperidone

 4. None of the above

55–13. What is the most important aspect of the initial treatment of individuals with trauma disorders?

 1. Establishing a sense of safety for the patient

 2. Getting to the intrusive memories

 3. Medicating the patient's somatic symptoms

 4. Telling the patient that he or she is in a dissociative state

55–14. The only source of systematic data on the treatment of dissociative amnesia and dissociative fugue is

 1. The literature on Vietnam War veterans.

 2. World War I literature on combat trauma.

 3. World War II literature on combat trauma.

 4. Field experience from the Gulf War combat trauma.

55–15. Which of the following is a common, striking feature in the history of patients with amnestic disorders?

 1. These patients recount histories of abuse with minimal affect and minimize the circumstances.

 2. These patients have no conscious memories of abuse.

 3. Frequently, the abuse is fabricated by these patients.

 4. None of the above.

■ **ANSWERS:**

55–1. **Answer: B (1 and 3).** Persistent dissociative amnesia after traumatic experiences occurs more frequently when the trauma involves interpersonal interactions, when it occurs at a young age, when it involves threat of death or when violence is prevalent, and when it is repetitive. Depersonalization is associated with single traumas, particularly natural disasters or those precipitated by nonhuman agents.

55–2. **Answer: C (2 and 4).** Physiological symptoms of posttraumatic stress disorder (PTSD) are addressed first, then the person is able to bear the feelings associated with the traumatic memories. Then the traumatic event(s) is placed in a coherent narrative, and reparation of self-esteem, damaged by the trauma(s), may occur. The person's relationships are reestablished in this phase. Finally, the person reconstructs a coherent system of meaning and belief that encompasses the trauma.

55–3. **Answer: E (All).** Patients coming to clinical attention after a dissociative fugue require careful evaluation for injuries sustained during the trauma, including closed head injury, fractures, damage to internal organs, sexually transmitted diseases, injury to the genitalia, and pregnancy.

55–4. **Answer: D (Only 4).** Acute dissociative amnesia or fugue states may resolve spontaneously once the patient is in a safe environment.

55–5. **Answer: B (1 and 3).** Viewing a patient's behaviors as attempts to master traumatic experiences, even if these attempts are highly maladaptive, may actually decrease the frequency of the behaviors. Positioning the patient in an adversarial role or as a "bad" person only serves to reinforce the role as victim.

55–6. **Answer: A (1, 2, and 3).** In general, the early stages of therapy, an unstable therapeutic alliance, current or ongoing abuse, acute external life crisis, extreme age, lack of ego strength, uncontrolled flashbacks, and severe primary alexithymia represent relative contraindications to uncovering dissociated memories. Many patients have a comorbid diagnosis of depression or of other anxiety disorders. The presence of a comorbid diagnosis does not preclude the exploration of memories.

55–7. **Answer: A (1, 2, and 3).** Grounding maneuvers are concrete, supportive techniques that move the patient from the past traumatic experiences to the present. Interpretations may be provided after the patient has stabilized.

55–8. **Answer: C (2 and 4).** In the rare circumstance when a new identity, occupation, and social relationships have been firmly established, the patient may resist treatment. A background of social, legal, and occupational problems does not bode well for the patient's motivation to uncover his or her identity.

55–9. **Answer: A (1, 2, and 3).** Amytal narcosynthesis interviews are used most frequently in general medical settings with patients who have conversion disorders and acute amnesias. Such interviews can be used for other patients with dissociative fugue states, although they are less productive and should be avoided if the patient is involved in legal proceedings.

55–10. **Answer: E (All).** Traumatic experiences are composed of multiple dimensions, including sensory, affective, cognitive, and behavioral.

55–11. **Answer: B (1 and 3).** The goals of the final stage of treatment of dissociative disorders include the voluntary and conscious containment of memories of the trauma that have lost their special quality. Complete repression of traumatic memories is not necessarily a goal. Patients may meet the criteria for other psychiatric disorders even when their primary diagnosis of dissociative disorder no longer applies.

55–12. **Answer: 4.** There are *no* pharmacological agents that specifically target dissociative amnesia or fugue states.

55–13. **Answer: 1.** Acute amnesia and fugue states are frequently psychological alternatives to suicide. Thus, establishing a sense of safety and acceptance is crucial in the initial management of patients with trauma disorders.

55–14. **Answer: 3.** The systematic data on dissociative amnesia and dissociative fugue are in the literature from World War II combat trauma.

55–15. **Answer: 1.** Many patients with amnestic disorder will present an ability to clearly recount their abuse but will minimize obvious traumatic circumstances.

CHAPTER 56

Dissociative Identity Disorder

DIRECTIONS: For questions 56–1 through 56–4, match the therapy with the associated statement(s). Each statement may be used once, more than once, or not at all.

56–1. Strategic integrationalism

56–2. Tactical integrationalism

56–3. Personality-focused treatments

56–4. Adaptationalism

a. In one subgroup of this model, attempts are made to heal the pain of the past with highly tangible corrective emotional experiences.

b. Management of life activities is the main focus.

c. This approach is consistent with psychoanalytic principles.

d. This model is the best example of a series of short-term treatments imbricated within a long-term treatment.

e. This approach is frequently used in the first stages of therapy.

f. Boundary violations are frequently seen in one subgroup of this approach.

g. Integration of the various alters is one goal of this approach.

h. Attempts at problem solving of the inner group or family are characteristic of this modality.

i. This modality is indicated when the patient has limited emotional resources.

j. The patient must be stable for this approach to work.

k. Integration of the various alters is not a critical goal of this approach.

l. This therapy uses a series of discrete interventions.

■ **DIRECTIONS: For questions 56–5 through 56–11, indicate**

  A if answers 1, 2, and 3 are correct.

  B if answers 1 and 3 are correct.

  C if answers 2 and 4 are correct.

  D if only answer 4 is correct.

  E if all are correct.

56–5. There is a great deal of controversy surrounding the believability of allegations made by patients with dissociative identity disorder (DID). In the treatment process, what might characterize the recall of memories?

  1. Nearly photographic recall of events

  2. Willful misrepresentation

  3. Fantasy blurred with reality

  4. Highly improbable allegations

56–6. Which of the following "truths" are equivalent?

  1. Psychological truth

  2. Scientific truth

  3. Legal truth

  4. Each truth is unique.

56–7. Alters are not considered fused until there have been 3 stable months of which of the following?

  1. Subjective sense of unity

  2. The presence of only half the original number of alters

  3. Continuity of contemporary memory

  4. A 50% reduction in overt behavioral signs of DID

56–8. Medication-assisted hypnosis is **not** indicated for what type of patients?

  1. Those involved in legal proceedings or who plan to pursue legal discourse

  2. Patients who are "too eager"

  3. Patients who have a high level of paranoia

  4. Patients who expect that a medication-facilitated interview will succeed

56–9. What type of medications may be used to facilitate hypnosis?

  1. Sublingual lorazepam

  2. Amobarbital

  3. Intravenous lorazepam

  4. Hexobarbital

56–10. Which of the following statements are **true** regarding family therapy work with DID patients?

  1. Work with the family of origin is critical to understanding the patient in the context of his or her family system.

  2. Marital therapy may be necessary.

   3. Work with the family of origin is usually highly productive.

   4. Supportive family work with current significant family members may be constructive.

56–11. What treatment modalities may be useful in patients with DID?

   1. Pharmacotherapy

   2. Behavior therapy

   3. Cognitive therapy

   4. Individual psychodynamic therapy

■ **DIRECTIONS: For questions 56–12 through 56–19, indicate whether the statement is true or false.**

56–12. _____ The accuracy of one allegation made by a DID patient is sufficient to validate all other allegations.

56–13. _____ If a patient has undergone hypnosis to recall memories, then a court may decide not to admit the hypnotically recalled allegations as criminal evidence.

56–14. _____ The absolute truth must be discovered for a DID patient to achieve mental health.

56–15. _____ Pursuing legal action for allegations of past abuse may not be in a patient's best interest with respect to his or her treatment.

56–16. _____ Patients who achieve and sustain integration are more successful and experience relapse less frequently than those patients who opt for resolution.

56–17. _____ Patients who demand proof of the therapist's caring, such as hugs, should be gratified.

56–18. _____ History gathering about each alter is counterproductive to treatment.

56–19. _____ Fusion techniques may be carried out by themselves to bring about a complete resolution of DID.

■ **DIRECTIONS: For questions 56–20 through 56–28, select the single best answer.**

56–20. What percentage of patients alleging incest can produce good supporting documentation of their allegations?

   1. 10%

   2. 40%

   3. 50%

   4. 75%

56–21. What percentage of patients with documented abuse will have no conscious memories when follow-up interviews are conducted?

   1. 10%

   2. 20%

   3. 30%

   4. 40%

■ **DIRECTIONS: For questions 56–22 through 56–28, using the following clinical material, select the single best answer.**

Ms. K. is an unemployed, college-educated 36-year-old who has a well-documented history of sexual and physical abuse by multiple male family members. At least three alters have been identified. She has intrusive thoughts, autonomic overarousal, nightmares, and a history of self-mutilation.

56–22. What types of interventions may be made in the first stage of therapy with Ms. K.?

1. Creating an atmosphere of safety
2. Creating a personal autobiographical memory
3. Maintaining a future orientation
4. Mourning the past abuse

56–23. One of Ms. K.'s alters is particularly engaging. Which of the following statements is **true** regarding the treatment of each alter?

1. Because this alter is particularly engaging, then the therapist may elect to spend more time on this alter.
2. The therapist may shift his or her behavior according to whatever alter predominates at a moment in time.
3. The therapist must be evenhanded with all the alters.
4. A complex interpretation concerning the unconscious conflicts of the alter is warranted.

56–24. Ms. K. has just obtained a hard-won employment situation. The therapist makes a warm and generally supportive comment. Ms. K. may react in which of the following ways?

1. The self-mutilation may increase.
2. A particularly hostile alter may appear.
3. She may withdraw and become mute.
4. All of the above.

56–25. Ms. K. has asked how many times per week therapy is preferable. What is the correct response?

1. Once every 2 weeks
2. Once a week
3. Twice a week
4. Three times a week

56–26. Ms. K.'s insurance company would like an estimated time frame for treatment of DID. For a case like that of the patient in question, what is the time frame for therapy of optimal intensity?

1. 6 months
2. 12 months
3. 3 to 7 years
4. There is no recovery from DID; therapy is continued indefinitely.

56–27. Ms. K. is the first DID patient that the therapist has ever treated. What difficulty may the therapist encounter?

    1. The therapist may become a detective and demand that the patient demonstrate the absolute truth.

    2. The therapist may try to love the patient to health.

    3. The therapist may become overwhelmed with the patient's pain.

    4. All of the above.

56–28. Ms. K. would like to join a group therapy process in addition to her individual therapy. Which of the following statements is **true** regarding group therapy for DID patients?

    1. Group therapy with other stable DID patients may be beneficial.

    2. Support groups without professional leaders are the most useful.

    3. Any long-term, open-ended group therapy process is beneficial.

    4. Group therapy is never indicated for these patients.

▪ **DIRECTIONS: For questions 56–29 through 56–31, match the type of hospitalization with the appropriate statement(s). Each statement may be used once, more than once, or not at all.**

56–29.	Brief hospitalization	a.	Addressing the alters by name is standard treatment in the unit milieu.
56–30.	Short admissions	b.	Discrete problems are addressed.
56–31.	Long admissions	c.	The time frame is 2 to 8 weeks.
		d.	This type of admission is to address problems that threaten to overwhelm the patient.
		e.	This type of admission is for patients who are massively decompensated.
		f.	Patients with serious comorbid psychopathology may benefit from this type of admission.
		g.	The staff are expected to recognize the alters.

▪ **ANSWERS:**

56–1. Strategic integrationalism: **c, g, j**

56–2. Tactical integrationalism: **d, g, l**

56–3. Personality-focused treatments: **a, f, h, k**

56–4. Adaptationalism: **b, e, i, k**

56–5. **Answer: E (All).** In the treatment process with any given DID patient, a wide spectrum of memories and allegations may be recalled. Highly improbable and/or horrible allegations may serve important dynamic functions and disguise more mundane maltreatment.

56–6. **Answer: D (Only 4).** The criteria for determining psychological truth, scientific truth, and legal truth are unique for each type of truth. What may inform successful treatment and assist the patient to lead a productive life may be without scientific or legal credibility.

56–7. **Answer: B (1 and 3).** Fusion is not considered until there are 3 stable months of 1) subjective sense of unity, 2) an absence of overt behavioral signs of DID, 3) an absence of alters (or the particular alter) on reexploration, 4) modification of the transference phenomena consistent with the bringing together of the personalities, and 5) clinical evidence that the unified patient's self-representation includes acknowledgment of attitudes and awareness that previously were segregated in separate personalities.

56–8. **Answer: A (1, 2, and 3).** Patients who are currently involved or anticipate being involved with the judicial system should obtain legal advice on the admission of their testimony if hypnosis, medication-facilitated or not, is to be used in their treatment process. Patients who are overly eager or paranoid should not receive medication-facilitated hypnosis.

56–9. **Answer: E (All).** Barbiturates, such as amobarbital, pentobarbital, and hexobarbital, as well as intravenous and sublingual lorazepam, are useful for facilitating hypnosis.

56–10. **Answer: C (2 and 4).** Work with the family of origin is rarely helpful, and counterproductive outcomes are not uncommon. Marital work may be necessary and useful. Working with current significant family members may be productive if the relationships are reasonably solid.

56–11. **Answer: E (All).** Behavioral interventions can help DID patients modify dysfunctional interpersonal interactions before they are prepared to address the genetic aspects of their behaviors. Cognitive therapy may strengthen healthy ego functioning and reinforce cohesive reality testing. Pharmacotherapy is useful to provide brief symptomatic relief of anxiety. Individual psychodynamic psychotherapy is the primary treatment for patients with DID.

56–12. **False**   Each allegation made by a DID patient may or may not be independent of other allegations.

56–13. **True**   The legal system may or may not allow hypnotically retrieved memories to be introduced as evidence in criminal proceedings.

56–14. **False**   Truth is relative to legal, personal, historical, and scientific interpretations.

56–15. **True**   The decision to pursue legal action may be contraindicated in some DID patients.

56–16. **True**   Patients who achieve and sustain integration of their alters have a better overall prognosis.

56–17. **False**   Boundary violations may occur when patients' wishes are gratified.

56–18. **False**   History gathering about alters may lead to integration.

56–19. **False**   Complete integration requires more than fusion techniques.

56–20. **Answer: 4.** Approximately 75% of patients alleging incest obtain corroboration of their experiences.

56–21. **Answer: 4.** Nearly 40% of patients with previously documented abuse will have no recollections when interviewed 17 years after the abuse.

56–22. **Answer: 1.** Creating a sense of safety and being understood are crucial in the first step of therapy. Mourning and remembrance of the past abuse as well as creation of a personal autobiographical memory are useful elements of the second stage of therapy. A future orientation is not generally possible until DID patients have largely integrated their alters.

56–23. **Answer: 3.** The therapist must maintain consistency between alters. Communication should be clear and straightforward, with complex interpretations avoided.

56–24. **Answer: 4.** DID patients rarely can accept general supportive comments or encouragements. Their reactions may appear paradoxical and manipulative. Anticipating a response such as the ones illustrated may decrease the intensity of the response.

56–25. **Answer: 4.** Three sessions per week is the preferred frequency. Patients who are in crisis may require daily sessions.

56–26. **Answer: 3.** Recovery from DID is possible and may occur with 3 to 7 years of optimal treatment.

56–27. **Answer: 4.** Most therapists respond to their first encounters with DID patients with fascination, becoming overly invested in the process. The therapist may retreat into a detached, skeptical stance and demand that the patient produce the absolute truth. Usual and expected therapeutic and professional boundaries may be abandoned as the therapist attempts to love the patient back to health. The therapist may become an advocate, urging the patient to pursue justice through confrontation, regardless of the consequences for the patient. The therapist may become overwhelmed by the patient's pain and develop vicarious posttraumatic stress symptoms.

56–28. **Answer: 1.** Group therapy for stable DID patients has proven beneficial when conducted by experienced group therapists. Support groups that have little or no structure are generally not useful and may be counterproductive.

56–29. Brief hospitalization: **b, f**

56–30. Short admissions: **c, d, f**

56–31. Long admissions: **d, f**

CHAPTER 57

Depersonalization

DIRECTIONS: For questions 57–1 through 57–6, indicate

    A if answers 1, 2, and 3 are correct.

    B if answers 1 and 3 are correct.

    C if answers 2 and 4 are correct.

    D if only answer 4 is correct.

    E if all are correct.

57–1. Depersonalization may be a concomitant of which of the following in patients who have experienced some type of trauma?

    1. Shame

    2. Anger

    3. Social isolation

    4. Anxiety

57–2. What states of arousal are represented by depersonalization?

    1. Low arousal

    2. Hyperarousal

    3. Internal hyperarousal

    4. Internal low arousal

57–3. Electroconvulsive therapy (ECT) may produce what results in patients with depersonalization disorder?

    1. Improvement in symptoms with increased feelings of being whole

    2. No improvement in symptoms of depersonalization

    3. Worsening of symptoms in general

    4. Improvement only in depressive symptoms

57–4. Which of the following medications have shown the most promise in the treatment of depersonalization?

    1. Imipramine

    2. Diazepam

    3. Lithium

    4. Fluoxetine

57–5.   What types of therapy are reported to be beneficial for the treatment of depersonalization disorder?

    1. Object-relations–based individual therapy or analysis

    2. Family therapy

    3. Group therapy

    4. Classical psychoanalysis

57–6.   Depersonalization symptoms may be triggered by which of the following?

    1. Intimate relationships

    2. Developmental milestones

    3. Environmental cues

    4. Employment situations

■   **DIRECTIONS: For questions 57–7 through 57–10, match the therapeutic technique with the appropriate statement(s). Each statement may be used once, more than once, or not at all.**

57–7.	Grounding	a.	This technique is based on internal containment.
57–8.	Distraction	b.	The patient turns his or her thought to a distracting stimulus.
57–9.	Controlled dissociation	c.	The patient makes physical contact with his or her environment.
57–10.	Creative visualization	d.	The patient rates his or her symptomatology.
		e.	Spiritual imagery may be used.
		f.	The patient deliberately increases the intensity of feeling of depersonalization.
		g.	The patient may recite his or her name and other personal information to himself or herself.

■   **ANSWERS:**

57–1.   **Answer: B (1 and 3).** The loss of control associated with experiencing a traumatic event may elicit feelings of shame, leading to social isolation.

57–2.   **Answer: B (1 and 3).** Depersonalization as a state of low arousal is thought by some researchers to represent one pole of the continuum of the effects of trauma, with the states of hyperalertness and arousal representing the other pole. Other researchers characterize depersonalization as internal hyperarousal and a withdrawal of attention from external cues.

57–3. **Answer: E (All).** Patients with depersonalization disorder may improve, worsen, or remain unchanged when treated with ECT. ECT in patients with comorbid depression may lead to improvement in the depressive symptoms while leaving the depersonalization symptoms unaffected.

57–4. **Answer: D (Only 4).** The selective serotonin reuptake inhibitors (SSRIs), such as fluoxetine, have shown the most promise of all the psychopharmacological agents in the treatment of depersonalization.

57–5. **Answer: A (1, 2, and 3).** Group therapy with individuals who have experienced the same trauma, such as a hurricane, may serve to mitigate their social isolation and sense of shame. Family therapy has been beneficial in some cases. Object-relations theory views depersonalization as a defensive maneuver and has been reported to be successful in the treatment of depersonalization.

57–6. **Answer: E (All).** Depersonalization symptoms may have protean triggers, such as intimate relationships that remind the patient of a past abuser, developmental milestones, environmental cues that remind the patient of past events, or employment situations in which the patient may reexperience being denigrated or exalted or being held overly responsible for events.

57–7. Grounding: **c, g**

57–8. Distraction: **b**

57–9. Controlled dissociation: **d, f**

57–10. Creative visualization: **a, e**

CHAPTER 58

■

Adjustment Disorders

■ **DIRECTIONS: For questions 58–1 through 58–5, select the single best answer.**

58–1. Data from randomized controlled trial data for the treatment of adjustment disorders are available for which of the following treatment modalities?

1. Psychopharmacological management
2. Psychological modalities
3. Social interventions
4. None of the above

58–2. What is the most important factor in the treatment of adjustment disorders?

1. Understanding the unconscious conflicts
2. Obtaining a thorough grounding in the patient's development
3. Delineating the stressor
4. Understanding the family dynamics

58–3. What percentage of children seen in psychiatric settings—inpatient and outpatient—receive the diagnosis of adjustment disorder?

1. 70%
2. 50%
3. 20%
4. 10%

58–4. In psychotherapy for adjustment disorders, which of the following are linked together to effect a cure?

1. Unconscious motives and behaviors
2. Affect and conflict
3. Thought and action
4. Facial expression and response of others

58–5. Treatment variables for adjustment disorder include all of the following **except**

1. Brevity.
2. Immediacy.
3. Complexity.
4. Proximity.

■ **ANSWERS:**

58–1. **Answer: 4.** There are no randomized controlled studies of any treatment modality for adjustment disorders.

58–2. **Answer: 3.** Treatment of adjustment disorders rests on understanding that these disorders arise from an overwhelming psychological reaction to a stressor. This stressor must be identified, described, and, if possible, mitigated.

58–3. **Answer: 1.** Approximately 70% of children seen in psychiatric inpatient and outpatient settings receive a diagnosis of adjustment disorder. The diagnosis of adjustment disorder for many children represents a prodrome of a more serious psychiatric disorder.

58–4. **Answer: 2.** The role of verbalization and the linking of affects with conflicts over the stressor(s) may be curative for patients with adjustment disorders.

58–5. **Answer: 3.** Treatment parameters for adjustment disorder include brevity, immediacy, centrality, expectancy (for recovery), proximity (to the stressor), and simplicity.

SECTION 8

Somatoform and Factitious Disorders

CHAPTER 59

■

Somatization Disorder and Undifferentiated Somatoform Disorder

■ **DIRECTIONS: For questions 59–1 through 59–5, select the single best answer.**

59–1. Patients with somatization disorder tend to congregate in which of the following medical settings?

1. Family medicine
2. Psychiatric
3. Plastic surgery
4. Pediatrics

59–2. The Epidemiologic Catchment Area (ECA) data indicate that the female-to-male ratio for somatization disorder is

1. 1:1.
2. 3:1.
3. 5:1.
4. 10:1.

59–3. How frequently should appointments be scheduled for patients with somatization disorder?

1. Every week
2. Every 2 to 3 weeks
3. Every 4 to 6 weeks
4. Every 8 to 12 weeks

59–4. Which of the following approaches is most efficacious in the treatment of patients with somatization disorder?

1. Patients should be told that they are not ill and that they should not seek further medical treatment.
2. Patients should be told that they will be referred to a specialist.
3. Patients should be told that nothing is wrong and that they may return if they develop any new symptoms.
4. Patients should be reassured that they will be seen and examined on a regular basis, regardless of any symptoms.

59–5. What is the rate of disability in patients with somatization disorder?

1. 5%–10%
2. 15%–25%
3. 25%–85%
4. 100%

■ **DIRECTIONS: For questions 59–6 through 59–12, indicate**

A if answers 1, 2, and 3 are correct.
B if answers 1 and 3 are correct.
C if answers 2 and 4 are correct.
D if only answer 4 is correct.
E if all are correct.

59–6. The DSM-IV criteria for somatization disorder require which of the following?

1. Four pain symptoms
2. Two gastrointestinal symptoms
3. One sexual symptom
4. One neurological symptom

59–7. Which of the following disorders are in the differential diagnosis for somatization disorder?

1. Panic disorder
2. Conversion disorder
3. Somatized anxiety disorder
4. Multiple sclerosis

59–8. What conditions are frequently associated with somatization disorder?

1. Panic disorder
2. Posttraumatic stress disorder
3. Generalized anxiety disorder
4. Dysthymic disorder

59–9. Which of the following personality disorders are commonly diagnosed in patients with somatization disorder?

1. Avoidant
2. Paranoid
3. Obsessive-compulsive
4. Dependent

59–10. Patients with somatization disorder are noted for which of the following life events?

1. Work disability
2. Multiple divorces

3. Difficulty with friendships

4. Solid social support systems

59–11. Group therapy for patients with somatization disorder utilizes what types of techniques?

1. Didactic presentations

2. A session devoted to members making and receiving positive statements

3. Rotation of group facilitators among the group members

4. Ongoing groups without a fixed number of sessions

59–12. What type of examinations or procedures should routinely be performed on patients with somatization disorder?

1. Chemistry profile

2. Complete physical examination

3. Urine drug screen

4. Partial physical examination

■ **DIRECTIONS: For questions 59–13 through 59–16, match the disorder with the most appropriate answer(s). Each answer may be used once, more than once, or not at all.**

59–13. Somatization disorder

a. Patients with this disorder have a lifelong history of multiple somatic symptoms.

59–14. Somatoform pain disorder

b. There is no conscious attempt to be ill other than to gain the sick role.

59–15. Factitious disorder

c. Symptoms are all limited to pain.

59–16. Conversion disorder

d. Patients with this disorder view themselves as "sicker than the sick."

e. The symptom or deficit cannot be fully explained by a neurological or general medical condition.

■ **ANSWERS:**

59–1. **Answer: 1.** Patients with somatization disorder frequent primary-care settings and general hospitals.

59–2. **Answer: 4.** The ECA data indicate that the female-to-male ratio for somatization disorder is 10:1.

59–3. **Answer: 3.** Regular outpatient visits for patients with somatization disorder should be scheduled every 4 to 6 weeks.

59–4. **Answer: 4.** The patient should be reassured and seen on a regular basis, even if no new symptoms have developed. This will keep the patient from having to develop any new symptoms to justify a visit. These patients should not be regularly referred to specialists because this only creates more symptoms and frustrates both physicians and patients.

59–5. **Answer: 3.** Disability rates among patients with somatization disorder range from 25% to 85%.

59–6. **Answer: A (1, 2, and 3).** DSM-IV contains a major revision of the diagnostic criteria for somatization disorder. Rather than requiring a certain number of positive symptoms from a list of 35, as was specified in DSM-III-R, the new diagnostic criteria require four pain symptoms from different sites, two gastrointestinal symptoms, one sexual symptom, and one pseudoneurological symptom.

59–7. **Answer: E (All).** The differential diagnosis for somatization disorder includes panic disorder, conversion disorder, somatized anxiety disorder, somatized depressive disorder, hypochondriasis, chronic pain disorder, factitious disorder, and general medical problems, such as multiple sclerosis, systemic lupus erythematosus, and hyperparathyroidism.

59–8. **Answer: B (1 and 3).** Comorbid conditions commonly found in patients with somatization disorder include major depression, panic disorder, and generalized anxiety disorder.

59–9. **Answer: A (1, 2, and 3).** The personality disorders most commonly diagnosed in patients with somatization disorder are avoidant, paranoid, and obsessive-compulsive personality disorders.

59–10. **Answer: A (1, 2, and 3).** Patients with somatization disorder are noted to have chaotic social lives, multiple divorces and remarriages, work disability, and marked interpersonal difficulties.

59–11. **Answer: A (1, 2, and 3).** Group therapy for patients with somatization disorder is time-limited. These groups are cognitively and behaviorally oriented. Didactic presentations are regularly used to increase assertiveness skills, improve coping methods for physical problems, and increase positive aspects of life. One session is devoted to members making and receiving positive statements about themselves. Group facilitators are selected among the group members on a rotating basis.

59–12. **Answer: D (Only 4).** A partial physical examination of the organ system that is the object of the patient's complaints should be conducted during each visit. Invasive diagnostic or therapeutic procedures should be avoided, as the risk of false positives and complications usually outweighs any benefits.

59–13. Somatization disorder: **a, d**

59–14. Somatoform pain disorder: **c, d**

59–15. Factitious disorder: **b**

59–16. Conversion disorder: **e**

CHAPTER 60

Conversion Disorder and Somatoform Disorder Not Otherwise Specified

■ **DIRECTIONS: For questions 60–1 through 60–14, indicate**

    A if answers 1, 2, and 3 are correct.

    B if answers 1 and 3 are correct.

    C if answers 2 and 4 are correct.

    D if only answer 4 is correct.

    E if all are correct.

60–1. What type of personality disorders are most frequently associated with patients who have conversion disorder?

    1. Borderline

    2. Dependent

    3. Narcissistic

    4. Histrionic

60–2. Historically, treatments for hysterical phenomena included which of the following?

    1. Marriage

    2. Burning at the stake

    3. Attracting the uterus back to its position

    4. Hypnosis

60–3. Which of the following patients would be particularly vulnerable to developing a conversion disorder?

    1. An adolescent girl with borderline intellectual functioning who is extremely concerned about not having a boyfriend

    2. A recent immigrant from rural Southeast Asia who has just lost her child

    3. An adolescent patient who has average intellect but is failing academically because he has missed so much school because of his seizure disorder

    4. A female business executive who has received a hard-won promotion

60–4. When Axis I pathology and conversion disorder coexist, the conversion disorder may be more of a symptom than a diagnosable primary disorder. What Axis I conditions are commonly associated with conversion disorder?

1. Major depressive disorder
2. Panic disorder
3. Schizophrenia
4. Generalized anxiety disorder

60–5. Which of the following characteristics are frequently identified in patients with conversion disorder?

1. La belle indifférence
2. Psychological conflict
3. Symbolic meaning of the symptom
4. Secondary gain

60–6. Patients with acute conversion symptoms tend to be seen more often by emergency room physicians. In an emergency room setting, which of the following are contraindicated in the treatment of a patient with a conversion disorder?

1. Hypnosis
2. Appropriate suggestion
3. Amytal interview
4. Multiple examinations

60–7. Anxiety surrounding the conversion symptoms may eventually subside, and increased resistance to treatment may occur. Which of the following statements are **true** regarding resistance to treatment?

1. The patient's symptoms serve as a focal point of concern, allowing other family conflicts to fade into the background.
2. Resistance to treatment may increase if the patient detects attitudes of contempt among the staff.
3. Patients may receive so much secondary gain from their symptoms that relinquishing the symptoms entails a significant loss.
4. Patients with conversion disorder are not psychologically minded and are less susceptible to resistance.

60–8. Which therapy is appropriate in treatment of patients with conversion disorder?

1. Family therapy
2. Physical therapy
3. Nonconfrontational supportive psychotherapy
4. Speech therapy

60–9. Which of the following disorders may be exacerbated by administration of Amytal?

1. Psychosis NOS
2. Major depressive disorder
3. Schizophrenia
4. Dysthymic disorder

60–10. Which medication may be used to maintain wakefulness in patients during an Amytal interview?

1. Lorazepam

2. Pemoline

3. Diazepam

4. Methylphenidate

60–11. Electroconvulsive therapy (ECT) has been reported to be effective in some patients with conversion disorder. Why is ECT effective in these patients?

1. ECT may have a direct effect on cortical inhibition.

2. ECT may work by treating an underlying depression.

3. The response may be the placebo effect of a dramatic treatment.

4. The production of a seizure may be an effective treatment.

60–12. Which of the following factors are related to a good prognosis for conversion disorder?

1. Symptoms are present for more than 6 months.

2. The patient is younger than 18 years of age.

3. The patient has a documented neurological disorder.

4. The patient does not have a documented neurological disorder.

60–13. Pseudocyesis will respond to which of the following techniques?

1. Confronting the patient with the fact that she is not pregnant.

2. Examining psychodynamically the patient's intrapsychic conflicts.

3. Exploring the patient's life situation and her hopes and fears surrounding the "pregnancy."

4. Encouraging the patient to publicly admit to her falsifying the pregnancy.

60–14. Which of the following statements are **true** regarding mass psychogenic illness?

1. The most symptomatic individuals should be removed from the group.

2. This disorder usually is seen in relatively closed social units.

3. The group should be given a task to perform to help reduce the contagion effect.

4. Adolescent girls are more vulnerable than adolescent boys.

■ **DIRECTIONS: For questions 60–15 through 60–23, indicate whether the statement is true or false.**

60–15. _____ Hypnosis may allow patients to reveal information regarding the precipitating event of the conversion disorder.

60–16. _____ An understanding of unconscious motivations and processes and the use of psychodynamic formulations in the development of treatment plans for patients with conversion disorder are outmoded.

60–17. _____ All patients with conversion disorder should be admitted to the psychiatric service.

60–18. _____ Patients with conversion disorder may be diagnosed with a neurological disorder at some point in the course of their illness.

60–19. _____ Many patients with conversion disorder know someone or have observed others with their particular symptom.

60–20. _____ Conversion disorder is less prevalent than in the past.

60–21. _____ Among children with conversion disorder, the male-to-female ratio is 1:1.

60–22. _____ Patients with conversion disorder have very little past medical history.

60–23. _____ The dramatic remission of a nonphysiological symptom effectively rules out the possibility of significant underlying disease.

■ ANSWERS:

60–1. **Answer: C (2 and 4).** Historically, histrionic personality disorder has been the personality disorder most often associated with conversion disorder. Currently, however, dependent personality disorder is noted at least as often. Frequently, no personality disorder is evident in patients with conversion disorder.

60–2. **Answer: E (All).** Since the disorder was first noted in 2000 B.C., sexual conflicts have been implicated in the etiology. Proposed treatments have included attracting the wandering uterus back to its position, marriage to cure the lack of sexual relationships, and incineration of the patient to rid him or her of demonic possession that resulted from, it was presumed, cohabitation with the devil. In the late 19th century, hypnosis became the cure for conversion disorder, and it is still utilized for diagnostic and treatment purposes.

60–3. **Answer: A (1, 2, and 3).** Individuals who are at greatest risk for developing conversion disorder are of lower intellectual functioning, poor education, and/or unsophisticated cultural background. Conversion disorder is found more frequently in patients with neurological disorders, especially seizure disorders. Traumatic events such as immigration and death of a loved one are also precipitating events in the development of conversion disorder.

60–4. **Answer: B (1 and 3).** Conversion disorder symptoms may be more socially acceptable than depressive symptoms and as such may be a "depressive equivalent." Effective treatment of the underlying depression may resolve the conversion symptoms. Conversion symptoms may occur in the context of schizophrenia.

60–5. **Answer: C (2 and 4).** La belle indifférence has long been a diagnostic marker of conversion. However, in systematic studies of conversion disorder patients, it is infrequent. Similarly, symbolic meaning of a particular symptom historically has been noted in patients but is not usually identified in systematic studies. Stress and/or psychological conflict are prominent findings in patients with conversion symptoms. Secondary gain as a cause and reinforcer is found in the large majority of conversion disorder patients.

60–6. **Answer: D (Only 4).** Rapid and accurate diagnosis of conversion symptoms is important to effect symptom relief and rule out concurrent disorders. The symptom may readily respond to a gentle, nonconfrontational suggestion; hypnosis; or, if available, an Amytal interview. Repeated examinations by different and/or inexperienced personnel will reinforce the symptom.

60–7. **Answer: A (1, 2, and 3).** The conversion disorder patient's symptoms may eventually become entangled with secondary gains that are less costly than the symptom and will be difficult for the patient to relinquish. The physical symptoms may serve as a focal point, allowing displacement of other family conflicts. Negative countertransference or contempt by the staff may lead the patient to feel an increased need to prove that he or she is sick. Patients with conversion disorder frequently are not psychologically minded, but they *are* prone to develop resistance to treatment.

60–8. **Answer: E (All).** Family therapy is a basic component in the treatment of children and adolescents with conversion disorder. When symptoms are highly reinforced by other family members, family therapy may be indicated even for adult patients. Nonconfrontational supportive psychotherapy encourages a more open expression of affects and reinforces positive coping skills. Physical therapy prevents or treats disuse atrophy and flexion contractures that may add significant morbidity to a conversion disorder. Speech therapy is indicated for patients with aphonia.

60–9. **Answer: B (1 and 3).** An Amytal-assisted interview may exacerbate psychosis in patients with psychosis, paranoia, or schizophrenia.

60–10. **Answer: D (Only 4).** Methylphenidate, a psychostimulant, may be used to maintain wakefulness and to facilitate verbal communication during Amytal interviews.

60–11. **Answer: A (1, 2, and 3).** In some patients with conversion disorder, ECT may be effective by treating an underlying depression or by directly affecting cortical inhibition or memory, or ECT may work because of the placebo effect of a highly dramatic treatment. The production of a seizure is probably not the reason ECT is effective.

60–12. **Answer: C (2 and 4).** Factors that indicate a good prognosis in conversion disorder are a precipitating event and good premorbid health without a comorbid psychiatric or neurological disorder. Symptoms in children and adolescents are usually responsive to treatment. Factors related to a poor prognosis include the presence of symptoms for more than 6 months, the presence of significant secondary gain, and older age.

60–13. **Answer: B (1 and 3).** Treatment of pseudocyesis includes gently confronting the patient with evidence that she is not pregnant, using supportive psychotherapy with a reality-based problem-solving approach rather than an intensive psychodynamic exploration, and treating any underlying psychiatric disorders. Providing a face-saving approach, such as attributing the absence of pregnancy to a miscarriage, is more helpful than encouraging the patient to publicly admit the disorder.

60–14. **Answer: A (1, 2, and 3).** Mass psychogenic illnesses are relatively rare and occur in closed social units, such as boot camp and schools. The most symptomatic members should be removed from the group, and the other members should be given a constructive task to prevent contagion. In the development of mass psychogenic illness, the setting is more important than gender.

60–15. **True** Hypnosis may reveal the event associated with the conversion symptoms.

60–16. **False** Psychodynamic formulations may guide the treatment of patients with conversion disorder.

60–17. **False** Patients with conversion disorder should be maintained in a suitable environment, but not necessarily a psychiatric unit.

60–18. **True** Many patients with conversion disorder have neurological disorders.

60–19. **True** Many patients with conversion disorder have a model for their symptom.

60–20. **False** Conversion disorder may be more complicated than in the past but is not less common.

60–21. **True** The male-to-female ratio for conversion disorder in prepubescent children is 1:1.

60–22. **False** Patients with conversion disorder frequently have an extensive past medical history.

60–23. **False** Several chronic disease processes may wax and wane on physical examination and in laboratory findings. The absence of positive findings does not rule out this disorder.

CHAPTER 61

Pain Disorders

■ **DIRECTIONS: For questions 61–1 through 61–11, indicate whether the statement is true or false.**

61–1. _____ There is a correlation between radiological findings on spinal roentgenogram and the severity of pain experienced by patients.

61–2. _____ For patients with chronic pain, the focus of treatment should be on relieving the pain.

61–3. _____ Depression lowers the pain threshold and predisposes patients to developing pain complaints.

61–4. _____ Chronic pain contributes to the development of depression.

61–5. _____ The traditional patient role as the passive recipient of cures as dictated by the physician is the most comfortable and efficacious for patients with chronic pain disorders.

61–6. _____ Successful operant conditioning programs for the treatment of patients with chronic pain depend on the patient's social support system's being willing and able to actively participate in treatment.

61–7. _____ Opioids and other analgesics should be provided on an as-needed basis postoperatively, because this gives patients the most control over their medication.

61–8. _____ The risk of addiction is so high from opioid analgesics that administration should be curtailed in patients with acute pain.

61–9. _____ Diazepam may exacerbate pain symptoms.

61–10. _____ Malingering is a common problem among patients seeking treatment for pain.

61–11. _____ If the only sign of improvement for patients receiving opioids long term for chronic pain is their report of pain reduction and there is no improvement in functioning, then the opioids should be discontinued.

■ **DIRECTIONS: For questions 61–12 through 61–19, select the single best answer.**

61–12. How long must pain be present before it is considered chronic and not acute?

    1. 1 month

    2. 3 months

3. 6 months

4. 12 months

61–13. Mr. K. is a socially isolated young man who has generalized anxiety disorder. He recently underwent a cholecystectomy. You are consulted concerning his psychiatric status and management of his pain. Which of the following statements is **true**?

1. His social isolation will have no impact on the amount of analgesic required.

2. His psychiatric disorder will have no impact on the amount of analgesic required.

3. He will be a stoic patient and may require less analgesic.

4. He may require more analgesic medication.

61–14. How long after the first dose of methadone will the onset of effective analgesia occur?

1. 2 to 3 hours

2. 6 to 8 hours

3. 1 to 2 days

4. 2 to 3 days

61–15. Mrs. Y. is a 65-year-old who has remained active despite her end-stage metastatic breast cancer. She complains of excessive sedation with her pain medication. Which of the following would be the most appropriate way of handling this situation?

1. Mrs. Y. should be reassured that she is near the end of her life and should enjoy the sedating peace afforded by the medications.

2. Mrs. Y. should be told that the excessive sedation is a consequence of her receiving too many opioids and using too much.

3. Methylphenidate may relieve some of her excessive sedation.

4. Mrs. Y. should receive trazodone to help with her excessive sedation.

61–16. Constipation is a common side effect of opioid analgesic medications. Treatment with laxatives should be initiated at what point in the treatment of a patient who requires more than one to two doses of opioid analgesics?

1. Treatment with laxatives should be started prophylactically.

2. Treatment with laxatives is not necessary.

3. Treatment with laxatives should not be started until the patient is constipated.

4. The statement is false; opioids do not cause constipation.

61–17. Which of the nonsteroidal anti-inflammatory drugs (NSAIDs) is available in parenteral form?

1. Ketorolac

2. Acetaminophen

3. Ibuprofen

4. Naproxen

61–18. Mr. K. is requesting a tapering off of his pain medication regimen. What is the most appropriate order in which the medications should be discontinued?

    1. Morphine, ibuprofen, and finally paroxetine

    2. Ibuprofen, morphine, and finally paroxetine

    3. Paroxetine, ibuprofen, and finally morphine

    4. Morphine, paroxetine, and finally ibuprofen

61–19. Which of the following is an appropriate step-wise progression of opioid analgesic medication?

    1. Codeine, then methadone

    2. Codeine, methadone, then morphine

    3. Methadone, then oxycodone

    4. Codeine, oxycodone, then morphine

■ **DIRECTIONS: For questions 61–20 through 61–29, indicate**

    A if answers 1, 2, and 3 are correct.

    B if answers 1 and 3 are correct.

    C if answers 2 and 4 are correct.

    D if only answer 4 is correct.

    E if all are correct.

61–20. For which of the following sites of pain may NSAIDs provide better pain relief than opioid analgesics?

    1. Muscle spasms after surgical procedures

    2. Neuropathic pain due to invasion of the nerve by cancer

    3. Abdominal pain due to metastatic invasion by cancer

    4. Bony pain due to metastatic invasion by cancer

61–21. What is the role of the psychiatrist in the treatment of patients with chronic pain?

    1. Assessing psychiatric comorbidity

    2. Assessing psychodynamic factors

    3. Acting as primary psychopharmacologist

    4. Developing a treatment plan that integrates behavioral, psychotherapeutic, and traditional medical plans

61–22. Migraine headaches may be treated with which of the following medications?

    1. Ergotamine

    2. Sumatriptan

    3. Morphine

    4. Lithium

61–23. Which of the following anticonvulsants are more efficacious than opioids in the treatment of patients with neuropathic pain?

    1. Phenytoin

    2. Carbamazepine

3. Sodium valproate

4. Diazepam

61–24. Which of the following antidepressants are effective in the treatment of diabetic neuropathy?

1. Amitriptyline

2. Paroxetine

3. Desipramine

4. Fluoxetine

61–25. For which of the following disorders are tricyclic medications the first line of treatment for the symptom of pain?

1. Facial pain

2. Posttherapeutic neuralgia

3. Migraines

4. Diabetic neuropathy

61–26. Gastrointestinal distress is a common side effect of chronic use of NSAIDs. Which of the following medications has documented efficacy for the prophylactic treatment of gastrointestinal distress in patients who require chronic NSAIDs?

1. Cimetidine

2. Famotidine

3. Ranitidine

4. Misoprostol

61–27. What routes of administration may be used for opioid analgesics?

1. Oral

2. Nasal

3. Intravenous

4. Intrathecal

61–28. Which of the following therapeutic techniques may be efficacious in the treatment of patients with chronic pain?

1. Relaxation training

2. Biofeedback

3. Hypnosis

4. Cognitive-behavior therapy (CBT)

61–29. Patients with chronic pelvic pain have a higher incidence of which of the following disorders than patients with other types of pain or the general population?

1. Major depression

2. Panic disorder

3. Posttraumatic stress disorder

4. Social phobia

■ ANSWERS:

61–1. **False** No correlation between radiological findings on spinal roentgenogram and pain as reported by patients has been found.

61–2. **False** The focus of treatment for patients with chronic pain is on daily functioning.

61–3. **True** Individuals who are depressed have lower pain thresholds.

61–4. **True** Chronic pain may precipitate a depression.

61–5. **False** The traditional patient role may be the most comfortable for patients with chronic pain disorder, but it is not the most efficacious.

61–6. **True** The patient's support system must be involved for operant conditioning techniques to succeed.

61–7. **False** Postoperative pain management is best accomplished with a scheduled dosing of analgesics.

61–8. **False** Acute pain should be treated with opioid analgesics if indicated.

61–9. **True** Diazepam may actually increase pain symptoms.

61–10. **False** Contrary to common assumptions, malingering is relatively rare among patients seeking treatment for pain.

61–11. **True** Functional improvement in daily tasks must be documented for the continuation of opioids.

61–12. **Answer: 3.** The 6-month time frame is the one most often employed in the literature to distinguish between whether pain is acute or chronic, but this duration is arbitrary.

61–13. **Answer: 4.** Patients with higher levels of anxiety and less social support have higher levels of postoperative pain and require more analgesic medication.

61–14. **Answer: 4.** The half-life of methadone is 24 hours, thus effective analgesia may take 2 to 3 days after the patient receives the first dose of methadone.

61–15. **Answer: 3.** A psychostimulant such as methylphenidate may relieve some of the excessive sedation experienced by cancer patients who require high doses of opioids. Patients with cancer should be encouraged to remain as active as they feel comfortable during all stages of their treatment.

61–16. **Answer: 1.** Constipation is a common side effect of opioid analgesics. Treatment with laxatives should be initiated prophylactically to prevent constipation.

61–17. **Answer: 1.** Ketorolac (Toradol) is available in a parenteral form.

61–18. **Answer: 1.** The first medication to be discontinued should be the opioid analgesic. The long-term consequences of opioids in patients without cancer are more serious than those of NSAIDs or antidepressants. The selective serotonin reuptake inhibitors (SSRIs) have the fewest long-term side effects of all the medications used to treat patients with chronic pain and should be the last to be discontinued.

61–19. **Answer: 4.** Codeine, oxycodone, and hydrocodone are all relatively mild opioids and should be used first in the treatment of pain. Methadone is a long-acting opioid and should be reserved for the treatment of chronic pain or for patients with cancer. Morphine and hydromorphone are potent opioids and are used after the relatively mild opioids have failed to provide appropriate analgesia.

61–20. **Answer: D (Only 4).** NSAIDs are more efficacious than opioids in the treatment of pain due to bony metastases.

61–21. **Answer: E (All).** The psychiatrist is generally the ideal person to develop an integrated treatment plan of behavioral, psychotherapeutic, and traditional medical techniques. The psychiatrist should assess comorbidity and the impact of psychodynamic factors in patients with chronic pain. The complex integration of psychotropic medications and traditional pain medications may be within the psychiatrist's purview.

61–22. **Answer: E (All).** Morphine may be used to treat acute migraine headaches, but it is falling out of favor with the advent of newer medications. Ergotamine, an alpha-adrenergic blocking agent, and sumatriptan, a serotonin receptor agonist, are commonly used in the treatment of patients with migraines. Lithium is effective for prophylactic treatment of cluster migraine headaches.

61–23. **Answer: A (1, 2, and 3).** Phenytoin, carbamazepine, and sodium valproate are efficacious in the treatment of chronic pain, especially neuropathic pain. Diazepam is an anticonvulsant and a benzodiazepine, and it is not usually used in the treatment of chronic pain.

61–24. **Answer: B (1 and 3).** Amitriptyline and desipramine are both efficacious in the treatment of diabetic neuropathy. The SSRIs, such as paroxetine and fluoxetine, are not effective in the treatment of diabetic neuropathy.

61–25. **Answer: C (2 and 4).** All of the disorders listed—facial pain, posttherapeutic neuralgia, migraines, and diabetic neuropathy—may be treated with antidepressants. The tricyclic antidepressants are the first line of medications used to treat pain associated with neuropathies.

61–26. **Answer: D (Only 4).** Misoprostol, a prostaglandin analogue, has documented efficacy for the prevention of gastrointestinal distress in patients who require chronic NSAIDs. Histamine H_2 receptor antagonists, such as cimetidine, famotidine, and ranitidine, have been used, but there is little evidence supporting their efficacy.

61–27. **Answer: E (All).** The routes of administration for opioid analgesics are intravenous by bolus or continuous infusions, or patient-controlled anesthesia pumps; by epidural and intrathecal infusion; or by nasal, transdermal, and intramuscular infusion. The route selected depends on the severity and type of pain that the patient is experiencing and the patient's physical status.

61–28. **Answer: E (All).** Relaxation training has the most documented support in the literature for the treatment of patients with chronic pain. CBT, biofeedback, and hypnosis have less documented evidence of efficacy but may prove beneficial to a wide range of patients.

61–29. **Answer: B (1 and 3).** Patients with chronic pelvic pain have an increased likelihood of having past or current major depression and of having posttraumatic stress disorder associated with sexual abuse or rape.

CHAPTER 62

■

Hypochondriasis and Body Dysmorphic Disorder

■ DIRECTIONS: For questions 62–1 through 62–13, indicate whether the statement is true or false.

62–1. _____ Patients with body dysmorphic disorder are most frequently seen by plastic surgeons.

62–2. _____ In severe primary hypochondriasis, any attempts at traditional reassurances offered by physicians are ineffectual.

62–3. _____ The patient with hypochondriasis may improve in an environment that provides acceptance for the patient's symptoms.

62–4. _____ The first physician usually consulted by patients with hypochondriasis is a family practitioner or general internist.

62–5. _____ The focus of concern in body dysmorphic disorder is most often on the breasts.

62–6. _____ Surgical intervention is a viable form of treatment for patients with body dysmorphic disorder.

62–7. _____ Patients with hypochondriasis or body dysmorphic disorder are psychologically minded.

62–8. _____ The etiology of body dysmorphic disorder involves fixation on a "defective" body part as a defense against overwhelming anxiety.

62–9. _____ Physicians should not charge patients with hypochondriasis for the time spent in consultation.

62–10. _____ Patients with hypochondriasis should be referred to another physician in a timely manner.

62–11. _____ There is anecdotal evidence that hypochondriasis responds to psychoanalysis.

62–12. _____ Primary hypochondriasis is relatively rare.

62–13. _____ Group therapy is contraindicated in the treatment of patients with hypochondriasis because they are too preoccupied with their own bodies.

■ **DIRECTIONS: For questions 62–14 through 62–23, indicate**

     A   if answers 1, 2, and 3 are correct.

     B   if answers 1 and 3 are correct.

     C   if answers 2 and 4 are correct.

     D   if only answer 4 is correct.

     E   if all are correct.

62–14. Which of the following diagnostic categories preclude the diagnosis of body dysmorphic disorder?

     1. Anorexia nervosa

     2. Transsexualism

     3. Bulimia nervosa

     4. Fetishism

62–15. Patients with hypochondriasis who improve with reassurance have which of the following characteristics?

     1. Comorbid depression

     2. Relatively recent onset of the disorder

     3. Comorbid anxiety disorder

     4. Little evidence of character pathology

62–16. Which of the following are recommended principles for the care of patients with hypochondriasis?

     1. Appointments should be once a week for a full hour.

     2. Symptoms should be regarded as emotional communications.

     3. Diagnostic procedures and laboratory should be conducted on a regular basis.

     4. The physician should be the patient's primary caregiver.

62–17. Which of the following psychodynamic issues would predict that reassurance as a form of treatment would fail with patients with hypochondriasis?

     1. A need to punish others

     2. An internal conflict over gender identity

     3. A need to mother oneself

     4. A conflict of separation-individuation

62–18. Which of the following cognitive-behavioral techniques may be incorporated into the treatment of patients with disease phobia?

     1. Thought stopping

     2. Implosion

     3. Imaginal flooding

     4. Cognitive restructuring

62–19. Which type of antidepressant medications are the most efficacious in the treatment of patients with body dysmorphic disorder?

   1. Clomipramine
   2. Sertraline
   3. Fluoxetine
   4. Amitriptyline

62–20. Body dysmorphic disorder is associated with which of the following disorders?

   1. Schizophrenia
   2. Obsessive-compulsive disorder
   3. Psychotic disorder NOS
   4. Social phobia

62–21. Which of the following are general guidelines for the treatment of patients with hypochondriasis?

   1. A thorough exploration of the patient's past treatment experiences with the medical community should be conducted.
   2. The patient's symptoms should be assertively confronted.
   3. A balance between creating a trusting therapeutic alliance and fostering independence to avoid a regression is of major importance in the treatment of patients with hypochondriasis.
   4. The patient should be immediately reassured that "nothing is wrong."

62–22. Which of the following disorders are frequently found in conjunction with hypochondriasis?

   1. Anorexia nervosa
   2. Major depression
   3. Bulimia nervosa
   4. Panic disorder

62–23. Which of the following medications have documented efficacy in the treatment of patients with hypochondriasis even in the absence of depression?

   1. Amitriptyline
   2. Paroxetine
   3. Nortriptyline
   4. Fluoxetine

■ **ANSWERS:**

62–1. **True** Plastic surgeons are the most frequently sought-out physicians by patients with body dysmorphic disorder.

62–2. **True** Patients with primary hypochondriasis will not accept reassurance.

62–3. **True** The symptoms of the patient with hypochondriasis may abate in a safe, accepting environment.

62–4. **True** Primary care physicians are usually the first physicians to see a patient with primary hypochondriasis.

62–5. **False** The focus of concern in body dysmorphic disorder is most often the face.

62–6. **False** Surgical interventions are rarely effective for patients with body dysmorphic disorder.

62–7. **False** Patients with hypochondriasis or body dysmorphic disorder are rarely psychologically minded.

62–8. **True** Body dysmorphic disorder is characterized by a fixation on a particular body part.

62–9. **False** Time spent in consultation represents patient care, especially for patients with hypochondriasis.

62–10. **False** Patients with hypochondriasis do best with a single treater.

62–11. **True** There are case reports of positive responses with psychoanalytic treatment for hypochondriasis.

62–12. **True** Primary hypochondriasis is a relatively rare condition.

62–13. **False** Group therapy in the treatment of patients with hypochondriasis may be beneficial.

62–14. **Answer: A (1, 2, and 3).** Body image disturbances, such as those found in anorexia nervosa, transsexualism, and bulimia nervosa, are excluded from the diagnosis of body dysmorphic disorder. Fetishism is not accompanied by body image disturbances.

62–15. **Answer: E (All).** Patients with hypochondriasis who respond to reassurance and education have several common characteristics: 1) usually a concomitant depression or anxiety disorder, 2) relatively recent onset of the disorder, and 3) little character pathology.

62–16. **Answer: C (2 and 4).** The physician should be the patient's primary and possibly only caregiver. Patients with hypochondriasis should be seen at regular and not overly frequent intervals. Appointments should be brief, and symptoms should be regarded as emotional communications. Diagnostic procedures, including laboratory testing and surgical interventions, for hypochondriacal symptoms should be judiciously avoided.

62–17. **Answer: B (1 and 3).** Reassurance is ineffective for patients who need to punish others and who have a need to mother themselves.

62–18. **Answer: A (1, 2, and 3).** Thought stopping, imaginal flooding, and implosion all have been used in the treatment of patients with hypochondriasis. Cognitive restructuring techniques are useful in the treatment of patients with depression, anxiety, and eating disorders.

62–19. **Answer: B (1 and 3).** Patients with body dysmorphic disorder experience the best pharmacological response to clomipramine or fluoxetine.

62–20. **Answer: E (All).** Body dysmorphic disorder is associated with schizophrenia, psychosis, depression, anxiety, social phobia, and a range of personality disorders.

62–21. **Answer: B (1 and 3).** A careful and thorough exploration of the patient's past experiences with the medical community and with types of treatment should be one of the first issues addressed in the treatment of patients with hypochondriasis. A balance between creating a trusting therapeutic alliance and fostering independence to avoid a regression is of major importance in the treatment of patients with hypochondriasis. The patient should be listened to with an open and nonconfrontational attitude. Reassurance should be used sparingly and not too hastily.

62–22. **Answer: C (2 and 4).** Major depression is the most common comorbid diagnosis with hypochondriasis, with 40% of patients experiencing this additional disorder. Panic disorder with agoraphobia is the next most frequent comorbid diagnosis.

62–23. **Answer: D (Only 4).** One study has documented the efficacy of fluoxetine in the treatment of patients with hypochondriasis even in the absence of depression.

CHAPTER 63

Factitious Disorders and Malingering

■ **DIRECTIONS: For questions 63–1 through 63–16, indicate whether the statement is true or false.**

63–1. _____ Patients with factitious disorders are honest and open about their disorder.

63–2. _____ External incentives are of primary importance in factitious and malingering disorders.

63–3. _____ Identification of a patient with a factitious disorder may save several thousands of health care dollars.

63–4. _____ Patients with Munchausen syndrome are amenable to psychiatric interventions.

63–5. _____ Patients with factitious disorders may be attempting to ward off a psychotic break.

63–6. _____ The presence of a comorbid major depression improves the prognosis for factitious disorders.

63–7. _____ Fevers of unknown origin may represent a factitious disorder.

63–8. _____ Psychoanalytic psychotherapy is contraindicated in the treatment of patients with factitious disorders.

63–9. _____ One-third of patients with a factitious disorder will admit to creating their symptoms.

63–10. _____ Most physicians do not expect patients to be deceiving them.

63–11. _____ The male-to-female ratio of patients with factitious disorders is 2:1.

63–12. _____ Patients with factitious psychological disorders have a high rate of suicide.

63–13. _____ Patients with factitious psychological disorders do not have a genuine psychiatric disorder.

63–14. _____ In Meadow's syndrome, the mother is usually the parent who produces symptoms in her children.

63–15. _____ Malingering patients are usually seen in outpatient settings.

63–16. _____ Forensic evaluations may be necessary in malingering patients.

■ **DIRECTIONS: For questions 63–17 through 63–23,
select the single best answer.**

63–17. Which of the following symptoms is seen in children with Meadow's syndrome?

    1. Bleeding

    2. Seizures

    3. Apnea

    4. All of the above

63–18. On the average, how many years elapse between the appearance of the first symptoms in a patient with a factitious disorder and the identification of the disorder?

    1. 1 to 2 years

    2. 3 to 5 years

    3. 6 to 10 years

    4. None of the above

63–19. Which of the following is **not** a theme that is frequently found in patients with factitious disorders?

    1. A childhood with consistent, nurturing parents

    2. A compulsive search for atonement for forbidden feelings

    3. A childhood characterized by deprivation and abuse

    4. A persistent search for mastery of a past illness

63–20. Which of the following is **not** generally useful in the treatment of patients with factitious disorders?

    1. Biofeedback

    2. Hypnosis

    3. Therapeutic double binds

    4. Confrontation

63–21. What is a typical reaction of medical and nursing staff to a patient with a factitious disorder?

    1. Staff are professionals and respond as such to a patient with a factitious disorder.

    2. Staff feel sorry for the patient.

    3. Staff respond empathically to the patient.

    4. Staff feel betrayed by the patient.

63–22. What is the mortality rate of Meadow's syndrome?

    1. < 1%

    2. 5%

    3. 10%

    4. 15%

63–23. If the diagnosis of Meadow's syndrome is confirmed, what treatment must be provided?

1. Family therapy to maintain an intact family system
2. Individual therapy for the perpetrator
3. Separation of the child from the abusive parent
4. There is no acceptable treatment.

■ ANSWERS:

63–1. **False** Patients with factitious disorders are *not* honest about their disorder.

63–2. **False** External incentives are of prime importance in malingering but not in factitious disorders.

63–3. **True** Extensive laboratory tests and surgical procedures are commonly performed on patients with factitious disorders.

63–4. **False** Patients with Munchausen syndrome are particularly recalcitrant to treatment.

63–5. **True** Somatic symptoms may be used to ward off psychosis.

63–6. **True** Treatment of the depression may ameliorate the factitious disorder.

63–7. **True** Fevers are a common factitious symptom.

63–8. **False** Psychoanalytic psychotherapy is an effective form of treatment of patients with factitious disorders.

63–9. **True** One-third of patients will eventually admit to creating their symptoms.

63–10. **True** Physicians tend to believe these patients.

63–11. **False** The male-to-female ratio of patients with factitious disorders is 1:2.

63–12. **True** The rate of suicide is high for patients with factitious disorders.

63–13. **False** Patients with factitious disorders are ill.

63–14. **True** The mother is usually the instigator of symptoms in Meadow's syndrome.

63–15. **True** Malingering patients do not usually subject themselves to painful, invasive procedures or restrictive settings such as a hospital.

63–16. **True** Malingering patients are frequently entangled with the legal system.

63–17. **Answer: 4.** Bleeding, seizures, apnea, diarrhea, vomiting, fever, electrolyte disturbances, and skin lesions, including burns, are frequently seen in children with Meadow's syndrome.

63–18. **Answer: 3.** Six to 10 years elapse before a factitious disorder is diagnosed.

63–19. **Answer: 1.** Childhood histories of physical abuse, sexual abuse, or general deprivation are frequent themes in patients with factitious disorders. Another common theme is one of a masochistic search for atonement for forbidden feelings. Patients who were traumatized by a medical illness during childhood may seek to master the past illness in the present by creating symptoms of various illnesses.

63–20. **Answer: 4.** Patients with factitious disorders may accept face-saving techniques such as hypnosis and biofeedback that can be utilized to reduce muscle spasm, increase blood flow to nonhealing wounds, and allow the patient to participate actively in treatment. In a therapeutic double bind, the patient is offered appropriate medical treatment but told that the diagnosis of factitious disorder will be made in the event that the treatment is unsuccessful. These techniques allow the patient to avoid the humiliation of being publicly discovered. Patients generally will not respond to confrontation, despite being presented with incontrovertible evidence.

63–21. **Answer: 4.** As part of the societal sick role, the patient is supposed to be honest, cooperate with treatment, and want to recover. When a patient is diagnosed with a factitious disorder, the staff feel betrayed and may react angrily toward the patient.

63–22. **Answer: 3.** A mortality rate of approximately 10% has been reported in children with Meadow's syndrome.

63–23. **Answer: 3.** If the diagnosis is confirmed, separation of the child from the abusive parent is necessary.

SECTION 9

Sexual and Gender Identity Disorders

CHAPTER 64

Sexual Desire Disorders (Hypoactive Sexual Desire and Sexual Aversion)

■ **DIRECTIONS: For questions 64–1 through 64–5, select the single best answer.**

64–1. Hypoactive sexual desire patients are characterized by which of the following attitudes toward sexual relationships?

1. They have no sexual appetite.
2. They are phobic about physical contact.
3. They have excellent marital relationships.
4. They have appropriate responses to sexually stimulating situations.

64–2. In which of the following situations would the use of fantasy for enhancing sexual desire be inappropriate?

1. For an older couple who enjoy each other's company but who no longer "turn each other on"
2. For postmastectomy or colostomy patients who have suffered a loss of their body image
3. For a partner who experiences overwhelming anxiety
4. None of the above

64–3. What comorbid psychiatric disorder is the most common among patients with sexual aversion disorder?

1. Major depressive disorder
2. Posttraumatic stress disorder
3. Panic disorder
4. Dysthymic disorder

64–4. Which of the following are reasons for why the use of fantasy with hypoactive sexual desire disorder patients fails to alleviate the disorder?

1. The partner is unable to tolerate the sexual fantasies.
2. Patients who are ambivalent about their partners become angry that fantasy-assisted intercourse is successful.

3. The underlying marital discord is not sufficiently addressed.

4. All of the above.

64–5. Which of the following medications may be used to treat patients with sexual aversions?

1. Alprazolam

2. Diazepam

3. Desipramine

4. Fluoxetine

■ DIRECTIONS: For questions 64–6 through 64–15, indicate whether the statement is true or false.

64–6. _____ Behavioral techniques are very important in the treatment of hypoactive sexual desire disorder and sexual aversion disorder.

64–7. _____ Behavioral techniques can be standardized, so that the same techniques will work for several couples.

64–8. _____ People who think that they do not have any sexual fantasies are among those fortunate individuals whose partner is their sexual fantasy.

64–9. _____ By the time individuals reach adulthood, their sexual fantasies are relatively impervious to outside influences.

64–10. _____ Suppression of sexual fantasy is a fairly common cause of partner-specific hypoactive sexual desire disorder.

64–11. _____ Treatment of infertility will enhance a couple's sexual relationship.

64–12. _____ Sexual skills training is never indicated in the treatment of hypoactive sexual desire disorder.

64–13. _____ Loss of control during sexual arousal is an issue for both men and women.

64–14. _____ Patients with sexual aversion disorder who do not respond to behavioral, cognitive, or pharmacological interventions are not amenable to treatment and should be considered "treatment failures."

64–15. _____ A thorough understanding of the patient's childhood sexual fantasies is critical in the treatment of every patient with sexual aversion disorder.

■ ANSWERS:

64–1. **Answer: 1.** Patients who have hypoactive sexual desire disorder experience little to no sexual appetite, even in sexually stimulating situations. They tend to have marital and relationship difficulties. Patients with sexual aversion disorder are intensely aversive to contact with their partners and phobically avoid sexual activity.

64–2. **Answer: 4.** The use of fantasy to enhance sexual relations is a principle treatment modality in hypoactive sexual desire disorder. Fantasy is useful for older couples who no longer turn each other on and for couples who have experienced a loss of body image through illness or surgery. Fantasy can be used to "bypass" anxiety about sexual performance and allow patients to function with their partners.

64–3. **Answer: 3.** There is a high rate of concordance between anxiety disorders and sexual aversions, with 25% of patients meeting the criteria for panic disorder.

64–4. **Answer: 4.** Marital discord is a frequent finding in patients with hypoactive sexual desire disorder. Hidden marital discord may sabotage any behavioral or cognitive therapeutic endeavors. Ambivalent patients may become angry or frustrated when they have a few good fantasy-assisted sexual experiences and may discontinue sexual relations. Overcoming a partner's inhibition or revulsion about the nature and content of the sexual fantasies represents a potential obstacle to successful treatment.

64–5. **Answer: 1.** Alprazolam may be used to acutely lower the patient's levels of anxiety to allow participation in a behavioral desensitization program. Fluoxetine is well known for inhibiting orgasm. Diazepam has a slower onset of action and is not as useful for acute panic states. Desipramine is not used for acute panic states.

64–6. **True**   Behavioral techniques are the mainstay of treatment for hypoactive sexual desire disorder and sexual aversion disorder.

64–7. **False**   Treatment, including behavioral techniques, should be individualized for each patient.

64–8. **True**   Sexual fantasies are nearly ubiquitous; some fortunate individuals have their partner as their fantasy.

64–9. **True**   Sexual fantasies become entrenched by adolescence.

64–10. **True**   Suppression of sexual fantasies because they are repulsive to the patient and/or partner or considered "wrong" is a common cause of hypoactive sexual desire disorder.

64–11. **False**   Infertility treatment may lead to sexual difficulties.

64–12. **False**   Sexual skills training may be beneficial for patients who have little practical knowledge of sexual techniques or anatomy.

64–13. **True**   Perceiving a loss of control during sexual activity is not a gender-specific issue.

64–14. **False**   A psychodynamic psychotherapeutic approach is frequently helpful with patients who are not responding to more typical sex therapy treatment.

64–15. **False**   A thorough understanding of the patient's childhood sexual fantasies may or may not be imperative for successful treatment.

CHAPTER 65

Male Erectile Disorder

■ **DIRECTIONS: For questions 65–1 through 65–11, indicate**

    A if answers 1, 2, and 3 are correct.

    B if answers 1 and 3 are correct.

    C if answers 2 and 4 are correct.

    D if only answer 4 is correct.

    E if all are correct.

65–1. Male erectile disorder is defined as a persistent or recurrent inability to obtain or maintain an adequate penile erection until completion of what type of sexual activity?

    1. Oral stimulation

    2. Anal intercourse

    3. Masturbation

    4. Vaginal intercourse

65–2. Which of the following statements are **true** regarding male erectile disorder?

    1. The prevalence ranges from 3% to 9% in community samples.

    2. Sufficient exercise will prevent the disorder.

    3. The incidence increases with age.

    4. The disorder only occurs in heterosexual men.

65–3. Which of the following medical conditions are associated with increased prevalence of erectile disorders?

    1. Diabetes mellitus

    2. Atherosclerotic peripheral vascular disease

    3. Hypertension

    4. Mumps

65–4. What psychiatric disorders may be associated with erectile dysfunction?

    1. Major depressive disorder

    2. Panic disorder

3. Generalized anxiety disorder

4. Schizophrenia

65–5. Who should be interviewed or involved in a comprehensive assessment of sexual problems?

1. The patient's parents should be interviewed to provide critical information on child-rearing practices.

2. The patient's partner should be interviewed.

3. The assessment should be a family process involving the children and both parents.

4. The patient should be interviewed.

65–6. In the evaluation of a patient with suspected male erectile disorder, what type of physical assessments of the patient should be conducted?

1. Sensory testing of the perineum

2. Measurement of circulating hormone levels

3. Vascular evaluation of the lower extremities

4. Recordings of erections during sleep

65–7. What factors contribute to a good prognosis in the treatment of erectile disorders?

1. Evidence of inadequate sexual stimulation

2. Unrealistic demands for erectile performance

3. Overdependence on penile erections for female sexual satisfaction

4. Presence of a psychiatric disorder in the partner

65–8. What are the patient-reported difficulties associated with the use of external vacuum devices?

1. Lack of spontaneity

2. Inability to remove the device

3. Impaired ejaculation

4. Extreme pain

65–9. Intracavernosal injections have which of the following results in patients with erectile disorders?

1. Relief of performance anxiety

2. Improvement in naturally occurring erections

3. Improvement in intimacy

4. Improvement in sexual satisfaction

65–10. What types of therapy are useful in the treatment of patients with erectile dysfunction?

1. Cognitive therapy

2. Behavior therapy

3. Marital therapy

4. Individual psychotherapy

65–11. What type of vasoactive substances are used for intracavernosal injection?

    1. Papaverine

    2. Epinephrine

    3. Prostaglandin E_1

    4. Albuterol

■ **DIRECTIONS: For questions 65–12 through 65–18, indicate whether the statement is true or false.**

65–12. _____ Empirical evidence strongly implicates poor parental attitudes about sex as contributing factors to male erectile dysfunction.

65–13. _____ Changes in social or employment status, positive or negative, may affect sexual performance.

65–14. _____ Inadequate information is frequently a contributing factor in sexual dysfunction disorders.

65–15. _____ The sequence of behavioral steps in the treatment of patients with erectile disorders is first nongenital stimulation, then genital pleasuring (with erectile concerns minimized), and finally vaginal insertion.

65–16. _____ Sex therapy should not be attempted prior to penile prosthetic implants in patients who are suitable surgical candidates.

65–17. _____ Outcome studies consistently report excellent results for patients with erectile disorders.

65–18. _____ The dropout rates are the same for intracavernosal pharmacotherapy and external vacuum devices.

■ **ANSWERS:**

65–1. **Answer: E (All).** The definition of male erectile disorder encompasses behaviors of oral stimulation, anal intercourse, and masturbation, as well as vaginal intercourse.

65–2. **Answer: B (1 and 3).** The prevalence of erectile disorders is 3% to 9% in community samples. The incidence of the disorder increases with age. The disorder is found in homosexual, bisexual, and heterosexual males.

65–3. **Answer: A (1, 2, and 3).** Diabetes mellitus is perhaps the best-known disease associated with erectile disorders, with rates ranging from 27% to 71%. Atherosclerotic peripheral vascular disease and hypertension are associated with erectile disorders both as direct consequences of impaired blood flow to the penile vasculature and as a consequence of the medications used to treat the disorders. Mumps is associated with sperm dysfunction, but not with erectile dysfunction, if an adult male contracts the disease.

65–4. **Answer: A (1, 2, and 3).** Depressive disorder, generalized anxiety disorder, and panic disorder are all associated with an increased rate of male erectile dysfunction.

65–5. **Answer: C (2 and 4).** A detailed psychosexual assessment should include the patient and his or her partner. Children and parents are not necessarily included.

65–6. **Answer: A (1, 2, and 3).** The physical examination for a patient with suspected male erectile disorder should include evaluation of secondary sexual characteristics, palpation of the penis, sensory testing of the perineum, and vascular evaluation of the lower extremities. The need for an assessment of circulating hormones is well established. Recording erections during sleep is not usually part of such an assessment.

65–7. **Answer: A (1, 2, and 3).** Good prognostic indicators for the successful treatment of erectile disorders include evidence of inadequate sexual stimulation, overdependence on penile erections for female sexual satisfaction, unrealistic demands for erectile performance, and lack of accurate information on age-related changes in sexual functioning. The presence of a psychiatric disorder in the patient's partner is associated with a poorer outcome.

65–8. **Answer: B (1 and 3).** The most commonly reported difficulties with external vacuum devices are lack of spontaneity, difficulty applying the device, impaired ejaculation, and discomfort.

65–9. **Answer: D (Only 4).** Self-administered intracavernosal injections result in regular intercourse and greater sexual satisfaction. This treatment modality does not affect performance anxiety, naturally occurring erections, or intimacy.

65–10. **Answer: E (All).** Cognitive therapy to address irrational and negative thoughts; behavioral techniques to enhance sexual pleasure as well as performance; marital therapy to address issues of communication, intimacy, and sexuality; and individual psychotherapy to address intrapsychic conflicts—all are used to treat patients with erectile disorders.

65–11. **Answer: B (1 and 3).** Papaverine, prostaglandin E_1, and phenoxybenzamine are vasoactive substances that are injected into the corpora cavernosa, creating a relaxation of arterial and cavernosal smooth muscle with increased penile arterial inflow.

65–12. **False** There is no evidence to support poor parental attitudes as causal factors in erectile dysfunction.

65–13. **True** Major life events may affect sexual performance.

65–14. **True** Lack of basic information regarding sexuality, medical conditions, and anatomy all contribute to erectile dysfunction.

65–15. **True** The sequence of behavioral steps in the treatment of patients with erectile disorders is one aspect of treatment of sexual disorders that is standardized.

65–16. **False** Sex therapy is less invasive and associated with less morbidity than is surgical implantation; as such, it should be attempted prior to prosthetic implants.

65–17. **False** Outcome studies report highly variable results for patients with erectile disorders.

65–18. **False** External vacuum devices are accepted by 80% of patients, a proportion that is far higher than that for intracavernosal injection therapy.

CHAPTER 66

Female Sexual Arousal Disorder and Female Orgasmic Disorder

■ **DIRECTIONS: For questions 66–1 through 66–9, select the single best answer.**

66–1. Female sexual excitement is under the control of what neurochemical system?

    1. Adrenergic

    2. Cholinergic

    3. Dopaminergic

    4. Serotonergic

66–2. What is the prevalence of female sexual arousal disorder (FSAD)?

    1. 5%

    2. 10%

    3. 15%

    4. Prevalence unknown

66–3. The female orgasm is a genital reflex controlled by spinal neural centers. During orgasm, muscles contract rhythmically at what rate?

    1. 0.1 second

    2. 0.5 second

    3. 0.8 second

    4. 1.0 second

66–4. Women may achieve orgasm through

    1. Erotic fantasy.

    2. Coitus.

    3. Masturbation.

    4. All of the above.

66–5. Higher levels of satisfaction are reported by which group of heterosexual women?

    1. Women who experience orgasm simultaneously with their partner

    2. Women who experience orgasm after their partner

    3. Women who experience orgasm before their partner

    4. Women who experience orgasm without their partner

66–6. What percentage of the time do women achieve orgasm?

    1. 10% to 20%

    2. 30% to 50%

    3. 40% to 80%

    4. 75% to 100%

66–7. Which of the following medications is used to treat anorgasmia?

    1. Fluoxetine

    2. Cyproheptadine

    3. Paroxetine

    4. Sertraline

66–8. What type of stimulation is needed for women to maintain arousal?

    1. Intermittent

    2. One-shot

    3. Continual

    4. None

66–9. What are the goals of treatment of FSAD?

    1. Increased frequency of orgasm

    2. Improvement in the woman's sexual pleasure

    3. Pregnancy

    4. Improvement in the male partner's pleasure

■ **DIRECTIONS: For questions 66–10 through 66–20, indicate whether the statement is true or false.**

66–10. _____ Behavior therapy for FSAD is highly successful even when dynamic issues are not addressed.

66–11. _____ Sexual arousal varies systematically across the menstrual cycle.

66–12. _____ Women tend to have a more solid, flexible sense of gender identity than men.

66–13. _____ Girls and boys masturbate at the same frequency.

66–14. _____ Women can take part in a full range of sexual activities without being aroused.

66–15. _____ Reframing negative self-labeling is a critical element of cognitive therapy for FSAD.

66–16. _____ Group therapy is the preferred treatment of FSAD.

66–17. _____ Directed masturbation is an important element of treatment of FSAD.

66–18. _____ Sexual intercourse may be proscribed as part of therapy for FSAD.

66–19. _____ Sensate focus exercises should be individualized to each patient.

66–20. _____ Kegel exercises serve to weaken the pubococcygeal muscles and are not part of the treatment of FSAD.

■ ANSWERS:

66–1. **Answer: 2.** The sexual excitement phase is under the control of the parasympathetic nervous system, which consists mainly of cholinergic fibers.

66–2. **Answer: 4.** The prevalence of FSAD is unknown. This disorder rarely presents as a discrete problem.

66–3. **Answer: 3.** During orgasm, the muscles surrounding the vagina, the ischio- and bulbocavernosi and the pubococcygeal muscles, contract rhythmically at 0.8-second intervals.

66–4. **Answer: 4.** Achievement of orgasm for women occurs along a continuum. Some women achieve orgasm only via erotic fantasy. Others achieve orgasm through coitus alone or with added clitoral stimulation. Still others achieve orgasm through masturbation.

66–5. **Answer: 3.** Women who experience orgasm before their male partner generally report higher levels of satisfaction.

66–6. **Answer: 3.** Various studies have indicated that women are orgasmic between 40% and 80% of the time, regardless of the method of stimulation.

66–7. **Answer: 2.** The selective serotonin reuptake inhibitors (SSRIs) are strongly implicated in anorgasmia. Cyproheptadine has been successfully used to reverse this side effect of SSRIs.

66–8. **Answer: 3.** Women need fairly continuous stimulation, either tactile or mediated by imagery, to maintain arousal.

66–9. **Answer: 2.** The goals of treatment of FSAD include improvement in the woman's intimate relationship and increased enjoyment of sexual relationships.

66–10. **False**

66–11. **False**

66–12. **True**

66–13. **False**

66–14. **True**

66–15. **True**

66–16. **False**

66–17. **True**

66–18. **True**

66–19. **True**

66–20. **False**

CHAPTER 67

Premature Ejaculation and
Male Orgasmic Disorder

■ **DIRECTIONS:** For questions 67–1 through 67–8, indicate

    A if answers 1, 2, and 3 are correct.

    B if answers 1 and 3 are correct.

    C if answers 2 and 4 are correct.

    D if only answer 4 is correct.

    E if all are correct.

67–1. When the diagnosis of premature ejaculation is made, which of the following factors must be considered?

    1. Novelty of the sexual partner

    2. Age of patient

    3. Frequency of sexual activity

    4. Sexual experience of patient

67–2. To what part of the penis is pressure applied during the squeeze technique?

    1. The juncture between the shaft and the glans

    2. The midsection of the shaft

    3. The topmost portion of the shaft

    4. The tip of the glans penis

67–3. What are the advantages of using masturbation for treatment of premature ejaculation?

    1. Masturbation is less arousing to most patients.

    2. The patient is freed from any performance anxiety.

    3. The partner may be less frustrated if the initial phase of treatment is already accomplished.

    4. The technique may be used in patients who are without partners.

67–4. Which of the following drugs will delay ejaculation?

    1. Marijuana

    2. Cocaine

    3. Alcohol

    4. Methylphenidate

67–5. Increasing the levels of which of the following neurotransmittors inhibit ejaculation?

    1. Epinephrine

    2. Norepinephrine

    3. Dopamine

    4. Serotonin

67–6. Which of the following surgical interventions are associated with inhibited orgasm?

    1. Exploratory laparotomy

    2. Abdominoperineal resection of the rectum

    3. Femoral-popliteal reconstruction

    4. Aortoiliac reconstruction

67–7. Which of the following medications may be used to treat inhibited orgasm?

    1. Cyproheptadine

    2. Fluoxetine

    3. Yohimbine

    4. Clomipramine

67–8. Which of the following behavioral sequences are used to treat premature ejaculation?

    1. Stimulation with a dry hand until 7 to 10 minutes of stimulation is tolerated, then stimulation with a lubricated hand.

    2. Oral stimulation until 7 to 10 minutes of stimulation is tolerated, then stimulation with a lubricated hand until 7 to 10 minutes of stimulation is tolerated.

    3. Oral stimulation until 7 to 10 minutes of stimulation is tolerated. Then the partner stimulates the penis until erection and places the penis in her vagina.

    4. Stimulation with a lubricated hand until 7 to 10 minutes of stimulation is tolerated. Then the partner places the penis in her vagina, and movement by both parties is encouraged.

■ **DIRECTIONS: For questions 67–9 through 67–16, indicate whether the statement is true or false.**

67–9. _____ The most common error patients make when using the stimulation-squeeze/pause technique is to become too aroused before pausing and squeezing.

67–10. _____ By the frequency of orgasm being raised, some increase in latency to ejaculation occurs independently of the training effect.

67–11. _____ Premature ejaculation that is not lifelong is seen more frequently in older men and is associated with erectile dysfunction.

67–12. _____ Premature ejaculation is frequently seen in men with complex interpersonal and intrapsychic conflicts.

67–13. _____ Behavioral treatment of premature ejaculation has an 80% to 97% success rate.

67–14. _____ Treatment for premature ejaculation takes 6 to 12 months.

67–15. _____ Women generally have tried for several weeks to get their partner into treatment for premature ejaculation.

67–16. _____ Medical problems are rarely associated with premature or inhibited ejaculation.

■ ANSWERS:

67–1. **Answer: E (All).** The diagnosis of premature ejaculation is dependent on the age, sexual experience and frequency of sexual activity of the patient, and the novelty of the sexual partner. Lifelong premature ejaculation is more commonly found in sexually inexperienced men younger than age 30 years. Relatively infrequent sexual activity increases the likelihood of premature ejaculation, as does a novel sexual partner.

67–2. **Answer: B (1 and 3).** During the squeeze technique, the juncture between the shaft and the glans is typically squeezed for 10 to 30 seconds to decrease stimulation. An alternative approach is to squeeze the uppermost portion of the shaft while the penis is within the vagina.

67–3. **Answer: E (All).** The stimulation-squeeze/pause technique may be used by the patient during masturbation. There are several advantages to masturbation, including the following: 1) masturbation is less arousing to most patients, and a longer duration of stimulation may be tolerated, leading to a shortened amount of time required to achieve success; 2) the patient is freed from performance anxiety; 3) if the partner is frustrated by the patient's premature ejaculation, then he or she may be pleased to see that the technique works; and 4) a patient without a partner may use this variation of the technique, and there is good carryover when he does locate a partner.

67–4. **Answer: A (1, 2, and 3).** Alcohol, marijuana, cocaine, barbiturates, and heroin all delay ejaculation.

67–5. **Answer: D (Only 4).** Increasing the level of serotonin decreases ejaculation.

67–6. **Answer: C (2 and 4).** Surgical interventions that involve retroperineal approaches, abdominoperineal resection of the rectum, anterior resection of the rectum, aortoiliac reconstruction, and surgical procedures for bladder cancer are all associated with a risk of inhibited orgasm.

67–7. **Answer: B (1 and 3).** Cyproheptadine (4 to 12 mg) and yohimbine (2.7 to 12.8 mg) are sympathomimetic agents that are ingested 1 to 2 hours prior to sexual activity and may enhance orgasm. Fluoxetine and clomipramine are powerful serotonergic inhibitors that increase the serotonin levels and inhibit ejaculation.

67–8. **Answer: B (1 and 3).** The usual sequence in the treatment of premature ejaculation is stimulation of the penis with a dry hand until 7 to 10 minutes is tolerated, then stimulation with a lubricated hand. If couples engage in fellatio, then oral stimulation is the next step after manual stimulation. The following step is for the partner to stimulate the penis until erection and then, astride the patient, place the penis in her vagina; movement is proscribed. The final step is to allow movement.

67–9. **True**

67–10. **True**

67–11. **True**

67–12. **False**   Premature ejaculation is frequently seen in young men or in those who are sexually inexperienced.

67–13. **True**

67–14. **False**   Treatment of premature ejaculation takes 2 to 3 months.

67–15. **False**   Sexual partners have frequently tried for months to get their partners into treatment.

67–16. **False**

CHAPTER 68

Sexual Pain Disorders

■ **DIRECTIONS: For questions 68–1 through 68–5, indicate whether the statement is true or false.**

68–1. _____ Dyspareunia is the most common sexual complaint spontaneously reported to gynecologists.

68–2. _____ Like male orgasmic disorder, female dyspareunia is frequently associated with a specific organic etiology.

68–3. _____ Gonorrheal infections may be associated with painful intercourse in males.

68–4. _____ Laser surgery for the treatment of vulvar vestibulitis may cause dyspareunia.

68–5. _____ Patients should not be encouraged to provide their theories on the etiology of the disorder.

■ **DIRECTIONS: For questions 68–6 through 68–13, indicate**

A if answers 1, 2, and 3 are correct.
B if answers 1 and 3 are correct.
C if answers 2 and 4 are correct.
D if only answer 4 is correct.
E if all are correct.

68–6. Common physical causes for coital discomfort include which of the following?

1. Vaginal, cervical, or fallopian tube infections
2. Endometriosis
3. Ovarian cysts and tumors
4. Hymenal remnants

68–7. Estrogen deficiency may cause a decrease in lubrication during the sexual excitation phase, and this may cause pain with coitus. Which populations of women are particularly vulnerable to this cause of dyspareunia?

1. Postmenarchal young women
2. Lactating women

3. Multiparous women

4. Postmenopausal women

68–8. Which of the following historical information may be elicited in patients with dyspareunia and vaginismus?

1. Association of sexuality with sin

2. Poor self-esteem and body image

3. Subtle sexual abuse

4. Active sexual experimentation

68–9. What types of treatment are used for patients with dyspareunia?

1. Relaxation techniques

2. Cognitive reframing

3. Progressive dilatation of the vagina

4. Psychopharmacotherapy

68–10. What are the consequences of vaginismus?

1. Inability to procreate

2. Inability to obtain routine gynecological examinations

3. Inability to use tampons

4. Inability to marry

68–11. What factors figure prominently in the etiology of vaginismus?

1. Monilial infections

2. Pelvic inflammatory disease

3. Postradiation vaginal atrophy

4. Psychological conflicts

68–12. What characteristics are commonly seen in women with vaginismus?

1. Immaturity

2. Confidence

3. Dependency

4. Confident sexual partners

68–13. What are the essential components of treatment of vaginismus?

1. Gradual insertion of objects into the vagina

2. Kegel exercises

3. Masturbation

4. Involvement of the partner

■ **ANSWERS:**

68–1. **True**

68–2. **True**

68–3. **True**

68–4. **False**

68–5. **False**

68–6. **Answer: E (All).** Infections of the vagina, cervix, fallopian tubes, and lower urinary tract may cause significant pain with coitus. Endometriosis, surgical scar tissue, and ovarian cysts and tumors may contribute to pain with sexual intercourse. Anatomic conditions such as hymenal remnants can also cause coital pain.

68–7. **Answer: C (2 and 4).** Estrogen deficiency is seen in postmenopausal and in lactating women.

68–8. **Answer: A (1, 2, and 3).** The psychosexual histories of women with dyspareunia and vaginismus frequently reveal an association of guilt and sin with sexuality; poor self-esteem and body image; subtle or overt sexual abuse; and little sexual experimentation or early exploration.

68–9. **Answer: A (1, 2, and 3).** Psychopharmacotherapy is not available for the treatment of dyspareunia, although any underlying psychiatric disorders should, of course, be appropriately treated. Relaxation techniques involve relaxation and control of vaginal dilatation and penetration with vaginal dilators, tampons, the patient's or her partner's fingers, and finally her partner's penis. Cognitive reframing and exploration of beliefs and assumptions may free the woman of excessive guilt and fears.

68–10. **Answer: A (1, 2, and 3).** Vaginismus inhibits a woman's ability to procreate or use tampons. This disorder may lead to disease states (e.g., cervical cancer, ovarian cancer, and fibroid tumors) going undetected because of an inability to obtain regular gynecological examinations. The woman with vaginismus may be quite capable of becoming sexually aroused, and it is not unusual for her to have found a partner and to enjoy a sexual relationship.

68–11. **Answer: D (Only 4).** Unlike in the etiology of dyspareunia, in which physical factors such as monilial infections, pelvic inflammatory disease, and postradiation vaginal atrophy play a significant role, the etiology of vaginismus tends to involve psychological factors.

68–12. **Answer: B (1 and 3).** Women with vaginismus tend to be immature, insecure, and dependent; to appear younger than their stated age; and to have relatively insecure sexual partners who may have erectile dysfunction.

68–13. **Answer: E (All).** It is frequently assumed, incorrectly, that vaginismus is the woman's responsibility and that only the woman should receive treatment. The partner may sabotage treatment by placing undue pressure on the woman to perform, or he may have a sexual disorder. Both parties may have performance anxiety that should be addressed as part of the treatment. Gradual insertion of objects into the vagina, Kegel exercises, and masturbation are all important elements in the treatment of vaginismus.

CHAPTER 69

Nonpedophilic and Nontransvestic Paraphilias

■ **DIRECTIONS: For questions 69–1 through 69–13, indicate whether the statement is true or false.**

69–1. _____ Paraphilic disorders primarily afflict men.

69–2. _____ Paraphilic disorders are solely ego-syntonic.

69–3. _____ Individuals with paraphilic disorders choose to experience an "alternative lifestyle."

69–4. _____ Character pathology is always seen in conjunction with paraphilias.

69–5. _____ Some paraphilic disorders need not be treated.

69–6. _____ Individuals with paraphilic disorders can be cured.

69–7. _____ A "lovemap" is the generalized representation of a culturally determined lover.

69–8. _____ Five-year follow-up data revealed less than a 5% recidivism rate in individuals who have undergone a relapse prevention program as part of the treatment of their paraphilia.

69–9. _____ Changes in behaviors observed in laboratory settings will necessarily generalize to the community setting.

69–10. _____ There are several well-designed studies documenting the efficacy of a 12-step addictions-model program for treatment of persons with paraphilias.

69–11. _____ Of all the treatment modalities for paraphilias, incarceration results in the lowest recidivism rates.

69–12. _____ Inpatient treatment is never warranted in the treatment of individuals with paraphilic disorders.

69–13. _____ Many orchiectomized men are not left impotent.

■ **DIRECTIONS: For questions 69–14 through 69–20, indicate**

    A if answers 1, 2, and 3 are correct.

    B if answers 1 and 3 are correct.

    C if answers 2 and 4 are correct.

    D if only answer 4 is correct.

    E if all are correct.

69–14. What are the goals of relapse prevention in the treatment of individuals with paraphilias?

1. To develop insight about those internal stimuli that trigger a paraphilic response

2. To develop a social support system

3. To develop insight about those external stimuli that trigger a paraphilic response

4. To develop insight into the vandalization of the lovemap that created the paraphilia

69–15. Aversive forms of behavior therapy attempt to extinguish the patient's paraphilic urges directly. What types of aversive behavior therapy are currently practiced?

1. Masturbatory satiation

2. Moderate electrical shock

3. Thought blocking

4. Ammonia

69–16. What are the basic steps of cognitive restructuring?

1. Identifying the thoughts that lead to deviant behaviors

2. Examining the logic behind the distorted thinking

3. Analyzing the thoughts that lead to deviant behaviors

4. Teaching "victim empathy" to the patient

69–17. Which of the following medications are true antiandrogens?

1. Leuprolide acetate (LPA)

2. Medroxyprogesterone acetate (MPA)

3. Testosterone

4. Cyproterone acetate (CPA)

69–18. What are the advantages of group therapy in the treatment of individuals with paraphilic disorders?

1. Encouragement and support may be provided by the group members.

2. Denial and minimization of the paraphilic behaviors can be confronted by the group members.

3. Victim empathy may be taught and supported by the group members.

4. The group may provide a rationalization for the individual's paraphilic behaviors.

69–19. Treatment with which of the following medications will initially cause an increase in testosterone production?

1. Dihydrotestosterone

2. CPA

3. MPA

4. LPA

69–20. Which of the following medications are approved by the Food and Drug Administration (FDA) for the treatment of paraphilic disorders?

   1. LPA

   2. CPA

   3. MPA

   4. Testosterone

■ **ANSWERS:**

69–1. **True**

69–2. **False**

69–3. **False**

69–4. **False**

69–5. **True**

69–6. **False**

69–7. **False**

69–8. **True**

69–9. **False**

69–10. **False**

69–11. **False**

69–12. **False**

69–13. **True**

69–14. **Answer: A (1, 2, and 3).** Relapse prevention involves helping the individual with a paraphilic disorder develop insight about stimuli (internal and external) that trigger or increase the risk of acting improperly. Because paraphilic behaviors often occur in isolated and unsupervised settings, developing and maintaining a social support system is an integral part of relapse prevention. Destruction of the lovemap, a personalized idiosyncratic representation in the mind/brain of one's idealized lover, may be responsible for the existence of paraphilic imagery. Developing insight into the nature of the vandalism of the lovemap is not essential for treatment of paraphilia or relapse prevention.

69–15. **Answer: C (2 and 4).** Peeping or engaging in sadistic sexual acts may be treated by moderate electrical shock or by exposure to the noxious smell of ammonia. Masturbatory satiation involves having a patient repeat his or her paraphilic fantasies over and over again for a sustained period of time, beginning immediately after masturbation to orgasm. Thought blocking involves having the patient identify the insidious onset of paraphilic fantasizing and displacing these fantasies with healthier thoughts.

69–16. **Answer: A (1, 2, and 3).** Cognitive restructuring uses three basic steps: (1) identifying the thoughts that lead to deviant behaviors, (2) objectively analyzing those thoughts, and 3) creating interventions, such as examining the logic behind the distorted thoughts. Teaching "victim empathy" is part of a behavioral intervention program.

69–17. **Answer: D (Only 4).** CPA is a true antiandrogen. It acts at the androgen receptor sites in the brain to block the uptake of testosterone and dihydrotestosterone through competitive inhibition.

69–18. **Answer: A (1, 2, and 3).** Group members may confront the denial, minimization, and rationalization that are so often encountered in individuals with deviant behaviors. The group may also provide support and encouragement.

69–19. **Answer: D (Only 4).** Treatment with LPA initially causes an increase in testosterone that may have the effect of increasing the sex drive and paraphilic behaviors.

69–20. **Answer: B (1 and 3).** LPA and MPA have been approved by the FDA for treatment of paraphilic disorders. CPA is approved for use in Europe.

CHAPTER 70

Pedophilia

■ **DIRECTIONS: For questions 70–1 through 70–10, indicate**

    A if answers 1, 2, and 3 are correct.
    B if answers 1 and 3 are correct.
    C if answers 2 and 4 are correct.
    D if only answer 4 is correct.
    E if all are correct.

70–1. Which of the following are **not** synonymous with the term *pedophile*?

1. Child molesters
2. Ephebophiles
3. Sexual deviants involving children
4. Sex offenders against individuals younger than 18 years of age

70–2. What are the goals in the treatment of pedophilia?

1. To maintain and enhance adult sexual interest
2. To decrease distorted cognitions supporting pedophilic acts
3. To enhance prosocial behavior
4. To prosecute and incarcerate offenders

70–3. What factors are important for relapse prevention in the treatment of pedophilia?

1. Identifying high-risk situations
2. Limiting the pedophile's support network
3. Structuring the pedophile's time
4. Making society responsible for the individual

70–4. Who can be involved in the surveillance network that provides feedback for the pedophile?

1. Family members
2. Parole officers
3. Individuals with whom the pedophile works
4. The pedophile

70–5. Which of the following are essential elements in the treatment of pedophiles?

  1. Family therapy with a family systems approach
  2. Victim empathy training
  3. Sexual addiction treatment
  4. Normalization of cognitive distortions

70–6. Practical aversive therapy for the treatment of pedophilia involves which of the following?

  1. The individual must be trained to associate the chain of events leading to pedophilic acts with the pungent smell of ammonia.
  2. The individual must carry the ammonia capsules at all times.
  3. The therapist must monitor the in vivo use of the technique.
  4. Electrical stimulation is paired to sexual fantasies of pedophilic acts.

70–7. Pharmacotherapeutic interventions in the treatment of pedophilia involve reducing the individual's sexual drive. Which of the following medications have documented efficacy in the reduction of the sex drive in patients with pedophilia?

  1. Medroxyprogesterone acetate (MPA)
  2. Cyproterone acetate (CPA)
  3. Leuprolide acetate (LPA)
  4. Fluoxetine

70–8. Which of the following agents are available in a clinically applicable depot form?

  1. MPA
  2. Testosterone
  3. CPA
  4. LPA

70–9. What are the potential side effects of MPA?

  1. Cholecystitis with cholelithiasis
  2. Decreased sperm count and motility
  3. Thrombophlebitis with pulmonary embolism
  4. Initial increase in testosterone

70–10. Which of the following behavioral techniques are **not** used in the treatment of pedophilia?

  1. Fading
  2. Exposure
  3. Satiation
  4. "Scared straight"

■ DIRECTIONS: For questions 70–11 through 70–16, indicate whether the statement is true or false.

70–11. _____ The single factor that separates pedophiles from nonpedophiles is on-going, recurrent sexual fantasies or urges involving children younger than 18 years of age.

70–12. _____ Treatment of pedophiles frequently occurs in group settings.

70–13. _____ Non–sex offenders are more likely than sex offenders to have suffered sexual abuse as children.

70–14. _____ Most pedophiles are violent.

70–15. _____ Psychological tests can accurately discriminate individuals with sex addictions from non–sex-addicted individuals.

70–16. _____ Videotaping the pedophile in the act of molesting a child mannequin serves to shame the pedophile into prosocial behavior.

■ ANSWERS:

70–1. **Answer: E (All).** Sex offenders against individuals younger than 18 years of age, sexual deviants involving children, child molesters, ephebophiles, and pedophiles are *not* synonymous terms.

70–2. **Answer: A (1, 2, and 3).** Treatment of pedophilia involves 1) reduction of pedophilic arousal and maintenance of adult sexual interest, 2) enhancement of prosocial behavior, 3) reduction of faulty or distorted cognitions that support pedophilic acts, 4) normalization of other deficits (e.g., lack of victim empathy, concomitant drug use, pedophile's own abuse history), and 5) development of a check-and-balance system to enhance adherence to the program. Prosecution and incarceration of the pedophile are of concern to the judicial system, not the medical profession.

70–3. **Answer: B (1 and 3).** Relapse prevention involves 1) identifying high-risk situations, 2) putting together support networks to assist the pedophile in making a transition to a nonpedophile lifestyle, and 3) structuring the pedophile's lifestyle to minimize stressors antecedent to child molestation.

70–4. **Answer: A (1, 2, and 3).** Surveillance group members function as a source of external validation and reality checks for the pedophile. Group members may include family members, individuals with whom the pedophile works, individuals from the pedophile's social group, and the parole officer.

70–5. **Answer: C (2 and 4).** One of the difficulties in the treatment of pedophilia is that pedophiles are rarely present when their victims experience the negative consequences; consequently, they have virtually no empathy for their victims. They may also have the cognitive distortion that the child enjoys the activity. Normalization of this cognitive distortion is imperative to the treatment. Family therapy and sexual addiction treatment for pedophilia are controversial treatments.

70–6. **Answer: A (1, 2, and 3).** Early attempts at aversion therapy involved the use of electrical stimulation paired to in vitro sexual fantasies of pedophilic acts. This type of therapy is infrequently used because it cannot be applied in vivo. Training the individual to associate the pungent smell of ammonia with the chain of events that leads to the pedophilic acts, having the individual carry and use the ammonia capsules, and the therapist's monitoring of the technique are all elements of aversive therapy for the treatment of pedophilia.

70–7.   **Answer: A (1, 2, and 3).** MPA, CPA, and LPA are all hormonal agents that have documented efficacy in reducing the sex drive of patients with pedophilia. Fluoxetine and sertraline both have shown promise in the treatment of pedophilia, but the mechanism of action is not clear.

70–8.   **Answer: D (Only 4).** LPA is available in a clinically useful depot form.

70–9.   **Answer: A (1, 2, and 3).** Potential side effects from MPA include elevation of systolic blood pressure; weight gain; decreased sperm count and motility; alteration of sperm morphology; cholecystitis with cholelithiasis; an elevated risk for diabetes, depression, and insomnia; and the potential for thrombophlebitis with pulmonary embolism. LPA is associated with a delay in reduction of testosterone levels, and there may initially be an acceleration of sex drive until production of testosterone is diminished.

70–10. **Answer: D (Only 4).** Satiation generally involves training the pedophile first to masturbate to nondeviant sexual fantasies until ejaculation and then, promptly after ejaculation, to continue to masturbate while focusing on one aspect of his deviant fantasy. Fading is a treatment designed to gradually transform the pedophile's arousal from a deviant attraction to an attraction to adults. Exposure involves having the pedophile view adult erotic material. "Scared straight" is a form of behavior modification used to treat children and adolescents with delinquent behaviors.

70–11. **False**   Pedophilia is distinguished by fantasies involving prepubescent children.

70–12. **True**

70–13. **True**

70–14. **False**

70–15. **False**

70–16. **False**

CHAPTER 71

Transvestism

■ **DIRECTIONS: For questions 71–1 through 71–7, select the single best answer.**

71–1. What is **not** a characteristic of most transvestites who present for treatment?

   1. High level of education
   2. A history of cross-dressing that began after age 12 years
   3. Currently or previously married
   4. Age in 40s

71–2. What are the primary motivators for older transvestites?

   1. Sexual arousal
   2. Expression of the "girl within"
   3. Exasperation of acquaintances
   4. Financial rewards

71–3. What percentage of patients who cross-dress as a fetish will purge their closets of the fetishistic objects?

   1. 10%
   2. 20%
   3. 30%
   4. 40%

71–4. Which of the following are **not** conscious motivations for cross-dressing?

   1. To relieve tension
   2. To escape from pressures of traditional masculine roles
   3. To feel beautiful and more masculine
   4. To express traditional feminine aspects of the individual's personality

71–5. What percentage of patients report that their transvestism had clearly harmful consequences in at least one area of their life?

   1. 0%
   2. 10%
   3. 25%
   4. 50%

71-6. Which of the following are found at a higher rate in men with transvestism?

1. Depression
2. Erectile dysfunction
3. Psychotic disorders
4. Marital discord

71-7. Which of the following modalities may be used in the treatment of patients with fetishes?

1. Psychotherapy
2. Aversive conditioning
3. Hypnosis
4. All of the above

■ **DIRECTIONS: For questions 71–8 through 71–17, indicate whether the statement is true or false.**

71-8. _____ Fluoxetine has been proven efficacious in the treatment of paraphilic disorders in double-blind trials.

71-9. _____ Antiandrogen medications (cyproterone acetate [CPA] and medroxyprogesterone acetate [MPA]) may decrease severe paraphilic behaviors.

71-10. _____ One goal for the treatment of transvestite cross-dressing may be to lower the patient's anxiety and to help him avoid being publicly detected.

71-11. _____ Most women who cross-dress and present for treatment have a gender identity disorder.

71-12. _____ Cross-dressing by homosexual and bisexual men is associated with fetishistic arousal.

71-13. _____ Most individuals who are successfully treated will permanently cease to cross-dress.

71-14. _____ Men who are transvestites have a higher rate of alcoholism compared with the general population.

71-15. _____ Men who practice transvestite activities describe these activities as one of the most fulfilling aspects of their adult lives.

71-16. _____ A common transvestite activity is cross-dressing while being sexually dominated by a woman.

71-17. _____ Husbands who revealed their cross-dressing activities prior to marriage are more likely to have their behaviors tolerated by their wives and are less likely to get divorced.

■ **ANSWERS:**

71-1. **Answer: 2.** Most individuals who present for treatment or volunteer to participate in studies are in their 40s, are Caucasian, either are married or have been married, are highly educated, and have a history of cross-dressing that began before age 12 years.

71–2.   **Answer: 2.** During the first decade of transvestite behavior, sexual arousal is the most important motivator. Older transvestites report expression of the "girl within" as the primary motivator.

71–3.   **Answer: 3.** Three or more lifetime "purges" of all female attire occur in approximately 30% of patients.

71–4.   **Answer: 3.** Reported motivations for cross-dressing include 1) to feel more comfortable; 2) to relieve tension; 3) to escape from pressures of the traditional masculine role; 4) to feel sensuous, elegant, or beautiful; and 5) to express traditional feminine aspects of the patient's personality.

71–5.   **Answer: 3.** Approximately 25% of patients report that their transvestite behaviors had clearly harmful consequences socially, occupationally, or personally.

71–6.   **Answer: 4.** Marital discord is the most common comorbid condition found in transvestite men. Erectile dysfunction occurs at a rate comparable to that for the general population. Psychotic disorders are not found more frequently in transvestite populations. There is some evidence for a higher rate of mood disorders.

71–7.   **Answer: 4.** Multiple treatment modalities, including aversive conditioning with electrical stimulation, posthypnotic suggestion, and psychotherapy, have all been used with variable success in the treatment of transvestite fetishism.

71–8.   **False**

71–9.   **True**

71–10. **True**

71–11. **True**

71–12. **False**

71–13. **False**

71–14. **False**

71–15. **True**

71–16. **False**

71–17. **True**

CHAPTER 72

Gender Identity Disorder in Children

■ **DIRECTIONS: For questions 72–1 through 72–10, indicate whether the statement is true or false.**

72–1. _____ Children have a solid sense of their gender by 18 to 24 months.

72–2. _____ The play of children with gender identity disorder is usually typical of their gender until puberty.

72–3. _____ The primary concern of parents who bring their children with gender identity disorder for treatment is that their children will become homosexual.

72–4. _____ Most parents are, in general, fairly tolerant of homosexuality but do not want their children to be homosexual.

72–5. _____ Toddlers generally prefer to play with same-sex playmates.

72–6. _____ Since the advent of gender-neutral toys, children no longer play with traditional sex-stereotyped toys.

72–7. _____ Referral rates for boys compared with girls for gender identity disorder is approximately 9:1.

72–8. _____ Parents have the right to request treatment for their children whom they suspect of having gender identity disorder, even if the child objects to treatment.

72–9. _____ The response of society to gender identity disorder in girls is equally harsh as the response to the disorder in boys.

72–10. _____ Older boys with gender identity disorder have more psychopathology than do younger boys with the disorder.

■ **DIRECTIONS: For questions 72–11 through 72–20, select the single best answer.**

72–11. What is the typical response of grade-school–age boys to another boy who prefers music, art, or other activities that are not sanctioned by the group?

　　1. Children this age are open minded and egalitarian, and they will be completely accepting of the child.

　　2. The other children will grudgingly accept him as a peer, especially if they have been reared appropriately.

3. Children this age exhibit parallel play and as such will largely ignore any atypical play patterns.

4. School-age children are notorious for rejecting any atypical behaviors, and children who exhibit atypical behaviors may be ostracized and ridiculed by their peer group.

72–12. What percentage of children aged 4 years and older will draw their sex when asked to draw a person?

1. 25%

2. 50%

3. 80%

4. 100%

72–13. When the mannerisms, gestures, and patterns of speech of boys with gender identity disorder are rated by diagnostically blinded judges, what is the result?

1. There are no discrepancies between the boys with gender identity disorder and their same-sex peers.

2. The mannerisms, gestures, and patterns of speech of the boys with gender identity disorder are identical to those of same-age girls.

3. Boys with gender identity disorder tend to have hypermasculine characteristics.

4. The mannerisms, gestures, and patterns of speech of boys with gender identity disorder are intermediate between those of same-age boys and those of same-age girls.

72–14. What physical characteristic has been consistently observed in infants and young children who later develop gender identity disorder?

1. The children are physically very attractive.

2. The children are physically unattractive.

3. The children look identical to a sibling who died.

4. There are no special physical characteristics.

72–15. Children with gender identity disorder and comorbid separation anxiety are more likely to come from what type of family constellations?

1. Biological children who are reared in an intact family-of-origin household

2. Adopted children who are reared in a two-parent household

3. Children who are reared in a single-parent household

4. There is no relationship between family constellation and separation anxiety disorder in children with gender identity disorder.

72–16. What is the usual behavioral reaction of parents to their child's cross-gender behaviors?

1. Most parents are inconsistent in their responses to their child's cross-gender behaviors.

2. Most parents are remarkably consistent in their disapproval of their child's cross-gender activities.

3. Most parents are remarkably tolerant of their child's cross-gender behaviors.

4. Most parents are repulsed by their child's cross-gender behaviors and refuse to discuss the issue with the child.

72–17. What therapeutic modality would be appropriate for an 8-year-old boy with gender identity disorder whose father is a 38-year-old business executive who is away from the home for most of any given month and whose mother is a 27-year-old housewife who is afraid to be alone at night?

1. Individual therapy for the child and mother separately

2. Family therapy

3. Individual therapy for the child concurrently with family therapy

4. No therapy is necessary; this family is capable of working things out on their own.

72–18. What is the principal goal in the treatment of children with gender identity disorder?

1. To thwart any budding homosexual impulses

2. To reassure the parents that their child cannot be "fixed"

3. To stop any transsexual behaviors

4. To help the child develop into a competent adult

72–19. What type of paternal behavior is usually therapeutic for girls with gender identity disorder?

1. The father should give strong preference to his sons.

2. The father should actively praise his daughter only for conventional masculine behaviors.

3. The father should praise his daughter for conventional feminine and masculine activities.

4. The father should praise his daughter only for conventional feminine activities.

72–20. What is one documented effect of prenatal androgenic hormones on later sex-typed play behaviors in childhood?

1. There is no relationship between levels of prenatal androgenic hormones and children's play behaviors.

2. Girls who were exposed to high levels of prenatal androgen display typical female sex–typed play behaviors.

3. Girls who were exposed to high levels of prenatal androgen display more interest in male sex–typed play behaviors.

4. Boys who were exposed to high levels of prenatal androgen display more interest in female sex–typed play behaviors.

■ ANSWERS:

72–1. **True**

72–2. **False** The play of children with gender identity disorder is usually play typically found in the opposite-gender child.

72–3. **True**

72–4. **True**

72–5. **True**

72–6. **False**   Despite the advent of gender-neutral toys, children frequently prefer traditional gender-specific toys.

72–7. **True**

72–8. **True**

72–9. **False**   Society is more tolerant of gender identity disorder in girls.

72–10. **True**

72–11. **Answer: 4.** School-age children are remarkably closed-minded about tolerating any differences in the group or cultural norm, despite the best efforts of enlightened parents and teachers. Children who do not conform to the social norms are frequently subjected to cruel taunts and are social outcasts. Interactive and competitive play is characteristic of school-age children. Parallel play is observed in young toddlers.

72–12. **Answer: 3.** From age 4 years on, approximately 80% of children will draw their own sex first when asked to draw a person. Most children with gender identity disorder will draw the opposite-sex person first when the same request is made.

72–13. **Answer: 4.** Diagnostically blind raters judged the mannerisms, gestures, and patterns of speech of boys with gender identity disorder as intermediate between those of same-age male and female children without gender identity disorder.

72–14. **Answer: 1.** Many infants and young children who later develop gender identity disorder are physically attractive children. In particular, these male children have a preponderance of traditional feminine physical characteristics, such as pretty faces and large eyes.

72–15. **Answer: 3.** Children with gender identity disorder reared in a single-parent household are more likely to have a comorbid diagnosis of separation anxiety disorder.

72–16. **Answer: 1.** Most parents are inconsistent in their responses to their child's cross-gender behaviors. Initially, the behaviors are seen as cute (e.g., the child's dressing in mother's nightgowns when he is 2 or 3 years old) and are positively reinforced. As the child matures, parents may have conflicting feelings about their child's behaviors, on some occasions reprimanding him or her for the behaviors and on other occasions covertly encouraging the same behaviors.

72–17. **Answer: 3.** For some women, their child emerges as the principal source of their emotional sustenance and companionship. The family described is at risk for this scenario to occur. Goals of family therapy in this case would be to encourage the father to be more available to his son and wife, to encourage the mother to separate from her child and to mature, and to encourage the child to assume his role as the child in this family. Individual therapy would allow the child to work on his conflicts around his role in the family and with peers in addition to intrapsychic conflicts.

72–18. **Answer: 4.** There are no convincing data showing that the direction of the child's sexual orientation can be modified. Children with gender identity disorder are frequently unhappy and conflicted in their relationships with themselves, their peers, and their parents. These issues may be successfully dealt with in a therapy process.

72–19. **Answer: 3.** Fathers should praise their daughters for androgynous or feminine behaviors and activities as well as for traditional masculine behaviors. Brothers should not receive preferential treatment from either parent.

72–20. **Answer: 3.** Girls with congenital adrenal hyperplasia due to exposure to high levels of prenatal androgen display more interest in male sex–typed behaviors. A related hypothesis is that boys who are exposed to lower levels of prenatal androgen may display more female sex–typed play behaviors.

CHAPTER 73

Gender Identity Disorders
(Transsexualism)

■ **DIRECTIONS: For questions 73–1 through 73–15, indicate whether the statement is true or false.**

73–1. _____ Most clinicians will never treat a patient with a gender identity disorder.

73–2. _____ Gender identity disorders are a heterogeneous group of syndromes, with transsexualism being the most extreme.

73–3. _____ Cross-dressing is intimately connected with sexual orientation.

73–4. _____ Core gender identity is directly linked to gender role.

73–5. _____ Psychosocial histories of transvestites may be similar to those of transsexuals.

73–6. _____ Adults with gender dysphoria have higher rates of psychopathology.

73–7. _____ Laboratory tests are available to diagnose gender identity disorders.

73–8. _____ Cross-dressing dramatically accelerates during and after puberty.

73–9. _____ Psychiatric treatment for gender identity disorder in adolescence may be initiated by the child or the parents.

73–10. _____ Psychotherapy is required for the treatment of gender-dysphoric patients.

73–11. _____ Superior surgical results in sex reassignment surgery are correlated with psychosocial improvement.

73–12. _____ The neovagina created during sex reassignment surgery functions satisfactorily during intercourse and retains the capacity for orgasm.

73–13. _____ In female-to-male sex reassignment surgery, patients will usually select the phalloplasty type that remains semi-erect rather than the one that allows them to urinate while standing.

73–14. _____ Many female-to-male patients with gender identity disorder have masculine appearance but work in employment arenas traditionally associated with females.

73–15. _____ Hormonal abnormalities are unusual in male-to-female patients with gender identity disorder.

■ **DIRECTIONS: For questions 73–16 through 73–26, select the single best answer.**

73–16. What percentage of female-to-male patients with gender identity disorder have polycystic ovarian disease?

    1. 7.5%

    2. 15%

    3. 25%

    4. 80%

73–17. Which of the following is **not** a treatment option for patients with gender identity disorder?

    1. Ignoring the situation

    2. Living part time in the opposite role

    3. Cross-dressing unobtrusively

    4. Having cosmetic surgery without sexual reassignment surgery

73–18. Hormonal treatment will achieve maximal breast enlargement for male-to-female patients with gender identity disorder after what duration of time?

    1. 4 months

    2. 8 months

    3. 16 months

    4. 24 months

73–19. What is the prevalence of gender identity disorder in adult men?

    1. 1 in 10,000

    2. 1 in 30,000

    3. 1 in 50,000

    4. 1 in 100,000

73–20. What chromosomal abnormality results in hermaphroditism?

    1. 46, XXY

    2. 46, YYY

    3. 46, XX

    4. 46, XY

73–21. What is a major tool in the initial diagnostic interview for gender identity disorder?

    1. Beck Depression Inventory

    2. Structured Clinical Interview for DSM-IV

    3. Sex History Inventory

    4. No particular inventories or structured interviews for gender identity disorder are available.

73–22. What type of work experience is frequently found in individuals with gender dysphoria?

    1. Prostitution

    2. Factory work

   3. Professional careers

   4. Night shift work

73–23. Patients with gender identity disorder typically present for treatment during which age range?

   1. 2 to 5 years

   2. 5 to 13 years

   3. 13 to 40 years

   4. 40 to 65 years

73–24. What is the prescribed minimum length of time of ongoing psychotherapeutic contact required before sex reassignment surgery can take place?

   1. 2 months

   2. 4 months

   3. 6 months

   4. 12 months

73–25. How much clitoral elongation may be expected to occur in a female-to-male patient after 1 year of hormonal treatment?

   1. 1 cm

   2. 3 cm

   3. 6 cm

   4. No clitoral elongation occurs.

73–26. The "true life test" involves the patient's living in the preferred gender for what length of time prior to surgical intervention?

   1. There is no time requirement.

   2. 6 to 12 months

   3. 12 to 24 months

   4. 24 to 36 months

∎ **DIRECTIONS: For questions 73–27 through 73–37, indicate**

   A if answers 1, 2, and 3 are correct.

   B if answers 1 and 3 are correct.

   C if answers 2 and 4 are correct.

   D if only answer 4 is correct.

   E if all are correct.

73–27. In diagnosing adolescent gender identity disorder, what types of psychosexual problems are evident?

   1. Intractable cross-gender identity

   2. Gender identity distress

   3. Social ostracism

   4. Cross-dressing for purposes of sexual arousal

73–28. What types of extreme behaviors are observed in patients with gender identity disorder in their efforts to obtain surgical procedures?

    1. They may engage in hypermasculine activities.

    2. They may lie about complicating medical conditions.

    3. They may keep secret their cross-dressing behaviors.

    4. They may falsify their human immunodeficiency virus (HIV) status.

73–29. What are the goals of psychotherapy with gender-dysphoric patients?

    1. To help patients understand the incurable nature of their disorder

    2. To help patients understand that their disorder is a disease process

    3. To help patients understand that their disorder is an inborn error of hormonal metabolism

    4. To help patients learn reasonable and secure ways of conducting their lives

73–30. What are the consequences of inadequately trained surgeons performing sexual reassignment procedures on inappropriate patients?

    1. Permanent pelvic anesthesia

    2. Psychosis

    3. Poor aesthetic results

    4. Suicide

73–31. In particular circumstances, which individuals may need to be interviewed for the accurate diagnosis of gender identity disorder?

    1. The patient's significant other

    2. The patient's parents

    3. The patient's siblings

    4. The patient's employer

73–32. What types of self-treatment have frequently been used by patients with male-to-female gender identity disorder?

    1. Electrolysis

    2. Birth control pills

    3. Breast augmentation

    4. Cross-dressing

73–33. In what ways does the therapist become the permissive and accepting transference parent in the treatment of patients with gender identity disorder?

    1. By encouraging the patient to cross-dress in appropriate settings

    2. By using the patient's name of choice

    3. By using appropriate cross-gender pronouns when addressing the patient

    4. By encouraging the patient to tell everyone about the situation

73–34. Contraindications to estrogen therapy include which of the following?

    1. Ischemic heart disease

    2. Hepatic insufficiency

    3. Renal insufficiency

    4. Well-controlled migraine headaches

73–35. What hormonal parameters should be followed when treating a male-to-female gender identity disorder patient with hormonal therapy?

    1. Serum testosterone

    2. Serum follicle-stimulating hormone

    3. Serum prolactin

    4. Serum luteinizing hormone

73–36. What is the usual hormonal management of female-to-male patients with gender identity disorder?

    1. Spironolactone

    2. Medroxyprogesterone

    3. Ethinyl estradiol

    4. Testosterone ester

73–37. Which of the following are **not** side effects of androgen therapy?

    1. Increased erythropoiesis

    2. Decrease of low-density lipoprotein

    3. Liver enzyme abnormalities

    4. Increased carbohydrate tolerance

■   **ANSWERS:**

73–1. **False**

73–2. **True**

73–3. **False**

73–4. **True**

73–5. **True**

73–6. **False**

73–7. **False**

73–8. **True**

73–9. **True**

73–10. **True**

73–11. **True**

73–12. **True**

73–13. **False**   The social convention of males' standing to void appears to be an important aspect in the decision of what type of prosthesis is used.

73–14. **False**

73–15. **True**

73–16. **Answer: 3.** The incidence of polycystic ovarian disease in female-to-male patients with gender identity disorder is 25%, whereas the incidence in the general adult female population is 7.5%. In patients with hirsutism and/or oligomenorrhea, the incidence approaches 80%.

73–17. **Answer: 1.** A wide range of treatment options are available to patients with gender identity disorder. The one option that is not in the patient's best interest and is contraindicated is ignoring the situation.

73–18. **Answer: 4.** Maximal breast enlargement in male-to-female patients with gender identity disorder is usually attained after 2 years of hormonal treatment.

73–19. **Answer: 2.** The prevalence of gender identity disorder in adult males is 1 in 30,000 and in adult females, 1 in 100,000.

73–20. **Answer: 1.** Klinefelter's syndrome (46, XXY) results in hermaphroditism.

73–21. **Answer: 3.** The Sex History Inventory is the major tool for the initial interview. This inventory lends itself to the nonjudgmental and efficient assessment of sexual behavior, attitudes, and feelings in gender disorders and conditions.

73–22. **Answer: 1.** A history of prostitution experience is frequently found in the assessment of many gender-dysphoric individuals because without skills in other work areas, these individuals are greatly in need of earning large sums of money to support their living needs and their treatment.

73–23. **Answer: 3.** Patients with gender identity disorder typically present for treatment when they are between 13 and 40 years of age.

73–24. **Answer: 3.** Before sex reassignment surgery can take place, a minimum of 6 to 12 months of ongoing psychotherapeutic contact is required.

73–25. **Answer: 3.** After 1 year of hormonal treatment, the clitoris may elongate to 6 cm in length.

73–26. **Answer: 2.** The "true life test" requirement involves living in the preferred gender role for 6 to 12 months. The experience may have occurred before or may occur during the psychotherapy with a primary therapist.

73–27. **Answer: E (All).** In adolescent gender identity disorder, several types of psychosexual problems occur, including 1) relative intractability of cross-gender identity disorder and a desire to change sex, 2) gender identity distress with continued cross-gender identification and social ostracism, 3) distress about homosexual behavior or orientation and, in some cases, a history of gender identity disorder, and 4) cross-dressing for purposes of sexual arousal with or without a history of gender identity disorder.

73–28. **Answer: C (2 and 4).** In desperate attempts to obtain surgical interventions, patients may conceal the extent or presence of complicating medical conditions such as HIV status, diabetes, or cardiac conditions. Typically, adolescent and young adult patients may attempt to deny their gender identity disorder with a flight into hypermasculine activity. Patients whose social and professional lives would be destroyed if their disorder were to become known may elect to keep their cross-dressing secret.

73–29. **Answer: D (Only 4).** One goal of psychotherapy with gender-dysphoric patients is to help the patient understand that gender identity disorder itself is not a disease and that it is not the patient's or family's fault. Another goal of therapy is to help the patient learn reasonable and secure ways of conducting his or her life. The exact pathogenesis of gender identity disorder remains under debate and is currently being examined.

73–30. **Answer: E (All).** Disastrous outcomes such as permanent pelvic anesthesia, grotesque aesthetic results, requests for reversal of the procedure, psychosis, and suicide may occur when inadequately trained surgeons perform sex reassignment procedures on inappropriate patients.

73–31. **Answer: A (1, 2, and 3).** Many gender clinics and private practitioners who regularly see gender identity disorder patients have been known to encourage verification of important aspects of the patient's history by interviewing family members and friends.

73–32. **Answer E (All).** Patients with gender dysphoria of the male-to-female type may have already obtained birth control pills and/or undergone electrolysis and breast augmentation, and may routinely cross-dress.

73–33. **Answer: A (1, 2, and 3).** The therapist becomes the permissive parent by encouraging the patient to cross-dress in safe and appropriate settings as well as to inform appropriate individuals about the disorder. The therapist should also address the patient by gender-appropriate pronouns and use the patient's name of choice.

73–34. **Answer: A (1, 2, and 3).** There are numerous contraindications to estrogen therapy, including 1) severe diastolic hypertension, 2) ischemic heart disease, 3) thromboembolic disease, 4) cerebrovascular disease, 5) hepatic insufficiency, 6) renal insufficiency, 7) family history of breast cancer, 8) heavy cigarette consumption, 9) poorly controlled diabetes mellitus, 10) marked obesity, 11) hyperprolactinemia, and 12) refractory migraine headaches.

73–35. **Answer: B (1 and 3).** Hormonal parameters that should be followed when a male-to-female gender identity disorder patient is being treated with hormone therapy include serum testosterone, serum estradiol, and serum prolactin. Serum luteinizing hormone, serum follicle-stimulating hormone, and serum dihydrotestosterone are usually not followed.

73–36. **Answer: D (Only 4).** Testosterone ester is given intramuscularly every 3 weeks for the hormonal treatment of female-to-male patients with gender identity disorder. Spironolactone is an antiandrogen that is usually indicated at 6 to 12 months following the initiation of estrogen therapy in the treatment of male-to-female patients with gender identity disorder. Medroxyprogesterone is used in conjunction with estrogen therapy to enhance breast development in male-to-female patients with gender identity disorder.

73–37. **Answer: C (2 and 4).** The main side effects of androgen therapy include 1) increased erythropoiesis, 2) water and sodium retention, 3) decreased carbohydrate tolerance, 4) decreased serum high-density lipoprotein cholesterol and increased low-density lipoprotein, and 5) liver enzyme abnormalities.

SECTION 10

Eating Disorders

CHAPTER 74

General Principles of Outpatient Treatment

■ **DIRECTIONS: For questions 74–1 through 74–12, select the single best answer.**

74–1. Long-term follow-up of patients with anorexia nervosa reveals a mortality rate of

  1. < 5%.
  2. 5%–15%.
  3. 20%–25%.
  4. None of the above.

74–2. What is the prevalence of bulimia nervosa in women?

  1. 10%
  2. 5%
  3. 1%
  4. 0.05%

74–3. Males account for which percentage of cases of bulimia nervosa?

  1. < 5%
  2. 5%
  3. 10%
  4. 15%

74–4. What type of treatment program is generally **not** helpful in the treatment of patients with bulimia nervosa?

  1. Group therapy
  2. Individual expressive-supportive therapy
  3. Evoked-response prevention behavioral programs
  4. 12-step programs

74–5. Group therapy may initially be most efficacious in the treatment of patients with bulimia nervosa if it is conducted at what frequency?

  1. Once per month
  2. Once per week

3. Multiple times per week

4. Every other week

74–6. Group therapy is more advantageous than individual therapy in the treatment of bulimia nervosa in all of the following areas **except**

1. Decreasing the egocentric preoccupation with body weight.

2. Decreasing the intensity of power struggles.

3. Providing mutual support.

4. Effecting improvement in interpersonal functioning.

74–7. Patients with eating disorders may be treated by a team approach or by an individual. What is the main advantage of treatment being delivered by an individual?

1. Social skills training may be used.

2. Vocational concerns may be addressed.

3. Family issues may be addressed.

4. Splitting is decreased.

74–8. For patients with anorexia nervosa, which of the following forms of treatment is the most efficacious?

1. No treatment is more efficacious than another.

2. Interpersonal psychotherapy

3. Cognitive-behavior therapy

4. Expressive-supportive psychotherapy

74–9. The initial daily caloric intake in the refeeding process of patients with anorexia nervosa should be

1. 500 calories/day.

2. 1,000 calories/day.

3. 1,500 calories/day.

4. 2,000 calories/day.

74–10. Patients with anorexia nervosa or bulimia nervosa frequently ingest drugs to control their weight. What is the most commonly used drug for appetite control?

1. Over-the-counter diet pills

2. Dextroamphetamine

3. Synthroid

4. Caffeine

74–11. What is the most common form of purging used by patients with eating disorders?

1. Laxative abuse

2. Diuretic abuse

3. Emesis

4. None of the above

74–12. The menstrual threshold is often a phobic weight beyond which a patient must pass to be nutritionally rehabilitated. What is the percentage of matched population mean weight that is conducive to sustained menses in patients with anorexia nervosa?

1. 50%
2. 65%
3. 85%
4. 100%

■ **DIRECTIONS: For questions 74–13 through 74–16, indicate**

A if answers 1, 2, and 3 are correct.

B if answers 1 and 3 are correct.

C if answers 2 and 4 are correct.

D if only answer 4 is correct.

E if all are correct.

74–13. Which of the following symptoms are found in patients with anorexia nervosa, bulimia nervosa, and naturally occurring starvation?

1. Slow eating
2. Delayed gastric emptying
3. Cognitive changes
4. Binge eating

74–14. An evaluation of idiosyncratic beliefs about and practices around food is essential in the treatment of patients with eating disorders. Which of the following are commonly found in patients with eating disorders?

1. Ingestion of multiple vitamins
2. An extensive knowledge of caloric values
3. Food phobias
4. A comprehensive knowledge of human metabolism

74–15. Laboratory investigations in the initial workup of patients with eating disorders should include which of the following?

1. Complete blood cell count
2. Urine drug screen
3. Serum electrolytes
4. Creatinine phosphokinase

74–16. Compulsory treatment of patients with eating disorders is a highly contentious issue. Which of the following may be invoked to explain eating disorder symptoms and may influence the decision to treat patients against their own judgment?

1. The symptoms are a form of social communication.
2. The symptoms serve as a sociopolitical statement.
3. The symptoms are antisocial and deviant acts.
4. The cognitive disturbances seen in patients with eating disorders may disrupt their ability to think clearly.

■ ANSWERS:

74–1.   **Answer: 2.** The mortality rate for anorexia nervosa is from 5% to 15%.

74–2.   **Answer: 3.** The prevalence of bulimia nervosa is from 1.0% to 1.5% in women. Anorexia nervosa occurs in 0.5% of women between the ages of 15 and 40 years.

74–3.   **Answer: 2.** Males account for approximately 5% of cases of bulimia nervosa.

74–4.   **Answer: 4.** Twelve-step programs, such as Overeaters Anonymous, that invoke an addiction model and focus on abstinence from certain foods are not usually therapeutic in patients with bulimia nervosa.

74–5.   **Answer: 3.** Intensive and frequent (i.e., multiple times per week) group sessions early in treatment are more effective in establishing control over symptoms than the traditional once-per-week format.

74–6.   **Answer: 1.** Group therapy has the advantage of providing mutual support, decreasing the intensity of power struggles, protecting against relapse, and enhancing interpersonal functioning. Individual therapy is more efficacious in addressing the patient's inability to express feelings and the egocentric preoccupation with body weight and shape.

74–7.   **Answer: 4.** Individual treatment has the advantage of decreased fragmentation of care and splitting. Treatment by a team has the advantages of addressing vocational concerns and family issues and of social skills training. Splitting is reduced by regular contact and discussion among team members.

74–8.   **Answer: 1.** In the treatment of patients with anorexia nervosa, no one form of treatment has been shown to be superior to another.

74–9.   **Answer: 3.** In the refeeding process with patients who have anorexia nervosa, the initial daily caloric intake should be 1,500 calories.

74–10. **Answer: 4.** Caffeine is the most commonly used appetite suppressant. Over-the-counter diet pills are used by up to 25% of patients with bulimia nervosa. Synthroid is used by 7% of patients with eating disorders to regulate their appetites. Dextroamphetamine is an appetite suppressant that is used to treat individuals with attention-deficit/hyperactivity disorder.

74–11. **Answer: 3.** Self-induced vomiting is reported by 20%–94% of patients with bulimia. Laxative abuse is reported by 25% of patients with bulimia nervosa. Diuretics are used by 20% of patients with eating disorders to control their weight but are not used for purging.

74–12. **Answer: 3.** The weight threshold for sustained menses is approximately 85% of matched population mean weight.

74–13. **Answer: E (All).** Symptoms such as food preoccupation, food hoarding, slow eating, disturbances in gastric emptying, binge eating, cognitive changes, mood lability, apathy, irritability, decreased libido, and sleep disturbances are all common in naturally occurring starvation and in patients with anorexia nervosa or bulimia nervosa.

74–14. **Answer: A (1, 2, and 3).** Patients with eating disorders may hold strong beliefs about vegetarianism and the intake of multiple vitamin and mineral supplements. They may have specific food phobias and distorted beliefs about food allergies, lactose intolerance, and hypoglycemia. They are frequently well versed in the caloric value of individual foodstuffs but have idiosyncratic or inaccurate views on human metabolism.

74–15. **Answer: E (All).** Complete blood cell count, serum electrolytes, blood urea nitrogen (BUN), and creatinine should be obtained. A urine drug screen should be obtained because drug abuse to control weight is a frequent finding in patients with eating disorders. Creatinine phosphokinase (CPK) should be obtained for any patient suspected of abusing laxatives.

74–16. **Answer: E (All).** Eating disorders, specifically anorexia nervosa, may be viewed as a form of social communication, a sociopolitical statement, or an antisocial or deviant act, or as serving a role in the family system. Cognitive disturbances are well documented in patients with eating disorders and may impede their ability to think clearly.

CHAPTER 75

Cognitive-Behavior Therapy

■ **DIRECTIONS:** Using the following vignette, for questions 75–1 through 75–6, select the single best answer for each question.

Ms. C. is a 23-year-old college student who has regularly induced vomiting and binged on a wide variety of snack foods for the past 4 years. She rarely if ever eats a full meal and does not eat at regular intervals.

75–1. Eating at regularly scheduled intervals is an important element in the nutritional rehabilitation of patients with bulimia nervosa. Which of the following statements is **true** regarding this aspect of treatment?

1. Patients with bulimia nervosa are usually underweight and unconcerned about returning to a normal weight.

2. Patients with bulimia nervosa are usually overweight and will lose weight when they return to normal eating patterns.

3. Patients with bulimia nervosa are usually overweight, and most will not gain weight when they return to normal eating patterns.

4. Patients with bulimia nervosa are usually underweight and are concerned that returning to normal eating patterns will increase their weight.

75–2. Ms. C. has just entered a cognitive-behavior therapy (CBT) program for her eating disorder. Which of the following approaches may be helpful to Ms. C. in the initial stages of her therapy?

1. Explaining to Ms. C. that she may notice more uncomfortable thoughts and feelings when she ceases to use her bulimic behaviors.

2. Explaining to Ms. C. that she will be rid of her symptoms within 8 weeks.

3. Discussing with Ms. C. that CBT is designed as an exploratory therapy that seeks to understand the unconscious conflicts that led to her eating disorder.

4. Carefully explaining to Ms. C. that once-a-week therapy is ideal and cost-effective for the treatment of bulimia nervosa.

75–3. Ms. C. is reviewing her dietary intake with a nutritionist. What dietary recommendation or observation is usually made to patients with bulimia nervosa?

1. A diet that emphasizes counting calories is best.

2. A liquid diet is usually better tolerated than any other diet.

    3. Using prepackaged dietary foods is usually well tolerated.

    4. A diabetic exchange diet is well tolerated.

75–4. How often should Ms. C. weigh herself?

    1. Once a day

    2. Once a week

    3. Once a month

    4. Never

75–5. Like many individuals with bulimia nervosa, Ms. C. may have what type of perception about her body?

    1. She may accurately assess her physical attributes.

    2. She may perceive herself as being thinner than her actual size.

    3. She may perceive herself as being larger than her actual size.

    4. She may misperceive one body part as being particularly disfiguring.

75–6. Ms. C. has successfully completed her course of CBT. What should she be told about future stressful situations?

    1. She will never have any adverse reactions to stressful situations because she has been in therapy.

    2. Should she ever binge or purge again, she will immediately experience a complete relapse of her symptoms.

    3. She may experience difficulties with eating and preoccupation with weight, especially during times of stress.

    4. She should conscientiously avoid all "high risk" foods during times of stress.

■ **DIRECTIONS: For questions 75–7 through 75–15, indicate whether the statement is true or false.**

75–7. _____ Cognitive restructuring is just a way of sugar coating reality.

75–8. _____ Most patients with eating disorders overvalue weight and body shape.

75–9. _____ One element of CBT for eating disorders involves emphasizing the medical consequences.

75–10. _____ Anorexia nervosa patients are usually not told that food is like medicine.

75–11. _____ In a CBT approach, patients with anorexia nervosa are usually asked to gain 5 pounds per week.

75–12. _____ Patients with anorexia nervosa, but not those with bulimia nervosa, require assertiveness training as part of their treatment.

75–13. _____ An example of an unrealistic short-term treatment goal is that patients will learn to love their body.

75–14. _____ Cognitive-restructuring techniques are especially effective in helping patients challenge the belief that their personal value resides only in their weight.

75–15. _____ Patients may experience difficulty in changing negative cognitions about their size and shape because society frequently "confirms" their negative cognitions.

■ **DIRECTIONS: For questions 75–16 through 75–20, indicate**

    A if answers 1, 2, and 3 are correct.
    B if answers 1 and 3 are correct.
    C if answers 2 and 4 are correct.
    D if only answer 4 is correct.
    E if all are correct.

75–16. Which of the following are examples of cognitive errors made by patients with bulimia nervosa?

1. Binging really isn't that bad for me; after all, I only have six cavities from vomiting.
2. As long as my boyfriend likes my clothes, then what I think doesn't matter.
3. If I go off this diet, then I know I will simply die!
4. I feel like everything is going to be terrible tomorrow and that it's all my fault.

75–17. Obsessive-compulsive symptoms are commonly found in which of the following conditions?

1. Anorexia nervosa
2. Bulimia nervosa
3. Starvation
4. Obesity

75–18. Which of the following techniques may actually decrease the effectiveness of CBT in the treatment of patients with eating disorders?

1. Guided imagery
2. Cognitive restructuring
3. Decentering
4. Exposure and response prevention

75–19. What topics should be covered in the early sessions of CBT for patients with eating disorders?

1. Reviewing possible obstacles to treatment
2. Reviewing the importance of regular homework assignments and attendance
3. Exploring the patient's social support system
4. Stressing the importance of self-monitoring nutritional intake and binge/purge symptoms

75–20. Which of the following variables predict a poor response of bulimia nervosa patients to CBT?

1. Family dysfunction
2. Comorbid depressive disorder
3. Borderline personality disorder
4. Comorbid anxiety disorder

■ **ANSWERS:**

75–1. **Answer: 3.** Patients with bulimia nervosa are frequently overweight and fearful of gaining weight if they return to a regular pattern of eating. In fact, the majority of patients do *not* gain weight if they return to regular eating patterns.

75–2. **Answer: 1.** CBT is aimed at symptom reduction and focuses on factors that maintain the eating disorder rather than underlying unconscious conflicts or interpersonal issues that may have contributed to the pathogenesis of the disorder. Traditionally, CBT is conducted on a weekly basis; however, more frequent sessions are more efficacious for the treatment of patients with bulimia nervosa. As patients with bulimia nervosa relinquish their symptoms, they may experience an increase in uncomfortable thoughts and feelings. A thorough explanation of these factors may reduce attrition during the course of therapy.

75–3. **Answer: 4.** A diet that emphasizes counting calories or relies on prepackaged foodstuffs is not well tolerated by patients with any type of eating disorder. A liquid diet is useful for patients with severe anorexia nervosa. A diabetic exchange diet is a flexible dietary plan that is individualized to each patient and is usually well tolerated.

75–4. **Answer: 2.** Patients should weigh themselves weekly.

75–5. **Answer: 3.** Many individuals with bulimia nervosa overestimate the size and shape of their bodies. They develop cognitive misrepresentations about their bodies that may be corrected through CBT.

75–6. **Answer: 3.** Even when patients have successfully completed a course of therapy for their eating disorder, they remain at risk for lapses and relapses. A single episode of binging and/or purging does not constitute a total relapse. Patients should be informed that they may have difficulties with eating and preoccupation with weight when they are in stressful situations.

75–7. **False** Cognition restructuring is not a way of sugar coating reality. This treatment approach involves understanding and countering patients' ingrained misinterpretations and misperceptions about themselves and their environment.

75–8. **True**

75–9. **True** Most patients with eating disorders do not fully appreciate the medical risks involved in their eating disorder.

75–10. **False**

75–11. **False** Patients are usually asked to gain 1–2 pounds per week.

75–12. **False**

75–13. **True**

75–14. **True**

75–15. **True**

75–16. **Answer: A (1, 2, and 3).** "Binging really isn't that bad for me; after all, I only have six cavities from vomiting" is an example of minimizing. An example of relying too much on others' opinions is the thought "As long as my boyfriend likes my clothes, then what I think doesn't matter." Catastrophizing (e.g., "If I go off this diet, then I know I will simply die!") is a common cognitive error of patients with bulimia nervosa. Excessive guilt (e.g., "I feel like everything is going to be terrible tomorrow and that it's all my fault") is usually seen in patients with depression.

75–17. **Answer: B (1 and 3).** Obsessive-compulsive symptoms are commonly found in anorexia nervosa and other starvation states.

75–18. **Answer: D (Only 4).** The inclusion of exposure and response prevention in the treatment of patients with eating disorders is controversial. Several reports have indicated that including exposure and response prevention does not strengthen the effects of CBT and may actually have a negative impact. Guided imagery is useful in helping patients with alexithymia experience emotions. Cognitive restructuring involves challenging and replacing the patient's negative cognitions. Decentering focuses on helping the patient to use less critical judgment of himself or herself.

75–19. **Answer: E (All).** Early in treatment, possible obstacles to treatment, compliance issues centering on attendance and homework assignments, the patient's social support system, and self-monitoring of nutrition and binge/purge symptoms should all be addressed.

75–20. **Answer: A (1, 2, and 3).** There is some evidence that individuals with Cluster B personality disorders (i.e., borderline, histrionic, antisocial, narcissistic), family dysfunction, severe baseline symptoms, comorbid depression, and low self-esteem do not respond well to CBT for treatment of bulimia nervosa.

CHAPTER 76

Psychoanalytic Psychotherapy

■ **DIRECTIONS: For questions 76–1 through 76–9, indicate**

    A if answers 1, 2, and 3 are correct.

    B if answers 1 and 3 are correct.

    C if answers 2 and 4 are correct.

    D if only answer 4 is correct.

    E if all are correct.

76–1. For which groups of patients with anorexia nervosa is family therapy effective?

    1. Patients with anorexia nervosa of early onset who are younger than 18 years of age

    2. Patients with anorexia nervosa of late onset who are older than 18 years of age

    3. Patients with a history of anorexia nervosa of 3 years or less

    4. Patients with a history of anorexia nervosa of more than 3 years

76–2. Which type of young patients with anorexia nervosa will especially benefit from individual therapy?

    1. Patients who belong to an ethnic minority

    2. Patients who are adopted

    3. Patients who have a concurrent chronic medical illness

    4. Patients who are eldest children

76–3. Which of the following are limiting factors in the treatment of patients with anorexia nervosa who have engaged in therapy?

    1. The patient moves from the area to continue his or her education.

    2. The patient seeks new employment in another geographic area.

    3. The patient travels frequently and sometimes for extended periods.

    4. The patient falls in love with the therapist.

76–4. What theoretical orientation(s) would apply to the following statement: "Patients with anorexia nervosa fear a loss of the sense of the integrity of the self."

    1. Ego psychology

    2. Family systems theory

3. Learning theory (behaviorism)

4. Self psychology

76–5. Which of the following patients with anorexia nervosa would be predicted to have the best response to psychoanalysis?

1. Ms. N. is a 25-year-old graduate student whose early adulthood is characterized by intense emotional relationships and social phobia. She has a 2-year history of anorexia nervosa.

2. Ms. K. is a 22-year-old gifted violinist who has a long history of agoraphobia and has no intimate friends except her manager. She has a 5-year history of anorexia nervosa.

3. Ms. P. is a 28-year-old who had dropped out of college. She had been voted "most likely to succeed" in high school. She has never dated and has no hobbies. She has a 4-year history of anorexia nervosa.

4. Ms. L. is an 18-year-old high school senior who has never made below a perfect grade and is a promising young ballet dancer. She has an active social life and lives in an intact family. She has a 5-year history of anorexia nervosa.

76–6. Which of the following reactions are typical of young therapists and their patients?

1. The patient feels the therapist to be intrusive and threatening.

2. The therapist becomes discouraged and angry that the patient is starving himself or herself.

3. The therapist identifies with the patient's reactions toward his or her parents.

4. The patient believes that his or her parents and the therapist are "just alike."

■ **DIRECTIONS: For questions 76–7 through 76–9, use the following case example:**

Sally is a 15-year-old patient with a 2-year history of anorexia nervosa. She was an exceptionally well-behaved young child and has done well in her private girls preparatory school. Her parents report that until Sally developed her disorder, their marital relationship was satisfactory.

76–7. Which of the following statements are **true** regarding Sally?

1. She will probably display borderline character pathology.

2. She will probably display behaviors indicative of oedipal conflicts.

3. Her relationships with other family members are characterized by high levels of confrontation.

4. Her relationships with other family members are characterized by avoidant behaviors.

76–8. What type of life events are observed in adolescents such as Sally?

1. Sexual abuse

2. An extensive dating history

3. Witnessing violent crime

4. An older sibling's having left home

76–9.   Which issues in Sally's life may be focused on late in treatment?

   1. Her social interactions with her peer group

   2. Her ambivalence over her evolving relationship with her mother

   3. Her desire to attend a top university

   4. Her fearfulness over intimacy

■   ANSWERS:

76–1.   **Answer: B (1 and 3).** Patients with anorexia nervosa of an early onset (younger than 18 years of age) and a short duration of illness (3 years or less) are the most likely to benefit from family therapy.

76–2.   **Answer: A (1, 2, and 3).** Patients with anorexia nervosa who have issues that pose a challenge to identity formation in adolescence, such as belonging to an ethnic minority, having been adopted, or having a concurrent medical illness, may particularly benefit from individual therapy.

76–3.   **Answer: A (1, 2, and 3).** Patients with anorexia nervosa who are in their late adolescence may form an adequate therapeutic alliance and remain in treatment for 18 to 24 months without disruption. The task of adolescence is to move forward into one's own identity—both occupational and personal. Hence, even a functional therapeutic alliance may be disrupted by the adolescent's progression through school and employment opportunities. Erotic transferences are not unusual with adolescents, and this type of transference is not a reason for therapy to be interrupted.

76–4.   **Answer: D (Only 4).** The statement in the question (i.e., "Patients with anorexia nervosa fear a loss of the sense of the integrity of the self ") applies to the self psychology idea of loss of the sense of integrity of the self. In patients with anorexia nervosa, there is a continuum between the classical oedipal fear of being sexually overwhelmed and endangered and the loss of sense of integrity.

76–5.   **Answer: A (1, 2, and 3).** Young adult patients with anorexia nervosa are more amenable to psychoanalysis. Their premorbid personalities are more rigid. Frequently, there is a history of intense episodes of anxiety and social isolation in older patients with anorexia nervosa. Younger patients tend to do well in family therapy, have less rigid premorbid personality structure, and usually have a history of good prepubescent social adjustment.

76–6.   **Answer: A (1, 2, and 3).** Younger therapists tend to identify with their adolescent patients, and their patients may find this identification intrusive and threatening. Older therapists may elicit a parental transference in their adolescent patients. All therapists may struggle with feelings of anger and rejection regarding this group of patients who refuse to take in literal and psychic nourishment.

76–7.   **Answer: C (2 and 4).** Families such as the one illustrated in this vignette are frequently conflict avoiding. They have good qualities for parenting prepubertal children. Adolescents like Sally are most likely to display intense oedipal conflict rather than borderline character pathology.

76–8. **Answer: D (Only 4).** Adolescents like Sally usually have not been exposed to extremely traumatic events, such as sexual abuse, physical abuse, abandonment, or witnessing violence. They are usually popular with their peer group until adolescence and rarely have extensive dating histories. A history of loss by death of a parent or grandparent, a change in a parent's employment status, or the departure from home of an older sibling is frequently found.

76–9. **Answer: C (2 and 4).** Early in the treatment process a focus on here-and-now issues such as social and academic interactions is usually the most productive. Later in the process, interpretations and an exploration of the patient's ambivalence toward her parents and siblings, as well as her fearfulness surrounding sexuality and intimacy, can be the aim of treatment.

CHAPTER 77

■

Psychopharmacological Treatments

■ **DIRECTIONS: For questions 77–1 through 77–4, select the single best answer.**

77–1. Which of the following appetite-enhancing medications may be efficacious in the treatment of anorexia nervosa?

　1. Cyproheptadine

　2. Clonidine hydrochloride

　3. Methylphenidate

　4. Tetrahydrocannabinol

77–2. What percentage of patients with anorexia nervosa have a chronic course of illness characterized by remission and relapse?

　1. 10%

　2. 20%

　3. 30%

　4. 40%

77–3. Which of the following trace elements should be supplemented as part of the nutritional rehabilitation of patients with anorexia nervosa?

　1. Iron

　2. Zinc

　3. Aluminum

　4. A balanced diet will provide sufficient trace elements.

77–4. What dose of fluoxetine is the most efficacious for the treatment of bulimia nervosa?

　1. 20 mg/day

　2. 40 mg/day

　3. 60 mg/day

　4. 80 mg/day

■ **DIRECTIONS: For questions 77–5 through 77–7, indicate**

    A if answers 1, 2, and 3 are correct.
    B if answers 1 and 3 are correct.
    C if answers 2 and 4 are correct.
    D if only answer 4 is correct.
    E if all are correct.

77–5. Which of the following statements are **true** regarding the use of tricyclic medications in the treatment of bulimia nervosa?

    1. Imipramine is superior to psychotherapy.
    2. There is no association between depression at baseline and response to treatment.
    3. Desipramine is superior to psychotherapy.
    4. Regular contact with a psychiatrist is therapeutic, even in the absence of a structured psychotherapeutic intervention.

77–6. Which of the following statements apply to fluoxetine but not to imipramine?

    1. The medication is well tolerated.
    2. There is a correlation between clinical response and drug levels.
    3. There are clinically meaningful changes in specific attitudinal disturbances associated with bulimia nervosa.
    4. The medication is not as efficacious as psychotherapy.

77–7. Which of the following medications are not efficacious in the treatment of bulimia nervosa?

    1. Lithium
    2. Carbamazepine
    3. Fenfluramine
    4. Desipramine

■ **ANSWERS:**

77–1. **Answer: 1.** Cyproheptadine promotes weight gain in a minority of patients with anorexia nervosa. Clonidine hydrochloride, methylphenidate, and tetrahydrocannabinol (THC) do not increase appetite or enhance weight gain in patients with anorexia nervosa.

77–2. **Answer: 3.** Anorexia nervosa has a chronic course in approximately 30% of patients.

77–3. **Answer: 4.** Current evidence indicates that a balanced diet will sufficiently replace trace elements.

77–4. **Answer: 3.** The standard dose of 20 mg/day of fluoxetine is not efficacious for the treatment of bulimia nervosa. The most efficacious dose is 60 mg/day.

77–5. **Answer: C (2 and 4).** Imipramine and desipramine are both somewhat effective in decreasing bulimic symptoms. Neither medication is superior to psychotherapy. One study demonstrated that regular contact with a psychiatrist was effective, even in the absence of a structured psychotherapeutic intervention.

77–6. **Answer: B (1 and 3)** Fluoxetine is well tolerated and produces clinically meaningful changes in specific attitudinal disturbances associated with bulimia nervosa. For both fluoxetine and imipramine, there is a relationship between clinical response and drug levels. Imipramine is not as efficacious as psychotherapy.

77–7. **Answer: B (1 and 3).** Lithium and fenfluramine have no documented efficacy in the treatment of bulimia nervosa. Carbamazepine is effective for a minority of patients.

CHAPTER 78

Family and Marital Therapy

■ **DIRECTIONS: For questions 78–1 through 78–12, indicate whether the statement is true or false.**

78–1. _____ High levels of expressed emotion (EE) are found in all families of patients with anorexia nervosa.

78–2. _____ Patients who are older than 18 years of age are more likely to remain actively engaged in individual therapy.

78–3. _____ Patients with eating disorders are in general agreement that their symptoms are due to deeply ingrained family conflicts.

78–4. _____ Conjoint family therapy may be too confrontational for some individuals with eating disorders.

78–5. _____ Separation-individuation issues are critical in the treatment of adolescent patients with eating disorders.

78–6. _____ The presence of family crisis is indicative of family psychopathology.

78–7. _____ Siblings of patients with eating disorders are more likely to develop eating disorders.

78–8. _____ Parental criticism predicts a poor outcome for family therapy of patients with eating disorders.

78–9. _____ Sibling rivalry occurs most often in closely spaced sibling pairs of the opposite sex.

78–10. _____ Marital therapy is always indicated in the treatment of married patients with eating disorders.

78–11. _____ Incest between siblings is a more closely guarded secret than sexual abuse caused by parents.

78–12. _____ Family therapy is valuable for patients who are adults.

■ **DIRECTIONS: For questions 78–13 through 78–17, indicate**

A if answers 1, 2, and 3 are correct.
B if answers 1 and 3 are correct.
C if answers 2 and 4 are correct.
D if only answer 4 is correct.
E if all are correct.

78–13. Which of the following conditions are relative contraindications for conjoint family therapy?

    1. A parent has abused the patient.

    2. The parents are divorced.

    3. One of the parents has severe psychopathology.

    4. The patient is an adolescent.

78–14. Which of the following are guidelines for a flexible family-oriented approach to the treatment of eating disorders?

    1. Parents should not be regarded as guilty of causing the eating disorder, but rather as coresponsible.

    2. Parents are assumed to lack essential problem-solving capacities.

    3. Siblings should be involved in the process.

    4. The patient is considered to be both the victim and the architect of the current set of symptoms.

78–15. Siblings of patients with eating disorders may function in a variety of roles in the family. Which of the following are examples of these roles?

    1. Siblings may act as nurturers, providing mutual support to each other.

    2. The parentified sibling is usually selected as a cotherapist.

    3. A parentified sibling may be the sibling who brings the family into treatment.

    4. Siblings will inevitably tell the therapist secrets in a competitive sibling rivalry situation.

78–16. What types of marital difficulties are seen in patients with anorexia nervosa?

    1. Low levels of intimacy

    2. Poor communication skills

    3. Low levels of openness

    4. No difficulties

78–17. Which of the following are guidelines for marital therapy of patients with anorexia nervosa?

    1. Individual goals for each partner are more important than goals as a couple.

    2. The nature of the disorder should not be discussed.

    3. The goal of treatment is improvement in symptoms of the identified patient.

    4. The couple is urged to see the focus of the treatment as an improvement in the marital relationship.

■ **ANSWERS:**

78–1. **False**   High levels of EE are found in families of some patients with anorexia nervosa.

78–2. **True**   Adolescents are less likely than adults to maintain an alliance with an individual therapist.

78–3. **False** Patients generally do not report deeply ingrained conflict. However, the family may be episodically in conflict.

78–4. **True**

78–5. **True**

78–6. **False** A family crisis may or may not be an indication that the family is dysfunctional. Families that are *always* in crisis are usually dysfunctional.

78–7. **True**

78–8. **True**

78–9. **True**

78–10. **False** Marital therapy may be indicated for some patients.

78–11. **True**

78–12. **True** Adult patients may maintain close, even enmeshed, relationships with their family of origin. For these patients, family therapy is indicated.

78–13. **Answer: A (1, 2, and 3).** If a parent has abused the patient or has severe psychopathology, the patient may require some protection from the parent. When a parent has severe psychopathology, he or she may be too vulnerable to participate in classical family therapy. The fantasy to reunite divorced parents is frequently harbored by patients with anorexia nervosa, and this wish may be exacerbated by conjoint family therapy.

78–14. **Answer: E (All).** More important than rigid adherence to a single theoretical model is the use of general principles and flexibility in a family-oriented approach to the treatment of patients with eating disorders. Siblings should be included because they may function as cotherapists and may make valuable observations. Family members are not considered guilty of creating the eating disorder but are coresponsible. Family issues and conflicts can be both the cause and the consequence of the eating disorder, and thus the patient is both the victim and the architect of the symptoms. Essential problem-solving skills are frequently absent in parents of children with eating disorders.

78–15. **Answer: B (1 and 3).** Siblings may act as nurturers to each other, providing mutual support. These relationships are particularly valuable in families with deficient parenting. Parentified siblings may bring the family into treatment but simultaneously maintain family secrets. The ability of the parentified sibling to keep family secrets makes the sibling less likely to be selected as a cotherapist. Siblings usually maintain strong loyalties, despite strife-filled situations.

78–16. **Answer: E (All).** Patients with anorexia nervosa have relatively low levels of intimacy, poor communication skills, and low levels of apparent openness. Patients with anorexia nervosa may also have no apparent marital difficulties.

78–17. **Answer: D (Only 4).** In marital therapy of patients with anorexia nervosa, the goals for treatment are extensively reviewed with the couple. Individual goals as well as goals as a couple are selected. The focus of therapy is on overall improvement in the marital relationship and not symptomatic improvement in the identified patient.

CHAPTER 79

Inpatient Treatment of Anorexia Nervosa

■ **DIRECTIONS: For questions 79–1 through 79–11, indicate whether the statement is true or false.**

79–1. _____ Lenient behavioral programs for the treatment of patients with anorexia nervosa are less efficacious than strict programs.

79–2. _____ Staff members who have or have had eating disorders are good members to have on treatment teams for patients with eating disorders.

79–3. _____ Patients with anorexia nervosa demonstrate poor interpersonal skills, so social skills training is an important part of their treatment.

79–4. _____ The efficacy of outpatient treatment of anorexia nervosa is independent of weight status.

79–5. _____ A standard cookbook approach is the most practical one in designing a milieu therapy for patients with anorexia nervosa.

79–6. _____ A group therapy approach involving a psychoeducational component and social skills training is efficacious in the inpatient treatment of patients with anorexia nervosa.

79–7. _____ Men who develop eating disorders are generally overweight.

79–8. _____ Individuals with insulin-dependent diabetes have a higher risk of developing anorexia nervosa.

79–9. _____ Staff burnout is the major complication of staffing an inpatient unit for eating disorder patients.

79–10. _____ The cost of day treatment programs for anorexia nervosa is less than half that of inpatient treatment programs.

79–11. _____ Negative and positive reinforcement for the treatment of patients with anorexia nervosa is a rational approach.

■ **DIRECTIONS: For questions 79–12 through 79–20, indicate**

    A if answers 1, 2, and 3 are correct.

    B if answers 1 and 3 are correct.

    C if answers 2 and 4 are correct.

    D if only answer 4 is correct.

    E if all are correct.

79–12. What are indicators for good prognosis for the transfer of patients with anorexia nervosa from inpatient treatment to an outpatient setting?

   1. There is a decrease in rejection of their body type during the inpatient admission.

   2. Development of an identity as an eating disorder patient is solidified during the inpatient admission.

   3. There is improvement in perceptual distortion during the inpatient admission.

   4. The family is willing to relinquish the patient and his or her care to the treatment team.

79–13. What personality disorders are most commonly found in patients with anorexia nervosa?

   1. Avoidant

   2. Dependent

   3. Obsessive-compulsive

   4. Borderline

79–14. Which of the following are examples of positive reinforcers?

   1. Increased freedom to move off grounds

   2. Room isolation

   3. Time with staff

   4. Remaining on a tray diet

79–15. Activities of daily living are frequently incorporated into the treatment of patients with chronic disorders. Which of the following skills are part of the treatment of individuals with anorexia nervosa?

   1. Grocery shopping

   2. Meal planning

   3. Preparation of meals

   4. Determination of caloric content of each meal

79–16. Family therapy in the treatment of anorexia nervosa is most efficacious for which of the following patients?

   1. Those in whom onset of the disorder occurs before age 18 years

   2. Those in whom onset of the disorder occurs after age 18 years

   3. Those in whom the duration of illness is less than 3 years

   4. Those in whom the duration of illness is more than 3 years

79–17. Which of the following medical interventions may be used in the treatment of severely ill patients with anorexia nervosa?

   1. Hyperalimentation

   2. Intravenous fluids

   3. Tube feeding

   4. Electroconvulsive therapy (ECT)

79–18. Anorexia nervosa patients who respond to outpatient treatment have which of the following characteristics?

1. The duration of illness is less than 1 year.
2. Less than 25% of ideal body weight has been lost.
3. Binge or purge behaviors are not engaged in.
4. No family members are involved in the treatment.

79–19. Under what conditions is inpatient treatment of patients with anorexia nervosa warranted?

1. The illness has been ongoing for more than 12 months.
2. A weight loss of more than 25% of ideal body weight has occurred.
3. Outpatient treatment has failed after 12 to 16 weeks.
4. Medical complications are present.

79–20. What are the factors that herald a return to physically healthy weight for patients with anorexia nervosa?

1. Decrease in preoccupation with thoughts of food
2. Decrease in bone demineralization
3. Decrease in body temperature dysregulation
4. Decrease in menses

■ ANSWERS:

79–1. **False** Individualized behavioral programs are the most efficacious for the treatment of patients with anorexia nervosa.

79–2. **False** Staff members with a current or past history of an eating disorder are usually *not* good staff members in this context, because their own intrapsychic and interpersonal issues may seep into the patient's treatment.

79–3. **False**

79–4. **False** Patients who are in a state of starvation, with a weight loss of 25%, will not respond as well to outpatient treatment.

79–5. **False**

79–6. **True**

79–7. **True**

79–8. **False** Patients with insulin-dependent diabetes are not at greater risk for developing an eating disorder, although their treatment is highly complex.

79–9. **True**

79–10. **False** The cost of day treatment is one-third that of inpatient treatment.

79–11. **True**

79–12. **Answer: B (1 and 3).** Good indicators for transfer from an inpatient unit to an outpatient setting include decreased rejection of body type, development of an identity *not* centered around the eating disorder, and improvement in perceptual disturbance. An appropriately supportive family is important.

79–13. **Answer: A (1, 2, and 3).** Cluster C personality disorders (i.e., avoidant, dependent, passive-aggressive, and obsessive-compulsive) are the ones most commonly seen in patients with anorexia nervosa. Cluster B personality disorders, in particular borderline personality disorder, are seen in patients with bulimia nervosa.

79–14. **Answer: B (1 and 3).** Positive reinforcers include time with peers or staff, especially in the treatment of adolescent patients, and an increase in privileges.

79–15. **Answer: A (1, 2, and 3).** Normalization of behaviors associated with food is essential in the treatment of patients with eating disorders. Planning and preparing of balanced meals, including grocery shopping, are integrated into treatment. The emphasis is on balance and moderation rather than calorie counting.

79–16. **Answer: B (1 and 3).** Patients in whom onset of the disorder occurs before age 18 years and duration of the disorder is less than 3 years have significantly greater improvement with family therapy compared with older patients or patients with a more chronic course of the illness.

79–17. **Answer: B (1 and 3).** Hyperalimentation and tube feeding will result in weight gain in severely ill anorexia nervosa patients. Both procedures have serious potential complications and are reserved for gravely ill patients. Intravenous fluids are not generally indicated, and too aggressive rehydration may result in cardiac overload. ECT is no more efficacious than pharmacotherapy but may be used to treat an underlying or secondary depression.

79–18. **Answer: A (1, 2, and 3).** Patients who respond best to outpatient treatment have been ill less than 1 year, have lost less than 25% of ideal body weight, do not binge or purge, and have a well-functioning and intact family.

79–19. **Answer: E (All).** Indications for hospitalization of patients with anorexia nervosa include duration of illness of 12 months, weight loss of more than 25% of ideal body weight, comorbid conditions such as depression or medical complications, and failure of 12 to 16 weeks of outpatient treatment.

79–20. **Answer: A (1, 2, and 3).** Factors that indicate a return to a heathy body weight in patients with anorexia nervosa include a return of normal menstrual cycles, improvement in bone demineralization, cessation of feeling colder than others, a return to a normal cycle of hunger and satiety cues rather than chronic hunger or satiety, decreased preoccupation with food, and a decrease in obsessive planning about eating activities.

CHAPTER 80

Inpatient Treatment of Bulimia Nervosa

■ **DIRECTIONS: For questions 80–1 through 80–10, select the single best answer.**

80–1. What is the critical value for potassium that warrants hospitalization of a patient with bulimia nervosa?

1. 2.5 mmol/L
2. 3.0 mmol/L
3. 3.5 mmol/L
4. 4.0 mmol/L

80–2. Ipecac intoxication may result in all of the following **except**

1. Death.
2. Mallory-Weiss tears.
3. Electroencephalogram abnormalities.
4. Generalized muscle weakness.

80–3. What percentage of bulimia nervosa patients will experience major depression?

1. 25%
2. 30%
3. 40%
4. 50%

80–4. An indication for hospitalization in patients with bulimia nervosa is

1. Deterioration in school performance.
2. Deterioration in social relationships.
3. Failure of outpatient treatment.
4. All of the above.

80–5. What is the first goal of hospitalization for patients with bulimia nervosa?

1. Cessation of binge/purge behavior
2. Insight into the etiology of the disorder
3. Resolution of familial conflicts
4. Improvement in body image

80–6.   Which of the following laboratory values is frequently **elevated** in patients with bulimia nervosa?

   1. Serum bicarbonate
   2. Serum chloride
   3. Serum potassium
   4. Serum amylase

80–7.   In the middle phase of hospitalization, patients with bulimia nervosa relearn or learn normal patterns of eating behaviors. Which meal is the first one for which the patient freely selects items?

   1. Snacks
   2. Breakfast
   3. Lunch
   4. Dinner

80–8.   Psychological issues addressed during hospitalization for bulimia nervosa include all of the following **except**

   1. Appropriate expression of anger.
   2. Issues of dependency and individuation.
   3. An overly perfectionistic attitude.
   4. Appropriate expression of happiness.

80–9.   Personality disorders are frequently found in patients with bulimia nervosa. Which of the following is the most commonly occurring personality disorder in patients with bulimia nervosa?

   1. Dependent
   2. Histrionic
   3. Borderline
   4. Obsessive-compulsive

80–10. Which of the following statements is **true** regarding structure for patients with bulimia nervosa?

   1. These patients frequently arrive on the inpatient unit with no structure in their daily lives.
   2. These patients frequently arrive on the inpatient unit with only their binge/purge behaviors to structure their lives.
   3. These patients frequently arrive on the inpatient unit with a highly structured exercise routine as well as binge/purge behaviors.
   4. These patients frequently arrive on the inpatient unit with a tightly structured daily routine.

■ ANSWERS:

80–1.   **Answer: 1.** A potassium level below 2.5 mmol/L significantly increases the risk of potentially lethal cardiac arrhythmias. Patients whose potassium falls below this level should be hospitalized.

80–2. **Answer: 3.** Ipecac poisoning may result in death, precordial pain, dyspnea, generalized muscle weakness, hypotension, tachycardia, and electrocardiogram abnormalities. Mallory-Weiss tears (i.e., tears in esophageal veins) may result from prolonged emesis. Electroencephalogram abnormalities are not seen in Ipecac poisoning.

80–3. **Answer: 2.** Approximately a third of patients with bulimia nervosa will experience a major depression.

80–4. **Answer: 4.** Patients with bulimia nervosa who are no longer able to function at work or school, who have a marked deterioration in their social or family relationships, or who have experienced outpatient treatment failure will benefit from hospitalization.

80–5. **Answer: 1.** Gaining insight into the pathogenesis of their disorder, facilitating an understanding of their intrapsychic and interpersonal conflicts, and improving their body image are all potential goals of treatment for patients with bulimia nervosa. The first goal of hospitalization is to stop the binge/purge behaviors.

80–6. **Answer: 4.** Elevations in serum amylase are frequently seen in patients with bulimia nervosa who induce emesis. Low levels of serum bicarbonate, chloride, and potassium are seen in patients with bulimia nervosa because of laxative abuse or induced emesis.

80–7. **Answer: 2.** Breakfast is usually the first meal for which patients with bulimia nervosa freely select items. The next two, in order, are lunch and dinner.

80–8. **Answer: 4.** Appropriate expression of happiness is not usually an aspect of treatment for patients with bulimia nervosa. Psychological issues addressed include appropriate expression of anger; issues of dependency, individuation, and control; and a perfectionistic, overly critical attitude toward the self.

80–9. **Answer: 3.** Borderline personality disorder is the most frequently diagnosed personality disorder in patients with bulimia nervosa.

80–10. **Answer: 2.** Patients with bulimia nervosa frequently arrive with only the bulimic behaviors to structure their lives. Patients with anorexia nervosa may have rigidly structured their lives with respect to daily routines, exercise, and eating.

CHAPTER 81

Atypical Eating Disorders

■ **DIRECTIONS: For questions 81–1 through 81–9, indicate**

    A if answers 1, 2, and 3 are correct.

    B if answers 1 and 3 are correct.

    C if answers 2 and 4 are correct.

    D if only answer 4 is correct.

    E if all are correct.

81–1. A cognitive-behavior therapy approach has been used in bulimia nervosa and binge-eating disorder. Which of the following apply to binge-eating disorder but not to bulimia nervosa?

    1. Establishment of a regular pattern of eating

    2. Reduction in the degree of avoidance of "feared" foods

    3. Reduction in the degree of distorted thinking regarding the importance of weight and body shape

    4. Use of a group therapy approach

81–2. Which of the following characterize the relationship between interpersonal psychotherapy and binge-eating disorder?

    1. Interpersonal deficits are a common problem in patients with binge-eating disorder.

    2. Patients who comply with interpersonal psychotherapy treatment initially gain weight.

    3. Role disputes are a common difficulty in patients with binge-eating disorder.

    4. Interpersonal psychotherapy does not focus on eating and is therefore not useful in the treatment of binge-eating disorder.

81–3. Which of the following medications are useful in the treatment of **both** binge-eating disorder and bulimia nervosa?

    1. Imipramine

    2. Fluoxetine

    3. Desipramine

    4. Sertraline

81–4. What nutritional-deficit disease is associated with pica?

  1. Beriberi
  2. Calcium deficiency
  3. Rickets
  4. Iron-deficiency anemia

81–5. Which populations are historically associated with pica?

  1. Pregnant women
  2. Older men
  3. Young children
  4. Adolescents

81–6. Which of the following statements are examples of self-talk in a patient with a binge-eating disorder?

  1. "I'm an ugly person who can never do anything right."
  2. "No one would ever want to date me, so I might as well eat."
  3. "My hips are the size of the Atlantic ocean."
  4. "I feel responsible for everything that goes wrong."

81–7. Complications of rumination include which of the following?

  1. Aspiration pneumonia
  2. Anemia
  3. Dental decay
  4. Normal weight

81–8. What are the populations most prone to develop rumination?

  1. Bulimic patients
  2. Neglected infants
  3. Mentally retarded individuals
  4. Neglected elderly patients

81–9. What is the treatment(s) of choice for rumination disorder?

  1. Administering very small doses of electric shock when the behavior is observed
  2. Using high levels of attention
  3. Placing a drop of lemon juice on the tongue when the behavior is observed
  4. Using cognitive-behavior therapy

■ **DIRECTIONS: For questions 81–10 through 81–18, indicate whether the statement is true or false.**

81–10. _____ The majority of patients with binge-eating disorder are of normal or below-normal weight.

81–11. _____ Approximately 2% of adult women have binge-eating disorder.

81–12. _____ Aversive therapy is the most common treatment for pica.

81–13. _____ Cognitive-behavior therapy is the treatment of choice for laxative abuse.

81–14. _____ Individuals with moderate or severe obesity have an increased risk of psychiatric disorders, even if they do not have an eating disorder.

81–15. _____ Lead intoxication may lead to behavioral disturbances and learning disorders in children.

81–16. _____ A high-fiber diet is not part of the treatment of laxative abuse.

81–17. _____ Cognitive-behavior therapy is successful in eliminating binge eating in approximately half of affected patients.

81–18. _____ Relapse prevention is an important part of cognitive-behavior therapy in the treatment of binge-eating disorder.

■ ANSWERS:

81–1. **Answer: D (Only 4).** Elements of cognitive-behavior therapy that are shared between bulimia nervosa and binge-eating disorder are achieving normalization of eating, eating on a regular schedule, reducing cognitive distortions, and reducing the importance of weight and body shape. Unlike bulimia nervosa patients, patients with binge-eating disorder are usually seen in a group process, and their treatment tends to be of shorter duration.

81–2. **Answer: A (1, 2, and 3).** Interpersonal psychotherapy is at least as effective as cognitive-behavior therapy in the treatment of binge-eating disorder, despite the lack of focus on eating, body image, and behavioral techniques. It was found that patients who comply with interpersonal psychotherapy initially attained a 2-kg net weight gain but 1 year after termination of therapy showed a net loss of 3 kg. Interpersonal deficits and role disputes are the two most common interpersonal issues for patients with binge-eating disorder.

81–3. **Answer: B (1 and 3).** Imipramine does not decrease the frequency of binge behaviors, but it does significantly shorten the duration of the episode. Desipramine reduces the frequency and intensity of binge-eating episodes. Selective serotonin reuptake inhibitors have documented efficacy in the treatment of bulimia nervosa. At this time, however, there are no trials documenting their use in binge-eating disorder.

81–4. **Answer: D (Only 4).** Iron deficiency is frequently associated with pica, but it is unclear whether the pica is induced by the iron deficiency or causes the deficiency.

81–5. **Answer: B (1 and 3).** Historically, pregnant women, especially from rural areas, and young children have been at risk for developing pica because of nutritional deprivation and cultural norms.

81–6. **Answer: E (All).** All of the statements listed are examples of the critical and self-defeating comments made by patients with binge-eating disorder to themselves. Cognitive-behavior therapy aims to make patients aware of such comments and to analyze the comments for their accuracy.

81–7. **Answer: A (1, 2, and 3).** Complications of rumination include aspiration pneumonia, anemia, dental decay, malnutrition, and, in infancy, failure to thrive.

81–8. **Answer: A (1, 2, and 3).** Severely deprived infants may develop rumination. Approximately 20% of patients with bulimia develop rumination. This disorder is most frequently seen in mentally retarded patients.

81–9. **Answer: A (1, 2, and 3).** Aversive therapy, such as electric shock and lemon juice, are the most common methods of treating rumination disorder, a disorder that is potentially lethal. This type of treatment is warranted only in severe situations. Infants may respond to high levels of attention and stimulation.

81–10. **False** The majority of patients with binge-eating disorder are overweight.

81–11. **True**

81–12. **True**

81–13. **True**

81–14. **False** There is no evidence of increased psychopathology in obese individuals.

81–15. **True**

81–16. **False**

81–17. **True**

81–18. **True**

Personality Disorders

CHAPTER 82

Paranoid Personality Disorder

■ **DIRECTIONS: For questions 82–1 through 82–3, indicate**

    A if 1, 2, and 3 are correct.

    B if 1 and 3 are correct.

    C if 2 and 4 are correct.

    D if only answer 4 is correct.

    E if all are correct.

82–1. Which characteristics of persons with paranoid personality disorder make treatment extremely difficult?

    1. Guardedness and mistrust

    2. An ego-syntonic defensive organization

    3. Rigidity of paranoid defenses

    4. Impulsive acting out

82–2. The basic principles of psychotherapy of patients with paranoid personality disorder include which of the following?

    1. Establishment and maintenance of a meaningful therapeutic alliance

    2. Confrontation of paranoid ideas

    3. Respect for the patient's autonomy

    4. Conversion of depression into paranoia

82–3. Which of the following are common countertransference reactions to patients with paranoid personality disorder?

    1. Feelings of annoyance or impatience

    2. Playing aggressor to the patient's victim

    3. Feelings of frustration and discouragement

    4. Feelings of helplessness and worthlessness

■ **DIRECTIONS: For questions 82–4 and 82–5, select the single best answer.**

82–4. A litigious stance is a continued concern in the treatment of patients with paranoid personality disorder. Litigious behavior can generally be avoided by

    1. Interpretation of unconscious sexual feelings.

    2. Attention to the therapeutic alliance and arrangements for dealing with privacy and confidentiality.

    3. Letting the patient know that you have retained an attorney.

    4. Presenting an air of unflappable confidence.

82–5. Which of the following adjunctive therapies has no demonstrable role in the treatment of patients with paranoid personality disorder?

    1. Short-term psychotherapy

    2. Family therapy

    3. Pharmacotherapy

    4. Behavior therapy

■ ANSWERS:

82–1. **Answer: A (1, 2, and 3).** There has been little research or clinical literature on the treatment of paranoid personality disorder for a variety of reasons. Because of their difficulties with trusting others, paranoid patients tend to be guarded and do not reveal a great deal of information about themselves. Also, because their defensive organization is ego-syntonic, they generally do not have symptoms but see other people as creating problems for them. Patients with paranoid personality disorder tend to have highly rigid defenses that are not easily shifted, making it difficult for them to allow others to get to know them. Impulsive behavior is unusual in these patients, who tend to be overcontrolled and cautious.

82–2. **Answer: B (1 and 3).** The first principle in treating patients with paranoid personality disorder is to establish and maintain a meaningful therapeutic alliance. The inherent suspiciousness of such patients makes this first task a formidable one. A second basic principle is that the therapy is designed to convert the patient's paranoid stance into depressive issues. As externalizing defenses are gradually eroded, the patient's underlying feelings of vulnerability and defectiveness may come to the fore. A third principle involves maintaining respect for the patient's autonomy to counteract the patient's constant concern that his or her autonomy is being threatened. Confrontation of paranoid ideas is ill-advised because it puts the therapist in the role of a persecutor or enemy.

82–3. **Answer: E (All).** Countertransference difficulties play a major role in psychotherapy of patients with paranoid personalities. Because these patients are difficult, contentious, and guarded, the therapist may become annoyed and impatient. Also, the patient's continued self-perception as a victim may ultimately coerce the therapist into taking on the role of aggressor in response. Because paranoid patients are typically refractory to psychotherapy, feelings of frustration and discouragement are also evoked in these processes. Finally, when nothing seems to be working, the therapist may actually feel worthless, deskilled, and helpless. All countertransference feelings must be carefully monitored in terms of their impact on the therapy.

82–4. **Answer: 2.** Because paranoid patients are suspicious and overly sensitive, they frequently make legal threats. When threats arise, they should be viewed as disruptions of the therapeutic alliance and be worked with accordingly. Much of the litigious behavior relates to concerns about confidentiality and privacy. It is helpful at the beginning of the therapy for the therapist to explain to the patient how such matters as medical records, insurance reports, and so forth will be handled.

82–5. **Answer: 4.** Long-term individual psychotherapy is usually considered the preferred approach to treatment for those paranoid patients who are capable of forming a therapeutic alliance. Short-term psychotherapy may at times be the appropriate treatment, because many patients cannot tolerate more intensive or extended therapy. Family therapy is occasionally useful as well, especially for adolescent patients whose family dynamics and patterns of interaction interfere with the patient's difficulties. Although pharmacotherapy has a limited role, medications can at times be useful to modify specific target symptoms that occur because of the failure of characterological defenses. Behavior therapy is contraindicated because of the patient's suspiciousness.

CHAPTER 83

◾

Schizoid and Schizotypal Personality Disorders

◼ **DIRECTIONS: For questions 83–1 through 83–5, indicate whether the statement is true or false.**

83–1. _____ Schizoid personality disorder is closer conceptually to schizophrenia than is schizotypal personality disorder.

83–2. _____ There is considerable overlap among the three eccentric-cluster personality disorders (paranoid personality disorder, schizoid personality disorder, and schizotypal personality disorder).

83–3. _____ Psychotherapy with schizotypal personality disorder patients is somewhat easier if paranoid features are not prominent.

83–4. _____ In the treatment of schizoid personality disorder patients, dynamic therapy is best carried out three or four times a week.

83–5. _____ The balance between inherent deficit and conflict is at the core of the psychotherapist's task in treating a schizoid personality disorder patient.

◼ **DIRECTIONS: For questions 83–6 through 83–10, indicate**

A if 1, 2, and 3 are correct.

B if 1 and 3 are correct.

C if 2 and 4 are correct.

D if only answer 4 is correct.

E if all are correct.

83–6. What are the overarching goals in the treatment of schizoid personality disorder and schizotypal personality disorder patients?

1. With schizoid personality disorder patients, the major goal is to encourage the patient to have close relationships.

2. With schizotypal personality disorder patients, the goal is to help the patient achieve stability in a close personal relationship.

3. For schizotypal personality disorder patients, the goal is thoroughgoing personality change.

4. For schizoid personality disorder patients, the goal is to make the patient's solitary life more rewarding and endurable.

83–7. Supportive psychotherapy with schizoid personality disorder and schizotypal personality disorder patients consists of which of the following interventions?

1. Education

2. Advice giving

3. Problem solving

4. Interpretation

83–8. The negative attitudes and assumptions addressed in cognitive-behavior therapy with schizotypal personality disorder patients include which of the following?

1. "I feel like an alien in a frightening environment."

2. "Everyone wants to exploit me for my sexual attractiveness."

3. "Relationships are threatening."

4. "I need people to admire me."

83–9. Which of the following statements are **true** regarding group therapy for schizoid personality disorder and schizotypal personality disorder patients?

1. Most of these patients thrive in a group setting.

2. Their characteristic fearfulness and mistrust of others make most of these patients reluctant to participate in group therapy.

3. Schizotypal personality disorder patients with extreme eccentricities may do particularly well in groups.

4. Group therapy may serve to melt down negative assumptions and form more realistic ones.

83–10. Which of the following statements are **true** regarding pharmacotherapy of schizoid personality disorder and schizotypal personality disorder patients?

1. Schizoid personality disorder patients generally do not respond well to any medication.

2. Small doses of anxiolytic medication may benefit anxious schizotypal personality disorder patients.

3. Low doses of antipsychotic medication may be useful in schizotypal personality disorder patients who are prone to psychotic ideation.

4. Better-functioning schizotypal personality disorder patients who are not prone to brief psychotic episodes may never require medication.

■ ANSWERS:

83–1. **False** Schizotypal personality disorder is characterized by more proneness to peculiarities of thought and even to brief psychotic episodes and is thus closer conceptually to schizophrenia than is schizoid personality disorder.

83–2. **True** Many patients with one of these three principal diagnoses—paranoid personality disorder, schizoid personality disorder, and schizotypal personality disorder—will have comorbidity for, or at least have traits of, one or two of the others.

83–3. **True** Significant paranoid features make it more difficult for the schizotypal personality disorder patient to form an alliance and trust a therapist.

83–4. **False** Dynamic therapy for schizoid personality disorder patients should take place once or twice weekly because of the patient's difficulty with emotional closeness.

83–5. **True** If a schizoid personality disorder patient is shy based on innate temperament, the therapist must be more supportive and educative. On the other hand, if there is conflict about being close, the therapist can be more expressive.

83–6. **Answer: C (2 and 4).** The goals of psychotherapy with schizoid personality disorder and schizotypal personality disorder patients vary to some degree, depending on such issues as conflict versus deficit, presence or absence of paranoid traits, and motivation for treatment. As a general rule, schizotypal personality disorder patients may have a greater chance of achieving stability in a close personal relationship and should be helped to do so. On the other hand, many schizoid personality disorder patients are too terrified of closeness with others to overcome their fears and to attempt to form close relationships. A more reasonable goal with these patients is to make their solitary lifestyle a more rewarding one.

83–7. **Answer: A (1, 2, and 3).** The mainstay of treatment for most schizoid personality disorder and schizotypal personality disorder patients, particularly those who are more on the deficit end of the continuum, is supportive psychotherapy. In addition to giving advice and education, the supportive therapist also problem-solves, listens sympathetically, occasionally offers exhortation, and may establish a quiet form of relatedness through nonjudgmental acceptance and the regularity of sessions. Interpretation is an intervention associated with expressive psychotherapy.

83–8. **Answer: B (1 and 3).** Cognitive-behavior therapy for schizoid personality disorder and schizotypal personality disorder patients proceeds by isolating basic assumptions maintained by the patient. Common negative attitudes and assumptions found in persons with schizotypal personality disorder include feeling like an alien in a frightening environment, imagining that things never happen by chance, and viewing relationships as threatening. The fantasy of being exploited for one's sexual appeal is more typical of histrionic personality disorder. The need for constant admiration is more typical of narcissistic personality disorder.

83–9. **Answer: C (2 and 4).** Group therapy may be problematic for many schizoid personality disorder and schizotypal personality disorder patients because their fearfulness of others makes it difficult for them to function in group settings. However, certain patients may have negative assumptions altered as a result of group therapy. For example, they may feel that no one likes them, only to learn through the feedback of other group members that they are likeable. Those schizotypal personality disorder patients who are extremely eccentric may be regarded as so repugnant and bizarre by other group members that they are driven out of the group or drive others out of the group.

83–10. **Answer: E (All).** When a schizoid personality disorder patient has few schizotypal or paranoid qualities, there is little likelihood that he or she will have any
target symptoms that respond to pharmacotherapy. On the other hand, there
are empirical studies suggesting that schizotypal personality disorder patients
may respond to small doses of anxiolytic medication if they are intensely anxious and to small doses of neuroleptic or antipsychotic medication if they are
prone to psychotic ideation. Schizotypal personality disorder patients with
marked paranoid traits may react negatively to antipsychotic medication, so
these agents must be used judiciously. Many high-functioning schizotypal personality disorder patients never require medication.

CHAPTER 84

Antisocial Personality Disorder

■ **DIRECTIONS: For questions 84–1 through 84–5, indicate whether the statement is true or false.**

84–1. _____ *Psychopathy* refers to personality traits (as well as manifest antisocial behavior) and is characterized by the callous and remorseless disregard for the rights and feelings of others or by aggressive narcissism.

84–2. _____ Most patients with antisocial personality disorder (ASPD) are primary psychopaths.

84–3. _____ There is a large body of controlled empirical research demonstrating that primary psychopaths and ASPD patients can be effectively treated.

84–4. _____ The prognosis for a patient with ASPD is improved if there is a treatable anxiety or depressive disorder.

84–5. _____ In the psychotherapeutic treatment of males with ASPD, an ability to form an alliance with the therapist has been shown to be a positive prognostic marker.

■ **DIRECTIONS: For questions 84–6 and 84–7, choose all answers that apply.**

84–6. Which of the following characteristics are found on the Hare Psychopathy Checklist—Revised?

1. Grandiose sense of self-worth
2. Lack of remorse or guilt
3. Good impulse control
4. Failure to accept responsibility for one's own actions
5. Callous/lack of empathy
6. Concern for others

84–7. Which of the following are common psychological defenses used by psychopathic individuals with ASPD?

1. Projection
2. Intellectualization

3. Rationalization

4. Isolation of affect

5. Devaluation

6. Repression

7. Denial

■ **DIRECTIONS: For questions 84–8 through 84–11, indicate**

A if 1, 2, and 3 are correct.

B if 1 and 3 are correct.

C if 2 and 4 are correct.

D if only answer 4 is correct.

E if all are correct.

84–8. Which of the following countertransference reactions are common in clinicians working with ASPD patients or primary psychopathic patients?

1. Therapeutic nihilism

2. Fear of assault or harm

3. Denial and deception

4. Hatred and the wish to destroy

84–9. A rational pharmacotherapy for aggression and violence in ASPD patients includes which of the following agents?

1. Lithium

2. Propranolol

3. Carbamazepine

4. Desipramine

84–10. Which of the following are guiding principles for milieu and residential treatments of patients with ASPD?

1. Patients should be allowed to come and go as they please to prevent violence on the unit.

2. Issues related to criminal activity, such as antisocial values and attitudes, should be addressed as part of the treatment.

3. Milieu and residential treatments are most effective when they target low-risk individuals.

4. Treatment should teach and strengthen interpersonal skills and model prosocial attitudes.

84–11. Milieu or residential approaches that appear promising for the treatment of ASPD include

1. Token economy programs.

2. Therapeutic communities.

3. Wilderness programs.

4. Partial hospitalization with group therapy.

■ **ANSWERS:**

84–1. **True**   There is a long clinical tradition of a psychodynamic construct referred to as *psychopathy,* or *psychopathic personality,* which is based on characterological features rather than on behavior alone. A psychopathy checklist has been developed to assess this construct.

84–2. **False**   Only a minority of patients who meet the DSM-IV criteria for ASPD also have the characteristics of primary psychopathy.

84–3. **False**   There is no body of controlled empirical research that demonstrates the existence of successful treatments for either primary psychopaths or ASPD patients.

84–4. **True**   Research on antisocial patients suggests that presence of an Axis I condition involving anxiety or depression improves the prognosis.

84–5. **True**   The ability to form an alliance reflects some attachment capacity in the ASPD patient and serves as a positive prognostic marker. Attachment capacity has also been associated with decreased drug use and better employment records. Without attachment capacity, psychotherapy is likely to fail.

84–6. **Answer: 1, 2, 4, and 5.** The Hare Psychopathy Checklist—Revised assesses personality traits that are characteristic of primary psychopaths. These persons are frequently grandiose and lack any remorse or guilt about the effect of their actions on others. They have poor impulse control and no capacity for empathy. They tend to blame others for their own behavior and fail to accept responsibility for their own actions.

84–7. **Answer: 1, 3, 5, and 7.** Psychopathic individuals with ASPD use primitive psychological defenses, including projection, rationalization, devaluation, denial, omnipotence, projective identification, and splitting. They rarely show higher-level neurotic defenses, such as idealization, intellectualization, isolation, and repression.

84–8. **Answer: E (All).** A common countertransference problem encountered with antisocial patients is a sense of *therapeutic nihilism,* which refers to the rejection of all patients with an antisocial history as being completely untreatable. An opposite countertransference reaction, called *illusory treatment alliance,* is also common and involves the perception of a treatment alliance when there is none. ASPD patients are dangerous and may produce realistic fears of assault or harm and also countertransference fears that are not based in reality. Denial and deception are common reactions that can be understood as a defense against the anxiety generated by working with violent patients. Hatred and the wish to destroy can be experienced by clinicians working with antisocial patients either as an identification with or a reaction against the patient. Other countertransference reactions commonly experienced include helplessness and guilt, devaluation and loss of professional identity, and assumption of psychological complexity.

84–9. **Answer: A (1, 2, and 3).** Appropriate pharmacotherapy of violence with ASPD patients or psychopathic patients requires an analysis of the mode of violence in which the patient has engaged. Lithium or fluoxetine may inhibit affective and predatory aggression related to the serotonergic system. Carbamazepine or phenytoin may be useful when electrical kindling is involved. Lithium or propranolol may be a rational choice if the noradrenergic system is linked to the violence. Desipramine has not been shown to be useful in the treatment of violent patients.

84–10. **Answer: C (2 and 4).** Milieu and residential therapies appear to be most effective with moderately high-risk individuals. Two of the most important principles are that criminal issues must be addressed as part of the treatment and that interpersonal skills and prosocial attitudes should be taught and strengthened. A loose structure that allows the patient to come and go from the unit will make it difficult for acting out to be contained.

84–11. **Answer: A (1, 2, and 3).** Token economy programs have been useful because they have been shown empirically to shape patient and staff behavior within institutions. Unstructured programs promote more aggressive and dependent behaviors. Therapeutic communities, in which peer problem solving is encouraged and daily group meetings monitor the activities of the milieu, have shown modest positive effects. Although therapeutic communities have been shown to be effective in reducing recidivism with nonpsychopathic populations, there is no evidence that they are helpful for psychopaths, whom they may even make worse. Wilderness programs have not been subjected to controlled outcome studies; however, there are anecdotal data suggesting that these programs might be useful. No studies on partial hospitalization are available to assess the efficacy of such a program.

CHAPTER 85

Borderline Personality Disorder

DIRECTIONS: For questions 85–1 through 85–5, select the single best answer.

85–1. Individual psychotherapy remains the cornerstone of treatment for patients with borderline personality disorder (BPD). Which of the following is **not** considered an essential component of treatment for these patients?

1. Provision of a stable treatment framework

2. Silent and passive receptivity on the part of the therapist

3. Establishment of a connection between the patient's actions and feelings

4. Identification of adverse effects of self-destructive behaviors

85–2. Which of the following is considered the **optimal** approach to a comorbid substance abuse in BPD patients?

1. Treatment of the comorbid substance abuse should be a high priority in the comprehensive treatment plan.

2. Resolution of the comorbid substance abuse has no impact on the course of the illness.

3. The suicide rate in BPD patients is unrelated to substance abuse.

4. Twelve-step groups based on an addiction model, such as Alcoholics Anonymous (AA), are contraindicated for BPD patients.

85–3. Which of the following statements is **not** accurate regarding psychoanalytic psychotherapy of BPD patients who have a history of childhood trauma?

1. The therapist must establish a sense of safety for the patient early in therapy.

2. The therapist must acknowledge and empathize with the patient's experience of being victimized.

3. The therapist must reframe the patient's anger and manipulative behaviors as understandable based on the rage associated with the patient's feeling that parents or caregivers have failed to provide adequately for developmental needs.

4. The therapist should tell the patient that expressions of anger are inappropriate in the therapy because the therapist has not been involved in any form of the patient's abuse.

85–4. Which of the following statements characterizes the role of supportive psycho-therapy in the treatment of BPD patients?

   1. Few BPD patients are seen in supportive psychotherapy.

   2. The goals of supportive psychotherapy are explicitly directed at changing personality.

   3. Some research has indicated that supportive treatments are able to bring about basic changes in personality comparable to those derived from ex-pressive treatments.

   4. Insight is necessary for change in supportive psychotherapy.

85–5. Which of the following statements **best** captures the current thinking on the use of short-term psychotherapy with BPD patients?

   1. Short-term psychotherapy may be particularly well suited for BPD patients, who have a tendency to drop out of more ambitious treatments.

   2. Short-term psychotherapy is not suited for patients with a fear of being en-gulfed or overwhelmed.

   3. Clinical experience suggests that time-limited interventions are never justi-fied or useful in the treatment of patients with BPD.

   4. There is no research suggesting that BPD patients are likely to show more improvement in sustained psychotherapy processes.

▓ **DIRECTIONS: For questions 85–6 through 85–12, indicate**

   A if 1, 2, and 3 are correct.
   B if 1 and 3 are correct.
   C if 2 and 4 are correct.
   D if only answer 4 is correct.
   E if all are correct.

85–6. Which of the following statements are **true** regarding family therapy of patients with BPD?

   1. Therapists must be mindful of the degree and strength of persisting attach-ments, even in highly dysfunctional or abusive families.

   2. Premature separation may cause the patient to deteriorate and may encour-age a problematic idealization of the therapist.

   3. In families where neglect has been a problem, conjoint sessions should be ap-proached slowly, and psychoeducational approaches probably are preferable.

   4. In families where the patient has suffered abuse, helping the patient main-tain some distance from the family may be an important step in increasing feelings of safety in the patient.

85–7. Which of the following statements are true regarding group therapy for BPD patients?

   1. Many of these patients benefit from group therapy, but concurrent individ-ual therapy is generally necessary.

   2. Too many of these patients in one group may negatively affect the nonbor-derline patients in the group.

3. Other patients in the group may be more successful than the therapist at confronting maladaptive and impulsive patterns.

4. No empirical research on group therapy with these patients has been reported.

85–8. Dialectical behavior therapy (DBT) has been studied in a randomized controlled trial and has demonstrated which of the following results?

1. Great improvement in hopelessness

2. Significantly fewer and less severe episodes of parasuicidal behavior than in the control group

3. Large reduction in suicidal ideation

4. Fewer days of inpatient treatment compared with in the control group

85–9. Which of the following are **true** regarding the use of low doses of neuroleptic medication in the treatment of patients with BPD?

1. It results in highly specific improvements.

2. It appears to have no positive effects.

3. It should be continued for extended periods.

4. It appears to reduce the severity of a broad range of symptoms in acutely distressed patients.

85–10. Which of the following statements are **true** regarding treatment of affective dyscontrol in BPD patients?

1. Monoamine oxidase inhibitors appear to be particularly effective for patients with atypical depression.

2. Initial studies of the effectiveness of SSRIs, such as fluoxetine, with BPD patients are encouraging and suggest that a variety of different symptoms are improved with these agents.

3. Although a trial of tricyclic antidepressants may be warranted, they are not generally considered the first line of treatment with BPD patients who are having persistent depressive symptoms.

4. Major depression in the context of BPD may represent a different syndrome than major depression alone and therefore may not respond in a predictable way to antidepressant medication.

85–11. Which of the following agents have been useful in treating impulsivity and behavioral dyscontrol in BPD patients?

1. Lithium

2. Alprazolam

3. Carbamazepine

4. Desipramine

85–12. Which of the following principles are important in the management of suicidal behavior in BPD patients?

1. A determination must be made as to whether the suicidal behavior is acute or chronic.

2. The clinician must avoid becoming the patient's rescuer or savior.

3. Access to an inpatient unit and a readiness to hospitalize the patient are essential aspects of any treatment plan.

4. Suicidal behavior is almost always manipulative, and therefore hospitalization is hardly ever needed to prevent a suicide.

■ ANSWERS:

85–1. **Answer: 2.** The general consensus is that the therapist needs to be highly active and involved in the psychotherapy of patients with BPD. Silence and passivity may increase transference distortions of a paranoid nature and cause the patient to feel that the therapist does not care. Other central components of an effective psychotherapy process include provision of a stable treatment framework, establishment of connections between the patient's actions and feelings, identification of adverse effects of self-destructive behaviors, and careful monitoring of countertransference feelings.

85–2. **Answer: 1.** An effective treatment program for BPD patients should begin by aggressively treating Axis I disorders, including substance abuse or major depression. Follow-up studies indicate that resolution of comorbid substance abuse improves the overall course of the illness. In one follow-up study, the subsample of BPD patients with major affective disorder and untreated alcoholism had an alarmingly high suicide rate. Twelve-step groups, such as AA, may be beneficial to many patients with BPD.

85–3. **Answer: 4.** Much research has demonstrated that many patients with BPD have histories of childhood sexual and physical abuse. This research has led to a modification in the psychoanalytic psychotherapy used with such patients. Rather than interpreting the inappropriateness of the aggression manifested by the patient, the therapist must now understand such aggression in terms of an immature self that is rightfully full of rage at parents or parent substitutes for their failure to provide a secure base and address developmental needs. Early in therapy, much of the therapist's effort should be directed at establishing a sense of safety for the patient and helping the patient form a trusting alliance. To facilitate these developments, the therapist must validate and empathize with the patient's experience of being victimized and reframe angry and manipulative behaviors as understandable given the early life experiences of the patient.

85–4. **Answer: 3.** In recent years, there has been a growing awareness of the value of supportive individual psychotherapy, often on a once-weekly basis, for patients with BPD. The process usually requires several years, as in expressive psychotherapy, but is not explicitly directed at changing the patient's personality. Rather, the focus is on the patient's adapting to life circumstances, decreasing the likelihood of self-destructive responses to interpersonal frustrations, and accepting the other reality problems of daily living. The report of the Menninger Psychotherapy Research Project indicates that many treatments of BPD patients begin with highly expressive techniques but gradually shift to more supportive strategies and that supportive therapy may make basic changes in personality similar in kind to those resulting from psychoanalytically oriented psychotherapy. Currently, most patients with BPD probably receive some form of supportive psychotherapy.

85–5. **Answer: 1.** The early pessimism about the use of short-term psychotherapy with BPD patients has been modified over time. A great many patients drop out of long-term psychotherapy after a few months, so many patients end up returning to therapy for periodic "doses" of circumscribed treatment. This intermittent strategy of short-term therapy appears to be particularly well suited for those individuals who have a tendency to drop out of more ambitious treatments as well as for those who are concerned about becoming engulfed or overwhelmed by the therapist. Clinical experience suggests that some BPD patients can get by with this approach of short-term intermittent therapy. However, research by Hoch and by Howard indicates that those BPD patients who are able to remain in sustained therapies are likely to show more improvement.

85–6. **Answer: E (All).** There are two general patterns of family involvement in families of BPD patients: overinvolvement and neglect. When the family pattern is characterized by *overinvolvement,* the therapist should encourage active, ongoing family participation in treatment. Even when the families have been highly dysfunctional or abusive, therapists must understand that the patient may have persisting attachments to the family. When the family is profoundly enmeshed, premature separations may lead to the patient's decompensation and overdependence on the therapist. When the family pattern is characterized by *neglect,* the therapist must move cautiously toward conjoint sessions. Psychoeducational approaches may work best to ease the family's wariness and to facilitate development of an alliance with them. For families in which abuse has occurred, the patient may need distance to feel safe. Reconciliation in such families is a rare occurrence but may be powerful when it does happen.

85–7. **Answer: A (1, 2, and 3).** A broad consensus is that group therapy is useful for many BPD patients. The presence of other patients in a group provides benefits that are not available in individual therapy. For example, other patients may be able to confront maladaptive personality traits without being perceived as controlling the patient. A group also provides a supportive, holding environment for the patient. Recent empirical studies have supported the effectiveness of group psychotherapy for BPD patients. Too many borderline patients in one group, however, may cause difficulties for the non-BPD patients in the group. There is general agreement that concurrent individual therapy is necessary when BPD patients are assigned to group therapy.

85–8. **Answer: C (2 and 4).** Dialectical behavior therapy was specifically designed for BPD patients by Marsha Linehan and her colleagues. The treatment involves one session weekly of individual therapy and one session weekly of group therapy. Suicidal and parasuicidal behaviors are the primary focus of the treatment. In a randomized controlled trial comparing DBT with "treatment as usual," the patients receiving DBT had significantly fewer and less severe episodes of parasuicidal behavior as well as fewer days of inpatient hospitalization compared with those in the control group. However, the patients receiving DBT did not differ from the control group on measures of depression, hopelessness, or suicidal ideation.

85–9. **Answer: D (Only 4).** Based on a number of randomized controlled trials of neuroleptic medication in patients with BPD, it appears that these agents improve the severity of a broad range of symptoms in acutely distressed BPD patients. The effect seems to be nonspecific and varied across studies. There is no evidence that continuing neuroleptic medication after the acute symptoms subside is of any value, and the risk of serious side effects should make the clinician cautious about prescribing these agents for extended periods.

85–10. **Answer: E (All).** A number of randomized controlled trials with antidepressant agents have been tried with BPD patients. Monoamine oxidase inhibitors appear particularly useful for BPD patients who have atypical depression with symptoms such as rejection-sensitive dysphoria, hypersomnia, and hyperphagia. Early studies of fluoxetine indicate that it is useful in BPD patients whether or not there is comorbid depression. Fluoxetine appears to improve such varied symptoms as paranoia, anxiety, depression, interpersonal sensitivity, hostility, and global functioning. Some data suggest that major depression in the context of BPD may represent a different syndrome than major depression alone, which may account for the fact that the coexistence of depression is not necessarily a strong predictor of a patient's response to antidepressant medication. Fluoxetine or another SSRI is considered the first line of treatment for borderline patients with persistent depressive symptoms. The next choice would be a monoamine oxidase inhibitor, and the third choice would be a tricyclic antidepressant.

85–11. **Answer: B (1 and 3).** Impulsive actions and behavioral dyscontrol may include such behaviors as bingeing, promiscuity, recklessness, and impulsive suicide attempts. Lithium has been useful in the treatment of angry outbursts and suicidal symptoms. Alprazolam has been shown to significantly increase behavioral dyscontrol. Carbamazepine has been shown to reduce behavioral dyscontrol in a double-blind, crossover study. Desipramine has no effect on symptoms of impulsivity in BPD patients.

85–12. **Answer: A (1, 2, and 3).** A significant number of BPD patients commit suicide in the course of their illness. Suicidal behavior must be taken seriously. The clinician must determine whether the behavior is acute or chronic. With chronically suicidal patients, it is advisable to avoid the role of idealized rescuer or savior. However, hospitalizations will be needed during acute suicidal crises, and the clinician who is seeing the patient must have access to a hospital unit and be ready to admit the patient to the hospital.

CHAPTER 86

Histrionic Personality Disorder

■ **DIRECTIONS: For questions 86–1 through 86–5, indicate whether the statement is true or false.**

86–1. _____ The treatment recommendations for patients with histrionic personality disorder are based on empirical studies.

86–2. _____ The majority of successful treatment reports for histrionic personality disorder have come from a psychoanalytic (or psychoanalytic psychotherapy) perspective.

86–3. _____ Treatment approaches to histrionic personality disorder must be adjusted to the patient's underlying vulnerability to sudden and disorganizing deflations in self-esteem.

86–4. _____ Cognitive-behavioral approaches to patients with histrionic personality disorder are useful for identifying irrational cognitions and disruptions of clear conscious representation and expression.

86–5. _____ Psychodynamic approaches are useful for understanding levels of transference, counteracting resistance, and establishing a therapeutic alliance.

■ **DIRECTIONS: Using the following vignette, for questions 86–6 through 86–8, select the single best answer for each question.**

A 26-year-old woman with histrionic personality disorder came to her first consultation asking for psychotherapy. She was in a state of considerable agitation because she said her boyfriend had just "dumped" her. She said that she didn't know what she was going to do, and she wept continually as she told her account of her difficulties in romantic relationships in general. She told the therapist about three similar relationships that had broken up over the last 2 years. She said she was feeling out of control and was afraid she would do something that she would later regret. The therapist asked her if she had ever attempted to hurt herself, and she responded that she had not but that she was frightened by thoughts of doing something self-destructive. She lacked any significant symptomatology associated with major depression, but she said she did not know where to turn for support.

86–6.   Which of the following initial approaches would be most useful with this patient?

    1. Hospitalize the patient.

    2. Confront the patient with her infantile behavior.

    3. Empathize with the patient's suffering and collaborate with her in developing a careful step-by-step plan for dealing with her problems.

    4. Treat her only with medication because psychotherapy is contraindicated.

86–7.   As the therapy develops with this patient, which of the following would be a major focus of treatment?

    1. Shifting attention from an inclusively external focus to an internal one

    2. Assuming the role of rescuer with the patient

    3. Interpreting the patient's resistance to the awareness of erotic transference

    4. Directing the patient toward more mature ways of behaving

86–8.   In the opening phase of the psychotherapy, how might the therapist best deal with the overwhelming emotions expressed by the patient?

    1. The therapist must tell the patient that her feelings are volatile and shallow.

    2. The therapist may use clarification and repetition in a calm, gradual way that offers empathic support and slows down the patient's associations.

    3. The therapist must set limits on such behavior in the sessions.

    4. The therapist must interpret the manipulative quality of the exaggerated emotions.

■ **DIRECTIONS: For questions 86–9 through 86–11, choose all answers that apply.**

86–9.   Many patients with histrionic personality disorder use a variety of inhibitory control processes to avoid emotionally distressing facts about themselves or others. Which of the following are avoidant or inhibitory control processes commonly seen in these patients?

    1. Reaction formation

    2. Contempt

    3. Suppression

    4. Repression

    5. Disavowal

    6. Denial

86–10. Which of the following techniques are useful in modifying defensive control processes that are obstacles in psychotherapy with histrionic personality disorder patients?

    1. Counteracting the tendency to avoid or quickly drop a topic that contains conflicts and dilemmas

    2. Counteracting the tendency to leave unresolved topics in a cloudy matrix of loose associations

3. Reinforcing by approval acts of paying attention to observing the behaviors and intentions of oneself and others

4. Modeling how to stay with unresolved topics until rational choice points are reached

5. Discouraging efforts to rationalize impulsive decisions to exit from under-modulated states or to disavow personal responsibility for actions

86–11. After identification of role-relationship models and scripts that are involved in perpetuating repeated cycles of states, what are useful therapeutic approaches to dealing with such maladaptive patterns?

1. Assisting the patient in identifying the patterns and the reasons for their presence

2. Encouraging the patient to develop new schemas

3. Forbidding the patient from repeating the pattern

4. Offering advice on what the patient needs to do to change

■ **DIRECTIONS: For questions 86–12 through 86–14, indicate whether the statement is true or false.**

86–12. _____ Psychoanalysis is an effective treatment for patients with histrionic personality disorder who are motivated to obtain maximum possible understanding and self-development.

86–13. _____ Marital therapy is rarely useful with histrionic personality disorder patients.

86–14. _____ In brief psychotherapy with histrionic personality disorder patients, an initial focus can be derived from recent life events that have served as stressors.

■ **ANSWERS:**

86–1. **False** Rigorous research has not been performed on histrionic personality disorder, and treatment for patients with this disorder is based on clinical experience and case reports.

86–2. **True** The vast majority of case reports have been written by analysts or psychoanalytic therapists, and only recently have other forms of treatment begun to appear in the literature.

86–3. **True** Many patients with histrionic personality disorder are vulnerable to rather chaotic reactions to narcissistic injuries. Others have higher levels of impulse control and lack such vulnerability. This dimension of the patient must be carefully assessed before planning the treatment.

86–4. **True** Cognitive distortions are a primary focus of cognitive-behavior therapy, which can be combined with psychodynamic techniques.

86–5. **True** Psychodynamic approaches are extremely important for working with transference and understanding the unconscious conflicts lying behind resistance. They also are helpful in forming a good therapeutic alliance with the patient.

86–6. **Answer: 3.** Patients with histrionic personality disorder frequently come to therapy in the middle of a crisis and are frightened by thoughts of being out of control. If there is no history of suicide attempts and the patient does not appear to be imminently at risk, hospitalization is not indicated. Confrontation of the patient's infantile behavior will destroy the possibility of forming a therapeutic alliance. Empathy with the patient's suffering, on the other hand, and the development of a plan to deal with the problems can be restorative. Psychotherapy is the treatment of choice for such patients, and the therapist must attend to developing a therapeutic alliance. Medication is occasionally useful adjunctively but is not the primary treatment.

86–7. **Answer: 1.** An ongoing task in psychotherapy with histrionic personality disorder patients is to help them shift their attention from an exclusively external focus to an internal one. For example, the patient needs to come to grips with the notion that her pattern of relationships with men has to do with internal factors that perpetuate the long-standing pattern. Prematurely interpreting erotic transference may sound seductive to the patient and may cause the patient to flee the therapy. The patient may be provocative and demanding and want the therapist to become a rescuer, but the therapist should model a calm persistence that suggests to the patient that answers will come through collaboration of both parties.

86–8. **Answer: 2.** Although the emotional displays of patients with histrionic personality disorder may appear volatile and shallow, they are felt by the patient to be unbearably intense and out of control. States of mind shift rapidly early in treatment, and the therapist must be prepared to help the patient understand these shifts. By calmly and gradually clarifying and repeating what is observed in the way of shifting states of mind, the therapist will help the patient feel empathized with and understood so that her associations will slow down enough to prevent continued rapid shifts. Interpretation of manipulative qualities would damage the developing therapeutic alliance.

86–9. **Answer: 3, 4, 5, and 6.** Defense mechanisms like suppression, repression, disavowal, and denial are useful control processes to avoid the experience of distressing thoughts or feelings. They work in the opposite direction of psychotherapy, which is designed to help the patient reflect on internal experience. Reaction formation and contempt are not common control processes found in patients with histrionic personality disorder.

86–10. **Answer: 1, 2, 3, 4, and 5.** Therapists must counteract the histrionic personality disorder patient's tendency to constantly shift the topic away from painful or disconcerting conflicts. The patient's attention can be redirected to the topic when the shift occurs. When concepts are left in a cloudy matrix of loose associations, the therapist can clarify the key issues and translate images into words. By reinforcing moments in the therapy when the patient is reflective and pays attention to the observation of his or her own behaviors, the therapist will bolster the patient's self-reflective attitudes. Tendencies to rationalize impulsive decisions, as well as to disavow personal responsibility for actions, must be discouraged. The therapist must always model how it is possible to stay with unresolved topics until points of rational choice are reached.

86–11. **Answer: 1 and 2.** It may take considerable time in the therapy before the role-relationship models and internal scripts within the patient have been clearly identified. The patient will be ambivalent about changing them, and offering advice about what to do to change them may simply heighten resistance. The therapist can be most useful by assisting in the identification of the patterns and the reasons for them. As the patient develops new schemas that lead to new role relationships, the therapist can be encouraging of these more adaptive developments. Attempts to get the patient to stop behavior patterns will be largely unsuccessful.

86–12. **True** Patients who are highly motivated for self-understanding and who have high levels of ego strength and low levels of narcissistic vulnerability may respond very well to psychoanalysis.

86–13. **False** Marital therapy is often a useful addition in the treatment of a histrionic personality disorder patient, especially when the patient's partner colludes in enacting the patient's role relationships and internal scripts.

86–14. **True** Often, the focus in the initial sessions of brief psychotherapy with histrionic personality disorder patients is diffuse. When recent psychosocial stressors are linked to other ideas and emotions, a focus can be developed and a brief psychotherapy process can occasionally be useful.

CHAPTER 87

Narcissistic Personality Disorder

DIRECTIONS: For questions 87–1 through 87–4, choose all answers that apply.

87–1. Narcissistic personality disorder exists on a continuum. The DSM-IV criteria stress the manifest exhibitionism and grandiosity of the overt or oblivious narcissistic individual. Which of the following characteristics are typical of patients at this end of the continuum?

1. Arrogance
2. Aggression
3. Easily invoked humiliation
4. Inhibition to the point of self-effacement
5. Self-absorption
6. Lack of empathy
7. A need to be at center stage

87–2. A pivotal concept in self psychology, a school of thought derived from the ideas of Heinz Kohut, is that narcissistic patients form particular types of transferences in the psychoanalytic setting. Which of the following characteristics apply to these transferences?

1. The analyst is viewed as a separate, autonomous individual.
2. The analyst is viewed as a "selfobject" who performs necessary functions that maintain a coherent and healthy sense of self in the patient.
3. The patient expects the analyst to provide a mirroring reaction of acceptance and confirmation to the patient's exhibitionistic wishes.
4. The patient idealizes the analyst.
5. The patient clings to the analyst excessively.
6. The patient sees the analyst as a mirror image or twin of himself or herself.

87–3. Kernberg's view of narcissistic personality disorder is based on the quality of object relations and the pattern of these patients' intrapsychic defenses. Which of the following are typical characteristics of narcissistic individuals in Kernberg's model?

1. They experience relationships with others as parasitic and exploitative.
2. They divide the world into those who are extraordinary and those who are worthless.

    3. They are incapable of relying or depending on others.

    4. They use the defenses of repression and reaction formation.

    5. They use the grandiose self to maintain their otherwise tenuously coherent sense of self.

    6. They have a well-developed capacity for empathy toward others.

87–4. Which of the following statements are **true** regarding narcissistic personality disorder?

    1. There are no controlled treatment studies.

    2. Treatment must be tailored to the individual case.

    3. Pharmacotherapy is generally a major part of the treatment.

    4. Individual dynamic psychotherapy or psychoanalysis is often the primary treatment modality.

    5. Marital, family, and group therapies are useful as adjunctive therapies in certain cases.

    6. Hospital treatment is known to have a profound, positive impact on the treatment.

■ **DIRECTIONS: For questions 87–5 through 87–8, indicate**

    A if 1, 2, and 3 are correct.

    B if 1 and 3 are correct.

    C if 2 and 4 are correct.

    D if only answer 4 is correct.

    E if all are correct.

87–5. The particular form of individual psychotherapy with narcissistic personality disorder patients is determined largely by the capacities and motivations of the patient as well as by the general level of ego strength and object relations. Which of the following statements are **true** regarding the task of tailoring the type of therapy to the individual patient?

    1. Most narcissistic patients with overt borderline or antisocial features should be assigned to psychoanalysis or intensive exploratory psychotherapy.

    2. Short-term psychotherapy is probably the preferred treatment when a narcissistic personality disorder patient has a reasonably satisfactory adaptation to life and limited neurotic symptoms.

    3. Supportive-expressive psychotherapy is not particularly useful with any narcissistic personality disorder patients.

    4. Patients who experience significant life impairments and have sufficient ego strength and object relations should be assigned to psychoanalysis or exploratory psychotherapy, with sessions occurring at least twice weekly.

87–6. Which of the following therapeutic approaches are characteristic of the technique derived from Kohut's self psychology?

    1. Understanding of "micro-empathic failures"

    2. Interpretation of idealization as a defense

3. Avoidance of critical interpretation of the patient's denigration or idealization of the analyst

4. Repeated interpretation of envy

87–7. Which of the following techniques reflect Kernberg's model of treatment with narcissistic personality disorder patients?

1. Consistent interpretation of the negative transference

2. Recognition in the countertransference of the hidden intention of the patient's behavior

3. Interpretation of idealization as a defense against feelings of rage and envy

4. Acceptance of idealization at face value

87–8. Which of the following statements are **true** regarding group therapy of patients with narcissistic personality disorder?

1. Group therapy is not useful for narcissistic patients.

2. Group therapy allows for the possibility that the patient's pathological behavior can be confronted firmly and supportively.

3. Patients with narcissistic personality disorder are ideal group therapy patients.

4. Group therapy with these patients must generally be accompanied by concomitant individual therapy.

■ ANSWERS:

87–1. **Answer: 1, 2, 5, 6, and 7.** The DSM-IV criteria for narcissistic personality disorder tend to focus on a type of narcissistic individual who is grandiose and exhibitionistic. These patients may be overbearing, boastful, completely absorbed in themselves to the point of not being aware of others' needs, and aggressive. They may try to be in the spotlight in all situations. The DSM-IV criteria do not capture patients on the other end of the narcissistic continuum—those who are often described as exhibiting covert or hypervigilant narcissism. These patients are ashamed of their grandiose and exhibitionistic wishes and may present as highly inhibited to the point of self-effacement. They are prone to shame and easily humiliated. They are overly tuned in to the reactions of others and are constantly feeling that they have been slighted. These two subtypes of narcissism have received support from empirical studies.

87–2. **Answer: 2, 3, 4, and 6.** Whereas Freud viewed narcissistic patients as incapable of being analyzed because of their inability to form transference attachments, Kohut stressed that the apparent absence of the intense transference relationships of neurotic patients *was* the narcissistic transference. Narcissistic patients are somewhat aloof and remote and treat the analyst as an extension of themselves rather than as a distinct and autonomous individual. Kohut referred to these transferences as "selfobject" transferences. In his view, the selfobject was an extension of the patient that provided the necessary functions to maintain a cohesive sense of self in the patient. Kohut delineated three primary selfobject transferences: 1) the mirror transference, involving the search for acceptance and confirmation of the child's early exhibitionistic wishes; 2) the idealizing transference, in which the patient feels an enhanced sense of self-esteem by being in the presence of an idealized figure; and 3) the twinship, or alter ego, transference, in which the patient perceives the analyst as just like him or her.

87–3.   **Answer: 1, 2, 3, and 5.** In Kernberg's conceptual model of narcissistic personality disorder, he views the narcissistic patient as employing defenses similar to those of the borderline patient—including devaluation, projective identification, omnipotence, and primitive idealization—all in an effort to preserve self-esteem and self-coherence as well as to combat underlying feelings of envy and rage. Repression and isolation of affect are defense mechanisms more associated with higher-level character neuroses. Narcissistic patients consider all of their relationships to be parasitic and exploitative. These patients envy those with fame, beauty, and wealth, and they divide the world into those who are extraordinarily successful and those who are not. The latter are then regarded as being either worthless or mediocre. Narcissistic patients have a great deal of difficulty depending or relying on others, so they rarely experience satisfying or mutually gratifying relationships. These patients are characterized as having a grandiose self that represents a pathological fusion of the ideal self, the ideal object, and the real self. Through this grandiose self, the patient maintains, although tenuously, a coherent sense of self.

87–4.   **Answer: 1, 2, 4, and 5.** Patients with narcissistic personality disorder vary widely in terms of the severity of their symptoms and the impairment of their functioning in interpersonal and vocational situations. No controlled studies of narcissistic personality disorder have been conducted, so treatment recommendations for patients with this disorder are based on clinical experience. Most of the literature focuses on the value of long-term individual psychotherapy or psychoanalysis as the primary modality. In some situations, however, marital, family, and group therapy also have been found to be useful. Pharmacotherapy is not effective for narcissistic personality disorder per se and is only used if there are comorbid Axis I conditions. Similarly, hospital treatment is recommended only when there are comorbid Axis I conditions that require hospitalization. Hospitalization is not known to have any direct benefit on the personality disorder itself.

87–5.   **Answer: C (2 and 4).** To tolerate the frustration inherent in psychoanalysis or exploratory psychotherapy, the patient must be experiencing severe-enough life impairments to have the motivation to persist. Reasonably adequate object relations and ego strength are also requirements for highly expressive treatments. Kernberg suggests that the depth of the patient's actual relationships with others rather than the extent of social interactions is most critical in determining the type of treatment. When narcissistic patients function on an overtly borderline level or have prominent antisocial features, supportive-expressive psychotherapy with limit setting is preferable to more expressive modalities. Finally, some patients have only limited neurotic symptoms and otherwise are satisfied with their adaptation to life. Short-term psychotherapy is useful for such patients because they may not be sufficiently motivated to tolerate the demands of an extended treatment process, such as psychoanalysis or expressive therapy.

87–6.   **Answer: B (1 and 3).** The self-psychological approach to narcissistic personality disorder designed by Kohut rests on the assumption of a developmental-arrest model. Kohut viewed the patient as requiring a primitive selfobject to maintain a cohesive sense of self. To help the patient build more stable self-structures, the therapist or analyst must allow the development of mirroring, idealizing, or twinship transferences. In that regard, empathy and an effort to understand "micro-empathic failures" are pivotal to the overall treatment strategy. Idealization is considered to be a normal developmental need and therefore is not interpreted. Critical interpretation of the patient's denigration or idealization of the analyst will cause the patient to feel a profound sense of shame, and thus such interpretations are avoided in this strategy. Interpretation of envy is not part of the self-psychological approach, because it is thought to increase the patient's sense of humiliation and shame.

87–7.   **Answer: A (1, 2, and 3).** The sine qua non of successful analytic work with narcissistic personality disorder patients, according to Kernberg, is consistent interpretation of the negative transference. He cautions, however, that if there is not also acknowledgment of the positive aspects of the transference, the patient may feel morally condemned by the analyst as "all bad." Kernberg also regards the monitoring of countertransference as crucial to the successful treatment of narcissistic personality disorder. Although he does not advocate bringing countertransference into the process by the analyst's self-disclosure, he *does* suggest that the analyst should be attuned to the hidden intention of the patient's behavior that is revealed by the countertransference. Idealization is viewed by Kernberg as a defensive projection of the patient's grandiose self. In contrast to Kohut, who suggests accepting idealization at face value, Kernberg advocates interpretation of idealization as a defense against envy or rage.

87–8.   **Answer: C (2 and 4).** Patients with narcissistic personality disorder present a number of problems in the group psychotherapy setting. They are likely to become scapegoated because of their sense of entitlement and wish for admiration. They also may devalue other members of the group and the therapist and therefore undermine cohesion in the group. On the other hand, certain narcissistic patients may benefit from being confronted by their peers in a supportive but firm manner. Their maladaptive interpersonal style can be dealt with through feedback from group members. If group psychotherapy is selected, however, individual psychotherapy must also be provided. Many narcissistic patients feel they do not get enough attention in the group so that individual therapy is necessary to keep them involved in the group psychotherapy process.

CHAPTER 88

Avoidant Personality Disorder

■ **DIRECTIONS: For questions 88–1 through 88–4, choose all answers that apply.**

88–1. Which of the following statements apply to the empirical studies on avoidant personality disorder?

1. Randomized controlled trials have demonstrated the efficacy of psychodynamic psychotherapy with avoidant personality disorder patients.

2. In three studies, avoidant personality disorder patients who received behavioral treatments showed significantly more improvement than did patients assigned to waiting-list control groups.

3. Social skills training alone or in combination with cognitive modification has been shown to result in significant improvement with avoidant personality disorder patients.

4. Both alprazolam and phenelzine have been found to be useful in treating avoidant personality traits of social phobia subjects.

5. Interpersonal psychotherapy has been proven to be effective with avoidant personality disorder patients.

88–2. Which of the following statements are **true** regarding cognitive and behavior therapies for patients with avoidant personality disorder?

1. Social skills training in conjunction with exposure techniques, systematic desensitization, and cognitive-behavior therapy is effective as treatment for social anxiety and avoidant behaviors.

2. Treatment gains should occur immediately after the therapy.

3. It appears to be important for many patients with avoidant personality disorder to engage in psychodynamic and/or interpersonal psychotherapy as an adjunct to a cognitive-behavioral approach.

4. The goal of cognitive therapy should be an understanding of unconscious conflicts about becoming close to others.

5. In cognitive therapy, the patient's tendency to negatively interpret social interactions can be followed by exposure experiences that contribute to an altered assessment of the experience of the world.

88–3. Which of the following statements are **true** regarding psychodynamic therapy for patients with avoidant personality disorder?

    1. Interpretive and uncovering approaches may be helpful in identifying unconscious fantasies related to these patients' fear that they will lose control and be criticized by others.

    2. The psychodynamic meaning of anxiety in these patients must be explored to understand the individual origins of the anxiety for each patient.

    3. Shame connected with self-exposure is often a central experience for avoidant personality disorder patients.

    4. Psychodynamic and exposure therapies appear to complement each other.

88–4. Which of the following statements are **true** regarding group therapy and family therapy for patients with avoidant personality disorder?

    1. Group therapy may be specifically effective for those patients who can endure the exposure inherent in such treatment.

    2. Group psychotherapy may reduce social embarrassment and increase social skills through a corrective emotional experience.

    3. Homogeneous groups appear to be better than heterogeneous groups for these patients.

    4. Family therapy may be useful when the avoidant behavior is reinforced by a family with overprotective tendencies.

    5. Even in the absence of family therapy, family members can be helpful to the patient by encouraging the patient to seek out new experiences.

    6. Family therapy is contraindicated in the treatment of these patients.

■ ANSWERS:

88–1. **Answer: 2, 3, and 4.** Psychodynamic psychotherapy has not been proven to be effective with avoidant personality disorder patients in randomized controlled trials. Although Cluster C personality disorders (i.e., avoidant, dependent, obsessive-compulsive) have been shown to improve with two forms of short-term psychodynamic therapy, the researchers did not report results specifically for avoidant personality disorder. Three different studies of avoidant personality disorder patients demonstrated that avoidant personality disorder patients who received behavioral treatments showed significantly greater improvement than did patients assigned to waiting-list control groups. Another study demonstrated that social skills training alone or in combination with cognitive modification produces significant improvements. Limited data exist regarding the pharmacotherapy of avoidant personality disorder. However, the literature on pharmacotherapy of social phobia may be useful and applicable to some avoidant personality disorder patients. Both alprazolam and phenelzine have shown promise in the treatment of avoidant personality traits of individuals with social phobia. Interpersonal psychotherapy has not been rigorously tested with avoidant personality disorder patients.

88–2. **Answer: 1, 3, and 5.** Several forms of behavior therapy, including cognitive-behavior therapy, social skills training in conjunction with exposure techniques, systematic desensitization, and rational-emotive therapy, have been effective in the treatment of social anxiety and avoidant behaviors. Treatment gains are often not impressive immediately after therapy because a longer period of exposure may be necessary for the gains to become evident. Psychodynamic and/or interpersonal psychotherapy may be needed as an adjunct to a cognitive-behavioral approach because, as studies have shown, there may be no generalization to in vivo intimate relationships. The goal of cognitive therapy is to alter the patient's self-critical cognitions and expectations of critical assessment by others; cognitive therapy does not deal with unconscious conflict. The combination of cognitive therapy to address the patient's tendency to negatively interpret social interactions and exposure experiences to positively alter the overall assessment of the world may be highly effective.

88–3. **Answer: 1, 2, 3, and 4.** The interpretation of unconscious fantasies is a key task in dynamic psychotherapy. Fantasies relating to loss of control that will result in criticism from others are particularly important. The individual meaning of anxiety for each patient varies, and the dynamic therapist must explore specific and unique meanings with each patient to understand the origins of the anxiety. Shame is a central affective experience in avoidant personality disorder patients and is often related to issues of self-exposure. Finally, psychodynamic therapies work in a complementary fashion with exposure therapies and appear to enrich the gains that are accomplished by the other modality.

88–4. **Answer: 1, 2, 4, and 5.** Although definitive data are not available, group therapy appears to have a specific beneficial effect on patients with avoidant personality disorder, provided they can tolerate the exposure associated with group treatment. A corrective emotional experience often occurs in the group, so that the patient's social embarrassment is reduced and social skills are enhanced. These changes may facilitate the patient's ability to pursue intimate relationships outside the group. There is no evidence that homogeneous groups are more effective than heterogeneous groups. In the same way that agoraphobic patients may become involved with a collusive family member, patients with avoidant personality disorder may have their avoidant behavior reinforced by the family context. Family therapy may be helpful when the family members are overprotective, and even when family therapy is not utilized, the family members can be encouraged to support the patient's seeking out of new experiences.

CHAPTER 89

Dependent Personality Disorder

■ **DIRECTIONS: For questions 89–1 through 89–5, indicate whether the statement is true or false.**

89–1. _____ Dependent personality disorder is common in the general population.

89–2. _____ Dependent personality disorder is often comorbid with Axis I conditions but rarely with Axis II disorders.

89–3. _____ Most of the treatment recommendations in the literature are based on large randomized controlled studies.

89–4. _____ Common precipitating factors involved in a dependent personality disorder patient's seeking treatment include loss of important relationships and situational or occupational changes.

89–5. _____ Dependent personality disorder patients who become depressed may respond to treatment, but some symptoms and social adjustment problems will remain.

■ **DIRECTIONS: For questions 89–6 through 89–10, choose all answers that apply.**

89–6. Which of the following countertransference difficulties can be expected in psychotherapy with patients with dependent personality disorder?

1. The therapist becomes frustrated because the patient makes no attachment to him or her.

2. The therapist may feel like withdrawing emotionally because of the patient's excessive demands for advice and succor.

3. The therapist may feel coerced to take over the patient's life and offer directives.

4. The therapist may begin to feel like punishing the patient for self-defeating patterns of behavior.

89–7. For which of the following does there appear to be a consensus in the psychotherapy literature concerning certain aspects of therapy with dependent personality disorder patients?

1. The therapist must allow the emergence of a dependent transference.

2. Early confrontation of dependency promotes growth.

3. The therapist must directly support and promote self-expression, assertiveness, decision making, and independence.

4. The therapist must allow ongoing dependence so that the patient is never expected to terminate.

89–8. Which of the following statements are **true** regarding dynamic therapy with dependent personality disorder patients?

1. Psychotherapy is usually helpful to these patients.

2. The efficacy of short-term versus long-term treatment has been extensively investigated.

3. Short-term therapies work best when the focus is circumscribed, the patient has the capacity to form a therapeutic alliance rapidly, and there is a limited tendency toward acting out.

4. Those patients without focal conflicts may require 2–4 sessions per week over several years to work through the dependent transference adequately.

89–9. Which of the following techniques are used in cognitive-behavior therapy with dependent personality disorder patients?

1. The therapist interprets the transference.

2. The therapist initially accepts the patient's dependent behavior.

3. The therapist encourages agenda setting for each session.

4. The therapist encourages independence by setting goals for treatment.

5. The therapist directs the patient's agenda.

6. The therapist uses a Socratic method in the psychotherapy.

7. The therapist continually challenges the patient's dichotomous thinking to improve self-evaluation.

89–10. Which of the following statements are accurate regarding the efficacy of medications in the treatment of patients with dependent personality disorder?

1. Imipramine and chlorpromazine have not shown more positive responses than placebo.

2. Some patients with dependent personality disorder may respond to antidepressants in the presence of an Axis I disorder.

3. When Axis I disorders are present, full recovery is generally less likely when there is comorbid dependent personality disorder compared with when no Axis II disorder is present.

4. Antipsychotic medication is the most effective of all psychopharmacological agents in the treatment of dependent personality disorder patients.

■ ANSWERS:

89–1. **True** In the Midtown Manhattan Study, dependent personality disorder was found in 2.5% of the entire sample.

89–2. **False** Empirical studies suggest that dependent personality disorder frequently occurs with other personality disorders, especially avoidant, histrionic, and borderline personality disorders.

89–3. **False** The treatment literature for dependent personality disorder is generally based on case descriptions and uncontrolled studies. A few controlled trials have examined various combinations of personality disorders, and some of the findings are relevant to dependent personality disorder.

89–4. **True** Patients with dependent personality disorder may not feel they need treatment unless a person on whom they are dependent has been lost or they have a new job or face another situation with greater demands for independent behavior.

89–5. **True** In the National Institute of Mental Health Treatment of Depression Collaborative Research Program, many patients (65%) had a Cluster C, or anxious, personality disorder. Of this group, a large number were patients with dependent personality disorder. Although there were lower attrition rates among patients with anxious-cluster personality disorders compared with among patients with other personality disorders, a lower percentage of patients with anxious-cluster personality disorders became symptom free in terms of depression compared with those without personality disorders. Two-thirds of the patients with anxious-cluster personality disorders continued to have some symptoms and problems even when they returned to baseline.

89–6. **Answer: 2, 3, and 4.** Many patients with dependent personality disorder expect the therapist to give advice and provide succor. They may approach the therapist with a sense of helplessness to encourage that the therapist take over for them. The therapist may be alienated or irritated by the excessive demands and, as a result, withdraw. The patient's protestations of helplessness may also lead the therapist to become highly directive and controlling. Particularly, when a therapist has a personal need to be an omniscient or idealized figure, he or she may collude with the patient's wish for such a figure. These countertransference behaviors on the part of the therapist may inhibit the patient from developing a sense of independence. Many dependent personality disorder patients engage in unsatisfying and self-defeating patterns of relationships. The therapist may become exasperated by the patient's behaviors and begin to act punitively toward the patient for not discontinuing the self-defeating patterns.

89–7. **Answer: 1 and 3.** Most therapists agree that in therapy with dependent personality disorder patients, the therapist must allow the development of a dependent transference so that it can be understood in the context of the here-and-now relationship with the therapist. Therapists also agree that some form of direct support is usually necessary to help the patient overcome fears of becoming assertive and independent. While supporting the patient's efforts toward becoming more self-reliant, however, the therapist should also clarify and interpret transference elements.

89–8. **Answer: 1, 3, and 4.** Few empirical studies have addressed the relative indications for short-term versus long-term dynamic therapy. The clinical impression from therapists who have worked extensively with dependent personality disorder patients, however, is that dynamic therapy is generally helpful. To be suited to short-term psychotherapy, patients should have a focal conflict and a capacity to form a therapeutic alliance relatively rapidly. They also must not be prone to severe episodes of acting out or extreme dependency. Patients who do not respond to short-term therapy or have extensive conflicts around dependency will require 2–4 sessions per week over several years before they are able to work through the dependent transference.

89–9. **Answer: 2, 3, 4, 6, and 7.** Cognitive-behavior therapy for dependent personality disorder is not based on interpretation of unconscious issues of the transference. Rather, a formulation is developed to foster accurate self-appraisal as well as independent decision making and behavior. The patient's dependent behavior is initially accepted, but independence is encouraged through the setting of goals with the patient. The therapist does not take over in the process of determining goals but, rather, allows the patient to develop them independently. The Socratic method is helpful in avoiding the risk of a directive approach to the patient's agenda. Dichotomous thinking (e.g., "If I am not fully successful, then I'm inadequate") is repeatedly challenged to improve the patient's self-evaluation. Diaries may also be used to monitor the patient's automatic thoughts.

89–10. **Answer: 1, 2, and 3.** One placebo-controlled study found imipramine or chlorpromazine no more effective than placebo with dependent personality disorder patients. Patients with Axis I disorders, such as depression, may show some improvement with antidepressants, but the benefits are not particularly impressive. In general, recovery from Axis I disorders is not as substantial as that in patients without personality disorders. There are no data suggesting that antipsychotics are helpful with dependent personality disorder patients.

CHAPTER 90

Obsessive-Compulsive
Personality Disorder

■ **DIRECTIONS: For questions 90–1 through 90–3,
select the single best answer.**

90–1. Which statement best characterizes the relationship between obsessive-compulsive disorder (OCD) and obsessive-compulsive personality disorder (OCPD)?

1. The two disorders are more or less identical.
2. The two disorders are part of a continuum.
3. The two disorders usually occur together in the same person.
4. Although a small portion of OCPD patients also have OCD, the two disorders are believed to be separate and distinct.

90–2. Which of the following statements is **true** regarding pharmacotherapy of OCPD?

1. The serotonin reuptake inhibitors used in the treatment of OCD have been rigorously studied in the OCPD population.
2. There are currently no medications available that are specific for the treatment of OCPD.
3. OCPD patients generally respond well to both anxiolytics and antidepressants.
4. Behavior therapy in conjunction with a serotonin reuptake inhibitor is the treatment of choice for OCPD.

90–3. The treatment of choice for OCPD is

1. Group psychotherapy.
2. Individual cognitive-behavior therapy.
3. Individual psychodynamic psychotherapy or psychoanalysis.
4. Pharmacotherapy.

■ **DIRECTIONS: For questions 90–4 and 90–5, indicate**

A if 1, 2, and 3 are correct.
B if 1 and 3 are correct.
C if 2 and 4 are correct.
D if only answer 4 is correct.
E if all are correct.

90–4. Psychodynamic psychotherapy and psychoanalysis with OCPD patients are organized around certain basic considerations, including

1. Attention to the typical defenses.

2. Softening and modification of morbid superego attitudes.

3. Identification and working through of underlying unconscious conflicts that generate symptoms.

4. Flamboyant displays of affect.

90–5. Which of the following are typical defenses of OCPD patients?

1. Repression and denial

2. Splitting and projective identification

3. Omnipotent control, devaluation, and contempt

4. Intellectualization, isolation of affect, undoing, displacement, and reaction formation

■ ANSWERS:

90–1. **Answer: 4.** For many years, OCD and OCPD were considered part of the same spectrum of illness. However, growing evidence suggests that they are separate and distinct. One study indicated that only about 6% of OCPD patients also have OCD. In differentiating the two, many clinicians have relied on the distinction that whereas OCPD traits are ego-syntonic, the obsessional thoughts and compulsive rituals of OCD patients are ego-dystonic. This distinction has some limitations because occasionally OCD symptoms *are* experienced as ego-syntonic.

90–2. **Answer: 2.** Few empirical data exist to guide the use of medication with OCPD. No medications specific for the treatment of OCPD are currently available. The SSRIs have not been rigorously studied in the OCPD population, as they have in OCD patients. Nonspecific anxiolytic agents are occasionally utilized, but the potential problem of dependency limits their usefulness. Antidepressants are only useful if the patient also has an Axis I diagnosis of depression. The current thinking is that pharmacological agents should be considered adjunctive at best with OCPD patients and should never be used as the primary treatment modality. Behavior therapy in conjunction with a serotonin reuptake inhibitor is usually considered the treatment of choice for OCD, not OCPD.

90–3. **Answer: 3.** Although rigorous empirical studies on the treatment of OCPD are lacking, the consensus of clinicians is that individual psychodynamic therapy or psychoanalysis is the best treatment. Because the thinking of patients with OCPD tends to be ego-syntonic, cognitive-behavioral approaches do not appear to be helpful. Group psychotherapy may be useful for some patients because it affords the opportunity for the patient to have his or her somewhat rigid defenses confronted by other patients. The peer pressure provided in group therapy may also lessen resistance. As noted in the answer to the previous question, pharmacotherapy has almost no role in the treatment of OCPD patients.

90–4. **Answer: A (1, 2, and 3).** The defenses of OCPD patients manifest themselves as resistances in the treatment process, so they need to be addressed early in the treatment to help the patient become aware of them. Because most of these patients are excessively harsh and critical of their thoughts and feelings, efforts to modify the superego attitudes are central to the treatment. Unconscious conflicts around aggression, sexuality, and competitiveness frequently emerge and must be identified in the transference as well as outside the therapeutic setting so that the patient can become aware of the relationship between symptoms and unconscious conflicts. Flamboyant affective displays are not characteristic of OCPD.

90–5. **Answer: D (Only 4).** In their efforts to prevent intense feelings, OCPD patients tend to intellectualize or isolate their affect. They also employ undoing, displacement, and reaction formation to prevent themselves from getting in touch with aggressive or sexual feelings. Repression and denial are more characteristic of patients with histrionic personality disorder. Splitting and projective identification are the typical defenses of patients with borderline personality disorder. Omnipotent control, devaluation, and contempt are most commonly found in patients with narcissistic personality disorder.

SECTION 12

Sleep Disorders

CHAPTER 91

Sleep Disorders

■ **DIRECTIONS: For questions 91–1 through 91–9, indicate**

    A if answers 1, 2, and 3 are correct.

    B if answers 1 and 3 are correct.

    C if answers 2 and 4 are correct.

    D if only answer 4 is correct.

    E if all are correct.

91–1. What are the specific targets of cognitive therapy for sleep disorders?

    1. Misconceptions about the causes of insomnia

    2. Misconceptions about the consequences of insomnia

    3. Misperceptions about sleep cycles

    4. Learned helplessness

91–2. Good sleep hygiene involves avoiding which of the following prior to going to bed?

    1. Alcoholic beverages

    2. Late-afternoon or early-evening exercise

    3. Coffee

    4. Warm milk

91–3. Large, well-controlled clinical treatment trials of behavioral/psychological and pharmacological treatments have been conducted for which of the following sleep disorders?

    1. Narcolepsy

    2. Restless legs syndrome

    3. Circadian rhythm sleep disorders

    4. Primary insomnia

91–4. Which of the following variables are **not** related to treatment outcome for treatment of patients with sleep disorders?

    1. Severity of the disorder

    2. Age of the patient

    3. Duration of the disorder

    4. Dependency on hypnotic medications

91–5. Treatment of narcolepsy involves which of the following modalities?

    1. Regularly scheduled naps

    2. Supportive group therapy

    3. Stimulant medication

    4. Maintenance of irregular sleep-wake cycles

91–6. Pharmacotherapy for the treatment of narcolepsy may include which of the following medications?

    1. Protriptyline

    2. Tranylcypromine

    3. Fluoxetine

    4. Pemoline

91–7. Which of the following are **not** part of stimulus control therapy for sleep disorders?

    1. The patient should arise in the morning at the same time, regardless of the amount of sleep obtained.

    2. The patient should go to bed only when he or she is sleepy.

    3. The patient should not lie in bed whenever he or she is unable to fall asleep.

    4. The bedroom should be used for all manner of activities, not only sleeping and sex.

91–8. Which of the following patients are most likely to develop obstructive sleep apnea?

    1. Mr. K. is a morbidly obese 55-year-old who has a long-standing history of hypertension.

    2. Sammy is a 1-year-old with Crouzon's syndrome.

    3. Mr. M. is a moderately overweight 63-year-old with a history of congestive heart disease.

    4. Kathy is a 1-year-old with cri du chat syndrome.

91–9. Patients with which of the following psychiatric disorders present with prominent disturbances in sleep?

    1. Posttraumatic stress disorder (PTSD)

    2. Mania

    3. Major depressive disorder

    4. Adjustment reaction

■ **DIRECTIONS: For questions 91–10 through 91–19, indicate whether the statement is true or false.**

91–10. _____ The patient is usually a passive recipient in treatment of sleep disorders.

91–11. _____ Patients are not requested to restrict their sleep below 4 to 5 hours per night when sleep restriction is used to treat insomnia.

91–12. _____ Poor sleepers are less well informed about good sleep hygiene and practice more unhealthy habits than good sleepers.

91–13. _____ Primary insomnia that persists longer than a month is considered chronic.

91–14. _____ Sleep hygiene alone is usually effective in the treatment of insomnia.

91–15. _____ Fewer than 10% of patients with sleep disorders increase their dose of benzodiazepines.

91–16. _____ The half-life of a particular benzodiazepine has little to no effect on the presence of rebound insomnia after discontinuation of the medication.

91–17. _____ Primary hypersomnia frequently occurs in conjunction with other sleep disturbances.

91–18. _____ Surgical intervention for obstructive sleep apnea is warranted when the patient is 50% over ideal weight.

91–19. _____ Shift rotation should proceed from days to evenings and then to nights to create the least disturbance in sleep-wake cycles.

◼ **DIRECTIONS: For questions 91–20 through 91–36, match the drug to the most appropriate statement(s). Each statement may be used once, more than once, or not at all.**

91–20.	Diazepam	a.	Suppresses stage 3 sleep.
91–21.	Amitriptyline	b.	Suppresses stage 4 sleep.
91–22.	Trazodone	c.	Suppresses REM sleep.
91–23.	Lorazepam	d.	Prolongs stage 3 sleep.
91–24.	Zolpidem	e.	Prolongs stage 4 sleep.
91–25.	Desipramine	f.	Increases REM sleep.
91–26.	Bupropion	g.	Is highly sedating.
91–27.	Diphenhydramine	h.	Is lethal in overdose.
91–28.	Cimetidine	i.	Causes memory impairment.
91–29.	Phenobarbital	j.	Suppresses stage 2 sleep.
91–30.	Meprobamate	k.	Prolongs stage 2 sleep.
91–31.	Alcohol	l.	Increases sleep spindles.
91–32.	Methylphenidate	m.	Activates gamma-aminobutyric acid.
91–33.	Fluoxetine	n.	Is an anxiolytic.
91–34.	Protriptyline	o.	Is an anticonvulsant.
91–35.	L-Dopa	p.	Has hepatotoxicity.
91–36.	Clonazepam	q.	Is used to treat nightmares.
		r.	Is used in the treatment of narcolepsy.
		s.	Suppresses appetite.
		t.	Has no effect on particular sleep stages.
		u.	Is used for intermittent short-term use.
		v.	Is used to treat cataplexy.
		w.	Is used to treat breathing-related sleep disorder.
		x.	Is used to treat restless legs syndrome.
		y.	Is used to treat intractable nightmares.
		z.	Is used to treat nocturnal movement disorders.

■   DIRECTIONS: For questions 91–37 through 91–41, match the stage of sleep with the associated disorder(s), electroencephalogram finding(s), or property. Each disorder, electroencephalogram finding, or property may be used once, more than once, or not at all.

91–37.	Stage 1	a.	Night terrors
91–38.	Stage 2	b.	Nightmares
91–39.	Stage 3	c.	Sleep spindles
91–40.	Stage 4	d.	Delta waves
91–41.	REM	e.	Enuresis
		f.	K complexes
		g.	Somnambulism
		h.	Alpha waves
		i.	Restless leg syndrome
		j.	Myocardial infarctions
		k.	Sleep paralysis
		l.	Amnesia for dreams
		m.	Asthma
		n.	Nocturnal erections
		o.	Decreases through the life cycle
		p.	Migraines

■   ANSWERS:

91–1. **Answer: E (All).** Cognitive therapy alters dysfunctional cognitions and perceptions about the causes and consequences of insomnia and about sleep cycles. The learned helplessness associated with the perceived unpredictability of sleep and the unrealistic expectations for sleep is addressed in the cognitive therapy process.

91–2. **Answer: B (1 and 3).** Good sleep hygiene includes avoiding caffeine and nicotine 4 to 6 hours prior to bedtime, as both are stimulants. Alcohol is a depressant and as such may facilitate the onset of sleep, but it often disrupts the sleep cycle. Late-afternoon or early-evening exercise, warm milk, minimizing noise and light, and appropriate temperature regulation will promote sleep.

91–3. **Answer: D (Only 4).** Large, well-controlled clinical treatment trials of behavioral/psychological treatments have been conducted for primary insomnia. Pharmacological treatments have been investigated for primary insomnia, narcolepsy, restless legs syndrome, periodic limb disorder, and simulated circadian rhythm sleep disorder.

91–4. **Answer: A (1, 2, and 3).** Age, gender, and severity and duration of the sleep disorder are *not* related to prognosis. The presence of psychiatric comorbidity and the dependence on hypnotic medications are related to a poorer treatment outcome in patients with a sleep disorder.

91–5. **Answer: A (1, 2, and 3).** Narcolepsy is best treated using multiple therapeutic modalities. Stimulant medication is the mainstay of pharmacological management. Behavioral treatments such as taking regularly scheduled 15-minute naps and maintaining a regular sleep-wake cycle are important components of treatment, as is supportive group therapy to assist the patient in adapting to a chronic illness.

91–6. **Answer: E (All).** Stimulant medications (e.g., pemoline, methylphenidate, dextroamphetamine, and methamphetamine) are the mainstay in the pharmacological management of narcolepsy. Tricyclic antidepressants (e.g., protriptyline and imipramine), monoamine oxidase inhibitors (e.g., tranylcypromine), and the selective serotonin reuptake inhibitors (e.g., fluoxetine) may be used to treat the accessory symptoms of cataplexy, sleep paralysis, and sleep-related hallucinations.

91–7. **Answer: D (Only 4).** Stimulus control therapy consists of a set of instructional procedures designed to curtail sleep-incompatible behaviors and to regulate sleep-wake schedules. The recommended procedures are that 1) the patient should use the bedroom only for sleep and sexual activity, 2) should go to bed only when sleepy, and 3) should arise at the same time every morning regardless of the amount of sleep the previous night. If unable to fall asleep, the patient should leave the bedroom and return in 15 minutes. This process should be repeated until the patient is sleepy.

91–8. **Answer: A (1, 2, and 3).** Obstructive sleep apnea tends to develop in overweight, middle-aged males who have a history of hypertension and/or cardiovascular disease. The disorder is also seen in individuals with craniofacial abnormalities such as Crouzon's syndrome. Cri du chat syndrome is caused by an absence of the short arm of one of the number 5 chromosomes; no major craniofacial abnormalities are associated with this disorder.

91–9. **Answer: A (1, 2, and 3).** Nightmares are a hallmark of PTSD. The absence of sleep is frequently noted in patients with mania or hypomania. Patients with major depressive disorder may experience hypersomnia or insomnia. Patients with adjustment reactions usually do not have prominent disturbances in sleep.

91–10. **False** Patients should be active participants in their treatment.

91–11. **True** Poor sleepers often increase their time in bed in an effort to induce sleep. Sleep restriction reduces the amount of time spent in bed.

91–12. **False** Poor sleepers are *better* informed about good sleep hygiene but practice more unhealthy habits than do good sleepers.

91–13. **True** The cut-off for acute primary insomnia is 1 month.

91–14. **False** Sleep hygiene alone is rarely effective in the treatment of insomnia.

91–15. **True** Fewer than 10% of patients with sleep disorders increase their dosage of benzodiazepine.

91–16. **False** Discontinuation of short-half-life benzodiazepines is more likely to produce rebound insomnia.

91–17. **False** By definition, primary hypersomnia cannot occur in conjunction with other sleep disturbances.

91–18. **False**   The weight cutoff for surgical intervention for the treatment of obstructive sleep apnea is 100% over ideal weight.

91–19. **True**   Rotating shifts that move from days to evenings to nights are easier to adapt to than shifts that rotate in the opposite direction.

91–20. Diazepam: **a, b, c, g, i, k, l, n, o, r, u, w, x, y, z**

91–21. Amitriptyline: **c, d, e, g, h, q, r, w, y**

91–22. Trazodone: **c, d, e, g, q, r, y**

91–23. Lorazepam: **a, d, e, g, k, q, r, y**

91–24. Zolpidem: **c, d, e, g, i, l, n, r, u, x, y, z**

91–25. Desipramine: **c, d, e, h, q, r, w, y**

91–26. Bupropion: **t**

91–27. Diphenhydramine: **c, d, e**

91–28. Cimetidine: **q**

91–29. Phenobarbital: **a, b, c, h, l, o**

91–30. Meprobamate: **p**

91–31. Alcohol: **a, b, c, d, e, f, h, i, q**

91–32. Methylphenidate: **a, b, c, r, s**

91–33. Fluoxetine: **c, r**

91–34. Protriptyline; **c, d, e, h, q, r, w, y**

91–35. L-Dopa: **c, f, x, z**

91–36. Clonazepam: **a, b, c, g, i, l, n, o, r, u, x, y, z**

91–37. Stage 1: **h**

91–38. Stage 2: **c, k**

91–39. Stage 3: **a, d, e, g, i, l, p**

91–40. Stage 4: **a, d, e, g, i , l, p**

91–41. REM: **b, j, k, m, n, o, p**

Disorders of Impulse Control

CHAPTER 92

Disorders of Impulse Control

DIRECTIONS: For questions 92–1 through 92–8, indicate whether the statement is true or false.

92–1. _____ Most patients with kleptomania are women.

92–2. _____ There are specific medications of choice for the disorders of impulse control.

92–3. _____ In the treatment of intermittent explosive disorder, there are several well-controlled efficacy studies documenting the use of anticonvulsants.

92–4. _____ Psychotherapy is rarely indicated in patients with intermittent explosive disorder.

92–5. _____ True pyromania is relatively rare in children.

92–6. _____ Alcoholism is frequently found in the family histories of patients with pyromania.

92–7. _____ Compulsive gambling is more common in men than in women.

92–8. _____ Treatment for compulsive gambling may follow a 12-step approach.

DIRECTIONS: For questions 92–9 through 92–14, indicate

A if answers 1, 2, and 3 are correct.

B if answers 1 and 3 are correct.

C if answers 2 and 4 are correct.

D if only answer 4 is correct.

E if all are correct.

92–9. Family therapy may be indicated for which of the following disorders?

1. Intermittent explosive disorder

2. Pyromania

3. Kleptomania

4. Trichotillomania

92–10. What personality disorder may not be diagnosed concurrently with intermittent explosive disorder?

1. Schizoid
2. Narcissistic
3. Paranoid
4. Borderline

92–11. Which medications have been used in the treatment of intermittent explosive disorder?

1. Carbamazepine
2. Propranolol
3. Phenytoin
4. Buspirone

92–12. What treatments are the most beneficial in the initial intervention for trichotillomania?

1. Clomipramine
2. Psychotherapy
3. Fluoxetine
4. Behavior therapy

92–13. What comorbid disorders are associated with trichotillomania?

1. Anxiety disorders
2. Psychosis
3. Depression
4. Substance abuse

92–14. What types of treatment may be used for patients with pyromania?

1. Fluoxetine
2. Behavior therapy
3. Valproic acid
4. Residential placement

■ ANSWERS:

92–1.   **True**   Kleptomania is more commonly found in women.

92–2.   **False**   There is no drug of choice for disorders of impulse control.

92–3.   **False**   In studies on the use of anticonvulsants in the treatment of intermittent explosive disorder, the medication trials have been largely uncontrolled.

92–4.   **False**   Patients with intermittent explosive disorder usually require psychotherapy to address the interpersonal and intrapsychic conflicts that arise from or form the basis of their behaviors.

92–5.   **True**   True pyromania is characterized by a fascination with fires without motive and does not usually occur in children.

92–6. **True** Alcoholism is frequently found in families of patients with pyromania.

92–7. **True** Two-thirds of compulsive gamblers are men.

92–8. **True** Treatment for compulsive gambling may include a 12-step self-help group approach.

92–9. **Answer: A (1, 2, and 3).** Legal and interpersonal conflicts are frequently complications of intermittent explosive disorder, pyromania, and kleptomania. Individuals with these disorders may function better with family therapy, and family involvement is frequently critical for the patient to avoid running afoul of the legal system.

92–10. **Answer: D (Only 4).** Borderline personality disorder may not be diagnosed concurrently with intermittent explosive disorder because the diagnostic criteria for borderline personality disorder include rage outbursts.

92–11. **Answer: E (All).** Anticonvulsant medications such as phenytoin, carbamazepine, and primidone may be used to treat patients with intermittent explosive disorder who have soft neurological signs and an "ictal" quality to their outbursts. Several researchers have reported decreased outbursts in patients with chronic brain syndromes, including mental retardation, who were treated with beta-blockers (e.g., propranolol). Buspirone has also been reported to decrease outbursts in a similar population.

92–12. **Answer: D (Only 4).** Behavior therapy is the most effective initial treatment for trichotillomania. Clomipramine, fluoxetine, and psychotherapy may also be useful.

92–13. **Answer: B (1 and 3).** Anxiety disorders and depression are comorbid conditions frequently associated with trichotillomania. Appropriate treatment of these disorders may alleviate the trichotillomania.

92–14. **Answer: E (All).** Of all the disorders of impulse control, pyromania is the most dangerous. Long-term containment of the patient may be indicated for the safety of the patient and society. Serotonin reuptake inhibitors (e.g., fluoxetine) and anticonvulsants (e.g., valproic acid) may decrease the impulse to set fires. Behavior therapy has met with some success in this population.

Continuing
Medical
Education
Self-Study Test

The American Psychiatric Association (APA) is pleased to offer you Continuing Medical Education (CME) credit for your participation in the self-study program. Please read the *Study Guide to Treatments of Psychiatric Disorders, Second Edition* and mark the correct self-study answers for each section.

The fee is $250 for the entire self-study test or $10 per credit hour for the individual sections. Complete the personal information required, and return the answer sheet with your check to the American Psychiatric Association, Office of Education, 1400 K Street, N.W., Washington, D.C. 20005. Make your check payable to the American Psychiatric Association.

This CME activity was planned and produced in accordance with the Essentials of the Accreditation Council for Continuing Medical Education.

> The APA is accredited by the Accreditation Council for Continuing Medical Education (ACCME) to sponsor continuing medical education for physicians.

> The APA designates this CME activity for up to 28 hours in Category 1 of the Physician's Recognition Award of the American Medical Association and for the CME requirement of the APA.

Release Date:	November 1996
End Date:	November 1998 (self-test will not be accepted for scoring/CME certificate after this date)
Estimated Time to Complete:	28 hours
Audience:	Psychiatrists, students, and other healthcare professionals who are preparing for examinations that test knowledge of psychiatric treatment

The American Psychiatric Association requires the disclosure of the existence of any significant financial interest or other relationship an author has with the manufacturer(s) of any commercial product(s) discussed in an educational presentation. The existence of such relationships does not necessarily constitute a conflict of interest, but the prospective audience must be informed of the author's affiliation with a commercial sponsor by way of an acknowledgment in this printed material.

Author	**Manufacturer**	**Relationship**
Sarah D. Atkinson, M.D.	None	None
Glen O. Gabbard , M.D.	Merck Pharmaceuticals	Manual Editorial Board

Educational Objectives for *Study Guide to Treatments of Psychiatric Disorders, Second Edition*

- To identify the key points in each chapter
- To organize the voluminous material into quantities that can be more easily assimilated
- To expand on key points by elaborating on material from the text in the answer key provided at the end of each chapter

Instructions: Each section consists of multiple choice and true-or-false questions. For all questions, select the **single best answer** and circle that answer on the answer sheet.

Section 1: General Considerations in Psychiatric Treatment

■   **DIRECTIONS: Answer the following 10 questions on the attached answer sheet. This section has been designated for 1.5 hours of CME Category 1 credit. The fee for Section 1 is $15.**

1. According to the American Psychiatric Association (APA) Practice Guideline on Depression (1993), psychotherapeutic management is

    1. Unnecessary in most cases.
    2. Only necessary when psychotherapy is a treatment of choice.
    3. Rarely useful.
    4. None of the above.

2. In comparison to Caucasians and African Americans, a much larger percentage of Asians are said to be "fast acetylators." This trait has an impact on the metabolism of which of the following drugs?

    1. Clonazepam
    2. Fluoxetine
    3. Haloperidol
    4. None of the above

3. In a study of 1,018 pairs of female twins, Kendler and co-workers examined the relationship between parental loss before age 17 years and adult psychopathology. These investigators found that

    1. There was no association between panic disorder as an adult and loss as a child.
    2. Paternal separation early in life was much more strongly associated with later development of panic disorder than was maternal separation.
    3. Parental death could not be linked with adult manifestations of panic disorder.
    4. The impact of parental loss was three times greater for panic disorder than for major depression.

4. A transfer or reassignment from a therapist of one gender to a therapist of the opposite gender

    1. May be a way of avoiding responsibility for failure or dealing with the embarrassment of a negative outcome.
    2. Is useful because gender itself is a highly significant variable in the majority of cases in which treatment is not successful.

3. May not be useful if a sexual interaction occurred with a previous therapist.

4. Should only be done if an erotic transference develops.

5. The term *emic* refers to

1. The conceptually narrow view by people in a given culture of a phenomenon occurring within that culture.

2. A presumed universal approach to the viewing of problems.

3. The biopsychosocial etiology of mental illness.

4. The imposition of a particular cultural perspective on observation about a different culture.

6. Which of the following biochemical changes has been associated with the early separation of infant rhesus monkeys from their mothers?

1. Lower levels of plasma cortisol and ACTH

2. Higher cerebrospinal fluid levels of norepinephrine

3. Higher levels of 3-methoxy-4-hydroxyphenylglycol (MHPG)

4. Lower levels of MHPG

True or False

7. _____ Women's physical complaints are more likely than those of men to be labeled psychogenic.

8. _____ The first modern proposal for a multidimensional approach to diagnosis came in 1947 from Essen-Möller and Wohlfahrt.

9. _____ The category *black* refers to a group of individuals who share the same cultural values.

10. _____ Mental retardation was first added to Axis II in 1987 with the publication of DSM-III-R.

Answers: 4,1,4,1,1,3,T,T,F,T

Section 2: Disorders Usually First Diagnosed in Infancy, Childhood, or Adolescence

■ **DIRECTIONS: Answer the following 15 questions on the attached answer sheet. This section has been designated for 5 hours of CME Category 1 credit. The fee for Section 2 is $50.**

1. Which of the following statements about group therapy for mentally retarded individuals is **false**?

1. There is an opportunity to directly practice social skills.

2. Adults, adolescents, and children do not benefit equally from group therapy.

    3. The therapist actively provides structure and facilitates communication.

    4. Participants feel less comfortable discussing topics with others who have similar disabilities.

2. Which of the following serotonin reuptake inhibitors has a Food and Drug Administration (FDA)–approved indication for its use in children and adolescents (10 years and older) for the treatment of obsessive-compulsive disorder (OCD)?

    1. Clomipramine

    2. Paroxetine

    3. Sertraline

    4. Fluoxetine

3. Which of the following statements is **true** regarding attention-deficit/hyperactivity disorder (ADHD)?

    1. There is a genetic origin for ADHD.

    2. Children will outgrow their ADHD.

    3. At least 30% of children with ADHD have concomitant learning disorders.

    4. Pharmacotherapy is curative.

4. Which of the following methods for suicide is the **least** common?

    1. Household poisons

    2. Hanging

    3. Gunshot

    4. Overdose

5. Which of the following statements applies to the alarm method of behavior therapy for enuresis?

    1. It is most successful for combined day and night enuresis.

    2. Significant relapse occurs in one-half of children despite an adequate 12-week course of treatment.

    3. A cure is defined as 14 consecutive dry nights and is usually achieved in the second month of treatment.

    4. It is as equally efficacious in the treatment of children who have additional psychiatric disorders as it is in the treatment of those who have only enuresis.

6. Which of the following statements is **true** regarding working with a child who is being maintained in an abusive home?

    1. Most abusive parents will never fully admit the abuse.

    2. Termination of parental rights should not be recommended.

    3. Work with the parent who is the perpetrator should be avoided.

    4. Involvement with the legal system should be avoided.

7. Disruptive behavior disorder is the most stable of all childhood disorders. The gender-specific rates are 9% for males and 2% for females. Which other statement is **valid** regarding disruptive behavior disorder?

    1. Punishment increases disruptive behaviors in a child with disruptive behavior disorder.

2. Parents of children with disruptive behavior disorder frequently request and follow through with treatment.

3. Approval and encouragement are sufficient rewards for the child with disruptive behavior disorder.

4. None of the above.

8. A sleep apnea event is an interruption of breathing while asleep that lasts what length of time?

1. 1 second

2. 5 seconds

3. 8 seconds

4. 10 seconds

9. What is the longest period of time between physical examinations acceptable for an evaluation of a child with a suspected anxiety disorder?

1. 6 months

2. 12 months

3. 18 months

4. 24 months

10. Which of the following medications has the fewest side effects and has proven efficacy in the treatment of Tourette's syndrome?

1. Haloperidol

2. Clonidine

3. Pimozide

4. Propranolol

11. Autism is a chronic and pervasive disorder; therefore, it is important to set realistic short-term and long-term goals. Which of the following statements is **true** about the treatment objectives?

1. Behavioral symptoms should be decreased, but attention to continued development is not critical.

2. Pharmacotherapy may be the sole treatment for temper tantrums, aggression, hyperactivity, and stereotypies.

3. Modification of the child's environment produces no lasting effects.

4. None of the above.

12. In a youth presenting with an initial episode of psychosis, which of the following should be considered as part of the workup?

1. Physical examination

2. Toxicology screen

3. Neuroimaging

4. All of the above

True or False

13. _____ The presenting signs and symptoms of sleep disorders in children may mimic those of attention-deficit/hyperactivity disorder.

14. _____ In substance abuse/dependence, relapse rates for adolescents and adults are roughly the same.

15. _____ The most frequent comorbid disorder in children with learning disorders is ADHD.

Answers: 4,1,3,1,4,2,4,1,1,3,1,3,1,4,4,7,7,7.

Section 3: Delirium, Dementia, Amnestic, and Other Cognitive Disorders

■ **DIRECTIONS: Answer the following 10 questions on the attached answer sheet. This section has been designated for 2 hours of CME Category 1 credit. The fee for Section 3 is $20.**

1. Which one of the following conditions is associated with ibuprofen overdose but not acetaminophen overdose?

    1. Comatose state
    2. Aseptic meningitis
    3. Death
    4. None of the above

2. The creation and use of a memory book is a complex process that has had some success in individuals with amnestic disorders. Which of the following statements regarding memory books is (are) **false**?

    1. The acquisition stage of the memory book process is dependent on some residual declarative memory skill.
    2. Prospective memory is essential for the memory book to have any practical application.
    3. The method of vanishing clues is essential to the creation of a memory book.
    4. All of the above.

3. Depression is a frequent clinical complication of dementia. The psychomotor retardation and pseudodementia associated with depression worsen the cognitive deficits of individuals with dementia. Which one of the following medications may be the most efficacious in the treatment of depression in patients with dementia?

    1. Fluoxetine
    2. Sertraline
    3. Paroxetine
    4. Amitriptyline

4. Treatment with physostigmine may result in improvement for which one of the following disorders?

    1. Fahr's disease
    2. Wilson's disease

3. Friedreich's ataxia

4. Olivopontocerebellar atrophies

5. Which of the following therapeutic modalities is (are) efficacious in the treatment of patients with Alzheimer's disease?

1. Cognitive therapy

2. Behavior therapy

3. Insight-oriented therapy

4. All of the above

6. What percentage of individuals with chronic alcoholism have some level of intellectual deterioration?

1. 25%

2. 50%

3. 75%

4. 100%

7. The dementia associated with systemic lupus erythematosus (SLE) may be treated by which of the following?

1. Placement of an intraventricular shunt

2. Propranolol

3. Corticosteroids

4. None of the above

True or False

8. —— Chlorpromazine is an anticholinergic agent.

9. —— Patients are frequently amnestic for the period of time that they were delirious.

10. —— Sensory deprivation alone is sufficient to cause delirium.

Answers: 2,3,2,4,3,4,2,3,T,T,F

Section 4: Substance-Related Disorders

■ **DIRECTIONS: Answer the following 10 questions on the attached answer sheet. This section has been designated for 2.5 hours of CME Category 1 credit. The fee for Section 4 is $25.**

1. Under which of the following conditions would the initial dose of methadone be 10 mg–20 mg?

1. The patient has used heroin 1 to 2 times a day for the past 3 weeks.

2. The patient has used heroin more than once a day for the past 3 weeks.

3. The patient has pupillary constriction and dry mouth.

4. None of the above.

2. Which one of the following drugs has **no** abstinence syndrome after repeated use?

1. Psilocybin

2. Alcohol

3. Benzodiazepines

4. Opioids

3. *Relapse* is defined by a return to substance use and secondary behaviors associated with substance use. Which of the following is a high-risk situation for relapse?

1. Being frustrated

2. Undergoing withdrawal and craving the substance

3. Experiencing the breakup of a significant relationship

4. All of the above

4. Which of the following is a sign of **early** problematic alcohol or drug use?

1. Disruptions of occupational functioning

2. Medical problems

3. Guilty feelings about the behaviors engaged in while using alcohol or drugs

4. Impaired relationships with family

5. Which one of the following statements is **true** regarding stimulant intoxication?

1. Hallucinations are common.

2. Medical emergencies are common.

3. Bipolar mania can be consistently distinguished from intoxication.

4. No treatment may be required.

True or False

6. _____ One goal of treatment in a therapeutic community is detoxification.

7. _____ The maximum starting phenobarbital dose for sedative-hypnotic withdrawal is 500 mg/day.

8. _____ Workplace testing for drugs and alcohol may be used to intimidate employees.

9. _____ Psychodynamic group therapy is therapy based on psychoanalytic principles.

10. _____ Protracted withdrawal syndromes of benzodiazepines and alcohol are similar.

Answers: 2,1,4,3,4,F,T,T,T,F

Section 5: Schizophrenia and Other Psychotic Disorders

■ **DIRECTIONS: Answer the following 10 questions on the attached answer sheet. This section has been designated for 2 hours of CME Category 1 credit. The fee for Section 5 is $20.**

1. Alcoholic psychotic disorder generally arises how long after the last intake of alcohol or significant reduction in intake?

   1. 8 hours
   2. 16 hours
   3. 24 hours
   4. 48 hours

2. What percentage of previously chronically hospitalized patients have returned to the community since the introduction of antipsychotic medications?

   1. 25%
   2. 50%
   3. 75%
   4. 90%

3. Job clubs were originally developed to train non–mentally ill individuals to help them locate and secure jobs. This concept has been adapted to individuals with severe mental illness. Which of the following factors is related to success in this form of rehabilitation?

   1. Having a diagnosis of schizophrenia
   2. Having been employed before the onset of the illness
   3. Receiving social security or other benefits
   4. None of the above

4. For patients who have persistent aggressive behavior, which one of the following is helpful in controlling the outbursts?

   1. Lorazepam
   2. Amoxapine
   3. Propranolol
   4. Clonidine hydrochloride

5. Which one of the following conditions or symptoms warrants long-term hospitalization?

   1. Severe antisocial behaviors
   2. A previous long-term hospitalization
   3. Cycling in and out of hospitals for brief hospitalizations
   4. Significantly below-average intelligence

6. What is the treatment of choice for shared psychotic disorder?

    1. Separation of the dyadic partners
    2. High-potency antipsychotics
    3. Low-potency antipsychotics
    4. None of the above

7. In a discussion of the pathogenesis of schizophrenia with family members, which one of the following statements may be constructive?

    1. The biomedical, psychophysiological, and behavioral determinants of schizophrenia are ubiquitous among individuals with schizophrenia.
    2. Vulnerability to this disorder is not shaped by the environment.
    3. The genetic transmission of schizophrenia is well documented and fully conceptualized.
    4. There is an association between stressful life events, the emotional quality of the environment, and the onset and course of schizophrenia.

8. Although dopamine is normally released from intracellular vesicles, it may be released from extravesicular pools. Which one of the following drugs can prompt such a release?

    1. Methadone
    2. Reserpine
    3. Haloperidol
    4. Methamphetamine

True or False

9. _____ One of the goals of long-term hospitalization is understanding of the symptoms relative to the individual's environment and self.

10. _____ Benztropine is used to treat acute extrapyramidal side effects.

Answers: 4,4,2,3,3,1,4,4,T,T

Section 6: Mood Disorders

◼ **DIRECTIONS: Answer the following 10 questions on the attached answer sheet. This section has been designated for 2.5 hours of CME Category 1 credit. The fee for Section 6 is $25.**

1. Which of the following is the best-studied psychological treatment for depression?

    1. Group therapy
    2. Cognitive therapy

   3. Interpersonal psychotherapy

   4. Behavior therapy

2. What is the mortality rate with electroconvulsive therapy (ECT)?

   1. 1 per 100 patients

   2. 1 per 1,000 patients

   3. 1 per 10,000 patients

   4. 1 per 100,000 patients

3. Which of the following unconscious meanings is associated with suicidal behavior?

   1. The wish to kill others

   2. The wish to appease an internalized sadistic tormentor

   3. The wish for a magical reunion with an idealized and unconditionally loving parental figure

   4. All of the above

4. You have made a decision to use a selective serotonin reuptake inhibitor (SSRI) in a patient with the following transaminase levels: SGOT 150 (14–50 U/L) and SGPT 250 (21–72 U/L). Which of the following SSRIs causes the most significant inhibition of the cytochrome P450 system?

   1. Paroxetine

   2. Fluoxetine

   3. Sertraline

   4. There is no difference in the degree of inhibition among the various SSRIs.

5. Which of the following factors influences (influence) in a **positive** manner or is (are) predictive of better adherence to treatment?

   1. A high socioeconomic status

   2. A college degree

   3. Past history of compliance with treatment

   4. All of the above

6. What percentage of patients will **not** respond to standard treatment for depression?

   1. 20%

   2. 30%

   3. 40%

   4. 50%

7. When should antidepressant medication be immediately used?

   1. When there is a strong family history of mood disorder.

   2. When the patient is most reluctant to take medication.

   3. When there is minimal suicide risk.

   4. When the patient is an adolescent.

True or False

8. _____ Severity of depression does **not** predict responsivity to medications.

9. _____ There are numerous long-term studies documenting the efficacy of light therapy.

10. _____ In general, 10 sessions should be allotted to a time-limited cognitive therapy.

Answers: 2,3,4,1,3,2,1,F,F,F

Section 7: Anxiety Disorders, Dissociative Disorders, and Adjustment Disorders

■ **DIRECTIONS: Answer the following 10 questions on the attached answer sheet. This section has been designated for 2.5 hours of CME Category 1 credit. The fee for Section 7 is $25.**

1. Psychotherapy is commonly prescribed for treatment of posttraumatic stress disorder (PTSD). Which of the following modalities has unequivocal documented efficacy in the treatment of PTSD?

    1. Systematic desensitization
    2. Cognitive-behavior therapy
    3. Psychodynamic psychotherapy
    4. None of the above

2. Which of the following is a common, striking feature in the history of patients with amnestic disorders?

    1. Frequently, the abuse is fabricated by these patients.
    2. These patients have no conscious memories of abuse.
    3. These patients recount histories of abuse with minimal affect and minimize the circumstances.
    4. None of the above.

3. Treatment variables for adjustment disorder include all of the following **EXCEPT**

    1. Brevity.
    2. Complexity.
    3. Proximity.
    4. Immediacy.

4. The overall orientation of psychotherapy for patients with acute stress disorder involves

    1. Intensely analyzing personality factors.
    2. Working through the intrapsychic and interpersonal aftermath of the traumatic experience.

3. Understanding intrapsychic conflicts that have arisen in the remote past.

4. None of the above.

5.   In the treatment of panic disorder, which is the **least** studied selective serotonin reuptake inhibitor (SSRI)?

    1. Sertraline

    2. Fluvoxamine

    3. Fluoxetine

    4. Paroxetine

6.   Which one of the following medications has shown the **most** promise in the treatment of depersonalization?

    1. Fluoxetine

    2. Diazepam

    3. Imipramine

    4. Lithium

7.   What percentage of patients with specific phobias prematurely discontinue treatment?

    1. 10%–25%

    2. 25%–50%

    3. 50%–75%

    4. None of the above

True or False

8. ——— *Adaptationalism* stresses the integration of the various alters as a critical goal of this approach.

9. ——— With clomipramine, the side effects correlate with the plasma level.

10. ——— Buspirone decreases apprehension.

Answers: 4,3,2,1,1,2,F,F,T

Section 8: Somatoform and Factitious Disorders

■ **DIRECTIONS: Answer the following 10 questions on the attached answer sheet. This section has been designated for 2 hours of CME Category 1 credit. The fee for Section 8 is $20.**

1.   What type of examination or procedure should routinely be performed on patients with somatization disorder?

    1. Chemistry profile

    2. Urine drug screen

3. Complete physical examination

4. Partial physical examination

2.   Which of the following symptoms is (are) seen in children with Meadow's syndrome?

1. Apnea

2. Vomiting

3. Seizures

4. All of the above

3.   Patients with acute conversion symptoms tend to be seen more often by emergency room physicians. In an emergency room setting, which of the following is contraindicated in the treatment of a patient with a conversion disorder?

1. Amytal interview

2. Hypnosis

3. Multiple examinations

4. Appropriate suggestion

4.   How long must pain be present before it is considered chronic and not acute?

1. 1 month

2. 3 months

3. 6 months

4. 12 months

5.   Which of the following medications has documented efficacy in the treatment of patients with hypochondriasis even in the absence of depression?

1. Nortriptyline

2. Paroxetine

3. Amitriptyline

4. None of the above

6.   How long after the first dose of methadone will the onset of effective analgesia occur?

1. 2 to 3 hours

2. 6 to 8 hours

3. 1 to 2 days

4. 2 to 3 days

True or False

7. _____ Conversion disorder is less prevalent than in the past.

8. _____ Forensic evaluations may be necessary in malingering patients.

9. _____ Chronic pain contributes to the development of depression.

10. _____ With factitious disorders, the symptoms or deficits cannot be fully explained by a neurological or general medical condition.

Answers: 4,4,3,3,4,4,F,T,T,F

Section 9: Sexual and Gender Identity Disorders

■ **DIRECTIONS: Answer the following 10 questions
on the attached answer sheet. This section has been
designated for 2.5 hours of CME Category 1 credit.
The fee for Section 9 is $25.**

1. Increasing levels of which of the following neurotransmittors inhibits ejaculation?

    1. Serotonin
    2. Dopamine
    3. Epinephrine
    4. Norepinephrine

2. What chromosomal abnormality results in hermaphroditism?

    1. 46, XXY
    2. 46, YYY
    3. 46, XX
    4. 46, XY

3. Who should be interviewed in a comprehensive assessment of sexual problems?

    1. The patient's partner should be interviewed.
    2. The patient's parents should be interviewed to provide critical information on child-rearing practices.
    3. The assessment should be a family process involving the children and both parents.
    4. None of the above.

4. Which of the following is **not** a conscious motivation for cross-dressing?

    1. To feel beautiful and more masculine
    2. To relieve tension
    3. To escape from pressures of traditional masculine roles
    4. To express traditional feminine aspects of the individual's personality

5. What percentage of children aged 4 years and older will draw their sex when asked to draw a person?

    1. 25%
    2. 50%
    3. 100%
    4. None of the above

6. Female sexual excitement is under the control of what neurochemical system?

    1. Adrenergic
    2. Cholinergic
    3. Dopaminergic
    4. Serotonergic

True or False

7. _____ Psychological tests can accurately discriminate individuals with sex addictions from non–sex-addicted individuals.

8. _____ Laser surgery for the treatment of vulvar vestibulitis may cause dyspareunia.

9. _____ Paraphilic disorders primarily afflict men.

10. _____ Infertility treatment may lead to sexual difficulties.

Answers: 1,1,1,4,2,F,T,T,T,T

Section 10: Eating Disorders

■ **DIRECTIONS: Answer the following 10 questions on the attached answer sheet. This section has been designated for 2 hours of CME Category 1 credit. The fee for Section 10 is $20.**

1. For which group of patients with anorexia nervosa is family therapy most effective?

    1. Those in whom onset of the disorder occurs after age 18 years
    2. Those in whom the duration of illness is less than 3 years
    3. Those in whom the duration of illness is more than 3 years
    4. None of the above

2. What is the prevalence of bulimia nervosa in women?

    1. 10%
    2. 5%
    3. 1%
    4. 0.05%

3. Which one of the following trace elements should be supplemented as part of the nutritional rehabilitation of patients with anorexia nervosa?

    1. Iron
    2. Zinc
    3. Aluminum
    4. A balanced diet will provide sufficient trace elements.

4. Ipecac intoxication may result in all of the following **EXCEPT**

    1. Death.
    2. Mallory-Weiss tears.
    3. Electroencephalogram abnormalities.
    4. Precordial pain.

5. Complications of rumination includes (include) which of the following?

1. Failure to thrive
2. Dental decay
3. Anemia
4. All of the above

True or False

6. —— Most patients with eating disorders overvalue weight and body shape.
7. —— Lenient behavioral programs for the treatment of anorexia nervosa patients are less efficacious than strict programs.
8. —— The presence of family crisis is indicative of family psychopathology.
9. —— Approximately 2% of adult women have binge-eating disorder.
10. —— Aversive therapy is the most common treatment for pica.

Answers: 2,3,4,1;F,F,F,T,T.

Section 11: Personality Disorders

■ **DIRECTIONS: Answer the following 10 questions on the attached answer sheet. This section has been designated for 2.5 hours of CME Category 1 credit. The fee for Section 11 is $25.**

1. The treatment of choice for obsessive-compulsive personality disorder is

1. Group psychotherapy.
2. Individual cognitive-behavior therapy.
3. Individual psychodynamic psychotherapy or psychoanalysis.
4. Pharmacotherapy.

2. Which one of the following therapeutic approaches is characteristic of the technique derived from Kohut's self psychology?

1. Interpretation of idealization as a defense
2. Repeated interpretation of envy
3. Understanding of "microempathic failures"
4. None of the above

3. A litigious stance is a continued concern in the treatment of patients with paranoid personality disorder. Litigious behavior can generally be avoided by

1. Interpretation of unconscious sexual feelings.
2. Attention to the therapeutic alliance and arrangements for dealing with privacy and confidentiality.
3. Letting the patient know that you have retained an attorney.
4. Presenting an air of unflappable confidence.

4. Which one of the following statements characterizes the role of supportive psychotherapy in the treatment of patients with borderline personality disorder (BPD)?

   1. Few BPD patients are seen in supportive psychotherapy.
   2. The goals of supportive psychotherapy are explicitly directed at changing personality.
   3. Some research has indicated that supportive treatments are able to bring about basic changes in personality comparable to those derived from expressive treatment.
   4. Insight is necessary for change in supportive psychotherapy.

5. Which one of the following adjunctive therapies has no demonstrable role in the treatment of paranoid personality disorder patients?

   1. Behavior therapy
   2. Pharmacotherapy
   3. Family therapy
   4. Short-term psychotherapy

True or False

6. _____ Marital therapy is rarely useful with histrionic personality disorder patients.

7. _____ Dependent personality disorder is common in the general population.

8. _____ Dependent personality disorder is often comorbid with Axis I conditions but rarely with Axis II disorders.

9. _____ In the treatment of schizoid personality disorder patients, dynamic therapy is best carried out three or four times a week.

10. _____ Schizoid personality disorder is closer conceptually to schizophrenia than is schizotypal personality disorder.

Answers: 3,3,T,1,F,T,F,F,F

Sections 12 and 13: Sleep Disorders and Disorders of Impulse Control

■ **DIRECTIONS: Answer the following 10 questions on the attached answer sheet. These two sections have, together, been designated for 1 hour of CME Category 1 credit. The total fee for Sections 12 and 13 is $10.**

1. Large, well-controlled clinical treatment trials of behavioral/psychological and pharmacological treatments have been conducted for which of the following sleep disorders?

   1. Restless legs syndrome
   2. Primary insomnia

    3. Narcolepsy

    4. Circadian rhythm sleep disorders

2.   What type(s) of treatment(s) may be used for patients with pyromania?

    1. Behavior therapy

    2. Valproic acid

    3. Fluoxetine

    4. All of the above

3.   Which one of the following is **not** part of stimulus control therapy for sleep disorders?

    1. The patient should go to bed only when he or she is sleepy.

    2. The patient should not lie in bed whenever he or she is unable to fall asleep.

    3. The bedroom should be used for all manners of activities, not only sleeping and sex.

    4. The patient should arise in the morning at the same time, regardless of the amount of sleep obtained.

True or False

4.   ———— Alcoholism is frequently found in the family histories of patients with pyromania.

5.   ———— Compulsive gambling is as prevalent in women as in men.

6.   ———— Patients are not requested to restrict their sleep below 4 to 5 hours per night when sleep restriction is used to treat insomnia.

7.   ———— Surgical intervention for obstructive sleep apnea is warranted when the patient is 100% over ideal weight.

8.   ———— Sleep hygiene alone is usually effective in the treatment of insomnia.

9.   ———— Residential placement can be used as a treatment for pyromania.

10.   ———— Primary hypersomnia cannot occur in conjunction with other sleep disturbances.

Answers: 2,4,3,T,F,T,T,F,T,T.

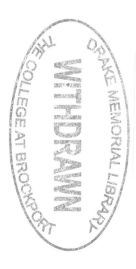